Developmental Epilepsy

From Clinical Medicine to Neurobiological Mechanisms

Developmental Epilepsy

From Clinical Medicine to Neurobiological Mechanisms

Editors

Carl E Stafstrom

The Johns Hopkins University School of Medicine, USA

Libor Velíšek

New York Medical College School of Medicine, USA

World Scientific

NEW JERSEY • LONDON • SINGAPORE • BEIJING • SHANGHAI • HONG KONG • TAIPEI • CHENNAI • TOKYO

Published by

World Scientific Publishing Co. Pte. Ltd.

5 Toh Tuck Link, Singapore 596224

USA office: 27 Warren Street, Suite 401-402, Hackensack, NJ 07601

UK office: 57 Shelton Street, Covent Garden, London WC2H 9HE

Library of Congress Cataloging-in-Publication Data
Names: Stafstrom, Carl Ernest, editor. | Velíšek, Libor, editor.
Title: Developmental epilepsy : from clinical medicine to neurobiological mechanisms / edited by, Carl E Stafstrom, Libor Velíšek.
Description: New Jersey : World Scientific, 2019. | Includes bibliographical references and index.
Identifiers: LCCN 2018051421 | ISBN 9789813277724 (hardcover : alk. paper)
Subjects: | MESH: Epilepsy | Brain--growth & development
Classification: LCC RC372 | NLM WL 385 | DDC 616.85/3--dc23
LC record available at https://lccn.loc.gov/2018051421

British Library Cataloguing-in-Publication Data
A catalogue record for this book is available from the British Library.

For any available supplementary material, please visit
https://www.worldscientific.com/worldscibooks/10.1142/11198#t=suppl

Typeset by Stallion Press
Email: enquiries@stallionpress.com

Dr. Stafstrom would like to thank his family — Jean,
Marit and Isaac — for their love and support.
Dr. Velíšek would like to thank his family — Jana,
Jana Jr., and Ivana — for their continuing years
of understanding, support, and love.

Preface

The adage "children are not just little adults" is quite appropriate when considering the developing brain. Indeed, the heightened susceptibility of the developing brain to seizures and epilepsy creates an immense clinical challenge: while the developing brain requires a bit more excitation for several aspects of its development, such as neuronal migration, synapse formation, and interneuronal connectivity, it comes at the price of increasing seizure susceptibility. When that observation is added to the multitude of developmental and acquired insults that can affect the developing brain, the perfect storm is created.

Over the past decade or so, our understanding of brain development, and in parallel, the predisposition of brain to epilepsy, has increased immensely. This volume provides an overview of current thinking and research on developmental epilepsy, aiming to review clinical aspects and the neurobiological basis. Our goal is to provide a taste of the spectrum of pathologies that can lead to epilepsy and identify age- and mechanism-specific treatments. The authors of these chapters, experts in the clinical and neurobiological aspects of developmental epilepsy, provide a sample of the important ongoing work that is attempting to decipher the mysteries of developmental epilepsy. The volume begins by considering normal brain development and how genetic and acquired pathologies can engender seizures at different developmental stages (Carrasco, Habela & Stafstrom) followed by a detailed review of mechanisms of seizures early in development (Worden & Staley). The next few chapters describe clinical aspects of early onset epilepsy syndromes (Cilio & El Kosseifi) and treatment opportunities (Ghusayni & Mikati). Burgeoning information about the role of fever as a substrate of increased seizure susceptibility (Curran & Baram) and roles of genetics (Greenberg & Pathak) and epigenetic factors (Boison) are explored in detail. Understanding the mechanisms of developmental epilepsy relies intimately on animal models, which are discussed from the point of view of developmental epileptic encephalopathies (Galanopoulou). Pre- or peri-natal stress appears to contribute significantly to developmental seizure susceptibility (Velíšek). The increasing recognition that inflammation plays a critical role in epileptogenesis and may offer unique treatment opportunities is covered comprehensively (Koh) as are the mechanisms of epileptogenesis caused by malformations of cortical development and cerebral dysplasia (Goodman). Discerning the molecular basis of aberrant cellular signaling pathways in individual disorders as well as the commonality of such pathways in multiple epilepsy etiologies is exemplified by the mTOR system (Wong). Comorbidities of developmental epilepsy are not only under-appreciated but are critical for comprehensive clinical care; understanding the neurobiological basis of epilepsy comorbidities could lead to improved psychosocial and educational function of affected children (Barry & Holmes). Finally, the role of sex differences in seizure predisposition is receiving increasing attention, as it may lead to sex-specific treatments (Velíšková).

We hope that these chapters instill critical thinking and new ideas about the developmental epilepsies, their neurobiological mechanisms and treatment options. There is hardly a more noble goal than to make inroads into these often devastating disorders that profoundly affect children, their families, and society as a whole.

Carl E. Stafstrom, MD, PhD
Libor Velíšek, MD, PhD

Contents

Chapter 1
Overview of Brain Development: Principles Relevant for Developmental Epilepsy

Melisa Carrasco, MD, PhD
Christa W. Habela, MD, PhD
Carl E. Stafstrom, MD, PhD

Division of Pediatric Neurology,
Departments of Neurology & Pediatrics,
The Johns Hopkins University School of Medicine,
Baltimore, MD, USA

1.1 Introduction

Brain development is a remarkable process — an almost miraculous one — when considering that after the initial conjunction of sperm and egg, over a mere several months, there emerges a structure so complex, so beautiful, and yet so prone to dysfunction as the human brain. Part of the miracle lies in the fact that brain development goes so well most of the time, a tribute to an exceedingly complex and intricate series of coordinated molecular and cellular steps that guide the developmental process. Molecular, genetic and cellular pathways that underlie brain development are regulated precisely at each stage of brain growth, yet these processes can also be influenced by environmental and epigenetic factors. This chapter describes brain development as a journey, at each step considering how genetic mutations or acquired errors can lead to deviations from normal development and provide useful clues for understanding the wide spectrum of developmental epilepsies.

1.2 Nervous system development

Brain development can be summarized as a series of sequential but overlapping steps (Table 1.1): (1) formation of the neural tube, (2) proliferation of neural progenitor cells, (3) neuroblast differentiation and

Table 1.1. Stages of human brain development and relevance to epilepsy.

Stage	Age (wga)	Representative disorders	Relevance to seizures
Neurulation	4	Encephalocele Myelomeningocele	Indirect via effect on subsequent neuronal migration
Neuronal proliferation, differentiation	7–27	Microcephaly	Imbalance between proliferation and apoptosis leads to abnormal neuronal circuits
Neuronal migration	12–24	Pachygyria Lissencephaly *ARX* mutations	Abnormal hyperexcitable circuits, excitation/inhibition imbalance
Neuronal organization	24–birth	Polymicrogyria Dysplasias Schizencephaly Ion channel mutations	Abnormal hyperexcitable circuits, excitation/inhibition imbalance
Synaptogenesis	24–birth	Autism spectrum disorders that include epilepsy	Abnormal hyperexcitable circuits, excitation/inhibition imbalance
Myelination	20 wga–20 yrs	Leukodystrophies (e.g., Alexander disease)	Abnormal propagation of neural activity

Abbreviations: *ARX*, Aristaless-related X-linked homeobox gene; wga, weeks gestational age; yrs, years.

migration, (4) cortical organization including axon and dendrite growth, (5) synaptogenesis, and (6) myelination. Each of these steps is summarized here; comprehensive coverage of these topics is available elsewhere [Stiles and Jernigan 2010; Lui *et al.*, 2011; Jiang and Nardelli, 2016; Silbereis *et al.*, 2016].

1.2.1 *Formation, closure, and regional development of the neural tube*

Brain development begins with a simple sheet of ectodermal cells that comprises the dorsal-most layer of the 3-layered embryo: endoderm, mesoderm, and ectoderm (Figure 1.1A). The ectodermal cells proliferate rapidly under the influence of secreted molecules from the underlying mesoderm (notochord). The proliferating ectodermal cells form a neuroectodermal sheet, or neural plate (Figure 1.1A, top and middle) that folds up into a tube with a central lumen (Figure 1.1A, bottom) and closes in a zipper-like fashion in both directions, from several sites along the neural tube (one site indicated by star in Figure 1.1B). Subsequently, the neural tube closes, first at the anterior end (rostral neural pore) on the 28th postconceptional day and then at the posterior end (caudal neural pore) one or two days later. The most caudal part of the neural tube becomes the spinal cord. Neural pore closure, a process called neurulation, creates a lumen that will form the ventricular system. The ectoderm overlying the neural tube becomes the skin (labeled epidermis in Figure 1.1A).

As the neural tube closes, a group of cells pinches off from the tube and forms the neural crest (Figure 1.1A, bottom). These motile neural crest cells migrate to various locations along the body and head of the embryo. Neural crest cells will form the majority of the peripheral nervous system (PNS), including neurons of the spinal and cranial sensory ganglia and autonomic ganglia, as well as enteric neurons within the gut lining and the Schwann cells that myelinate peripheral axons. The neural crest cells also form some important non-neural tissues such as the pia, arachnoid, and adrenal medulla. Finally, placodes are localized regions of ectoderm along the anterior neural crest and neural tube that will eventually form peripheral sensory neurons

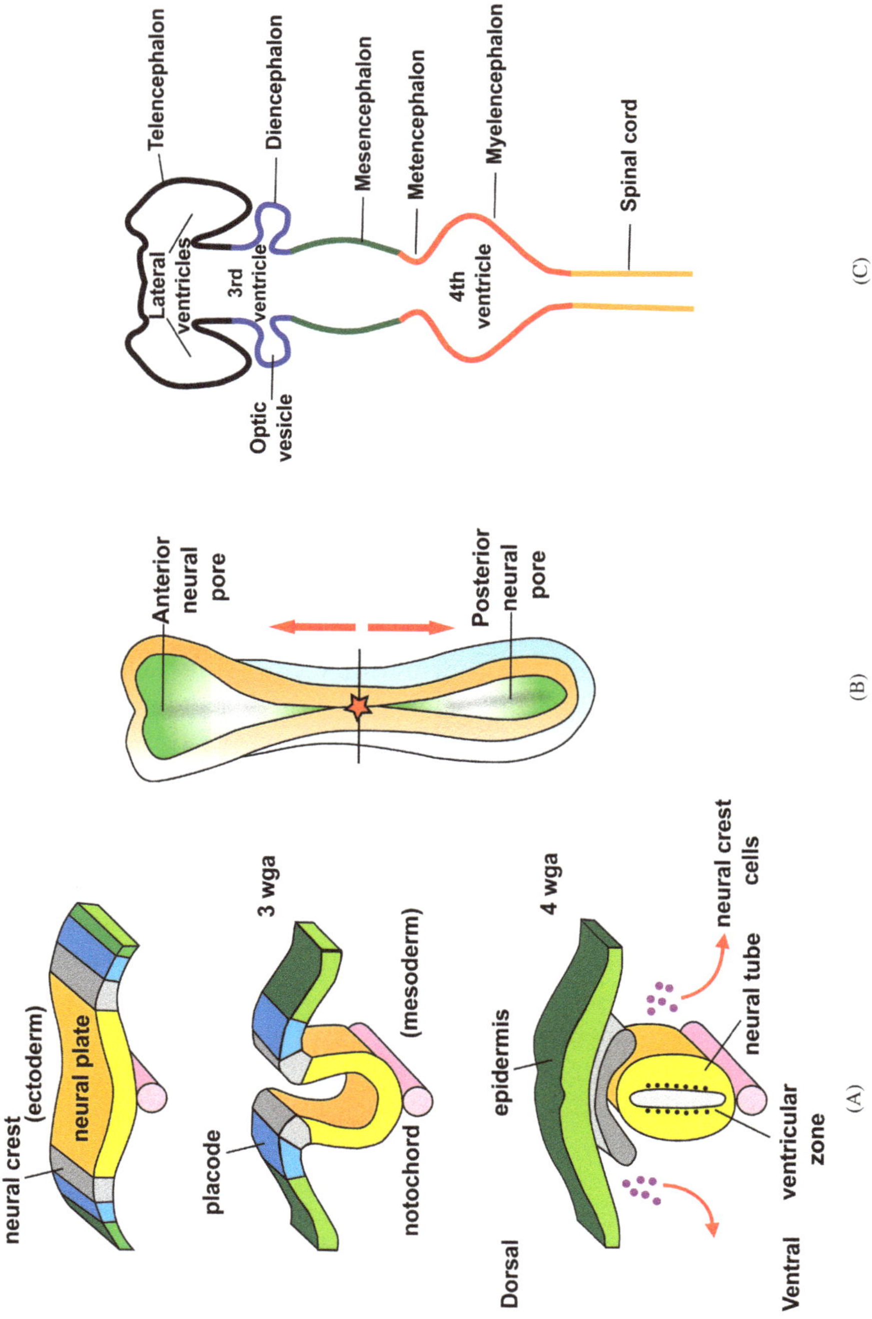
Telencephalon
Diencephalon
Mesencephalon
Metencephalon
Myelencephalon
Spinal cord
Lateral ventricles
3rd ventricle
4th ventricle
Optic vesicle
(C)
Anterior neural pore
Posterior neural pore
(B)
neural crest
(ectoderm)
neural plate
3 wga
placode
notochord
(mesoderm)
4 wga
epidermis
neural crest cells
neural tube
ventricular zone
Dorsal
Ventral
(A)

and their supporting glia. Seven pairs of placodes arise anteriorly along the neural tube, five of which give rise to sensory neurons (nasal, otic, ophthalmic, trigeminal, epibranchial), while the other two placodes form the lens of the eye and the anterior pituitary gland. Therefore, the nervous system derives from three embryonic sources: neuroectoderm, neural crest, and placodes. Some non-neural tissues also derive from these structures.

At the end of the 4th week of gestation (4 weeks gestational age or wga 4), after the neural tube has formed and closed, the next developmental step is the formation of several major divisions along the longitudinal axis. These divisions will eventually define the boundaries of the regions of the mature brain (Figure 1.1C). The neural tube undergoes contractions or expansions along its length as a consequence of rapid cell proliferation. The prosencephalon (forebrain) is the most anterior region, the mesencephalon (midbrain) is the next most caudal structure, then the rhombencephalon (hindbrain, which will become the pons, medulla, and cerebellum), and finally, the spinal cord is most caudal. At the fifth week of gestation, the cerebral hemispheres become distinguishable when the prosencephalon invaginates, dividing into the telencephalon (which will become the cerebral hemispheres) and the diencephalon (which will become the thalamus, hypothalamus, and retina). This is followed by the

Figure 1.1. Stages of early brain development.

A. Neural tube formation (neurulation). Brain formation begins as the trilaminar embryonic plates or sheets of cells (ectoderm, mesoderm, endoderm (not shown)). Under the influence of signals from a mesodermal structure, the notochord (pink), the neural plate folds and eventually pinches off to form the neural tube. In the ventricular zone adjacent to the ventricle surface, developing neurons (neuroblasts) proliferate rapidly. Cells derived from the neural crest (gray) migrate along the developing neural tube to form the components of the peripheral nervous system (see text). Overlying non-neural cells comprise the epidermis. B. At about 4 weeks of gestational age (wga), the neural tube closes, first at the anterior end (anterior neural pore) and 1–2 days later at the posterior end (posterior neural pore). Neural tube closure occurs in a zipper-like fashion from one or more sites along the longitudinal extent of the neural tube (for simplicity, one site is shown here, indicated by a red star). C. As neurons and glia proliferate rapidly, the neural tube undergoes regional expansions or contractions, and bends or flexures, eventually forming areas of the mature brain as indicated.

appearance of sulci and gyri on the cortical surface, which form to accommodate the rapid cell proliferation and allow cortical surface expansion without requiring a massively enlarged cranium.

1.2.2 *Neuronal proliferation, differentiation, and migration*

Neurons and glia are formed from neural stem cells. These are neuroepithelial cells that proliferate in vast numbers at the surface of the ventricle in the ventricular zone (VZ) (Figure 1.1A bottom, Figure 1.2). In the VZ, initial proliferation occurs via symmetric cell division, with each precursor producing two identical daughter cells. Later, around the 6th week of gestation, cell division becomes asymmetric — each parent cell divides to form one apical radial glial cell and either one post-mitotic neuron or an intermediate progenitor cell that divides further. The newly generated post-mitotic neurons leave the VZ and migrate to their target location in the cortical plate (CP) along the radial fibers of the radial glial cells, which extend to the pial surface. Above the VZ, the subventricular zone (SVZ) forms and is populated by intermediate progenitor cells and migrating young neurons [Ortega *et al.*, 2018]. The VZ and SVZ enlarge rapidly during fetal development, with all the future excitatory projection neurons of the cortex generated here, eventually forming the fully laminated neocortex (Figure 1.2). However, many neuronal precursor cells undergo programmed cell death (apoptosis), limiting the number of cells that ultimately migrate and reach functional maturity [Blanquie *et al.*, 2017].

The laminated architecture of the neocortex is the result of neuronal migration from the ventricular surface to the CP in an inside-outside manner. The earliest born neurons that migrate and arrive at the CP first become the deepest cortical layers (V and VI). Subsequent waves of migrating neurons attain their positions in more superficial cortical layers (II through IV). Layer I is the molecular layer, containing neurons originating from various origins, including the SVZ, and it contains a variety of cellular subtypes including neurons and interneurons such as Cajal-Retzius cells [Rakic and Zecevic, 2003].

Cajal-Retzius cells secrete reelin, which signals new projection neurons to bypass the earlier-born neurons to achieve the inside-out lamination pattern. Upon arriving at the CP, Reelin and other molecular signals dictate the end of migration but neural differentiation continues as neurons extend processes, specify axons and dendrites, develop ion channels, and form synaptic connections with other neurons [Wu *et al.*, 2014]. Superficial layers II and III contain neurons with exclusively intracortical connections whereas the neurons of layers IV, V, and VI project to the subcortical regions. Differentiation and migration of neurons is modulated initially by electrical synaptic transmission and later by chemical synaptic neurotransmission (discussed below). All radially migrating neurons from the VZ and SVZ will become glutamatergic.

In contrast to the glutamatergic cortical neurons just described, γ-amino-butyric acid (GABA)ergic interneurons are generated in the ventral telencephalon in the medial and lateral ganglionic eminences and migrate tangentially (rather than radially) into the CP where they form functional interneurons in different cortical laminae [Wichterle *et al.*, 1999; Luhmann *et al.*, 2014; Chu and Anderson, 2015]. Compared to the cortical excitatory neurons, interneurons have a longer path of migration and end up farther from their site of origin. A wide diversity of inhibitory interneurons, differing in synaptic targets, electrical properties, and function, segregate in appropriate cortical layers [DeFelipe *et al.*, 2013] (Figure 2). In these early developmental stages, the neurotransmitters GABA and glutamate exert trophic functions on neural progenitor cells, either stimulating or inhibiting their proliferation and migration [Luhmann *et al.*, 2015].

In summary, during and after a period of cell proliferation, neurons migrate to form the cortex by two routes: radial migration (excitatory neurons) and tangential migration (inhibitory interneurons). The general architecture of neocortex therefore consists of GABAergic (inhibitory) interneurons interspersed with glutamatergic (excitatory) projection neurons. These two classes of neurons are susceptible to different types of injury at different developmental time points, therefore resulting in different pathological outcomes [Back, 2014]. Aberrant neurogenesis or neuronal migration, from a genetic or acquired cause, are thought to underlie a variety of neurodevelopmental

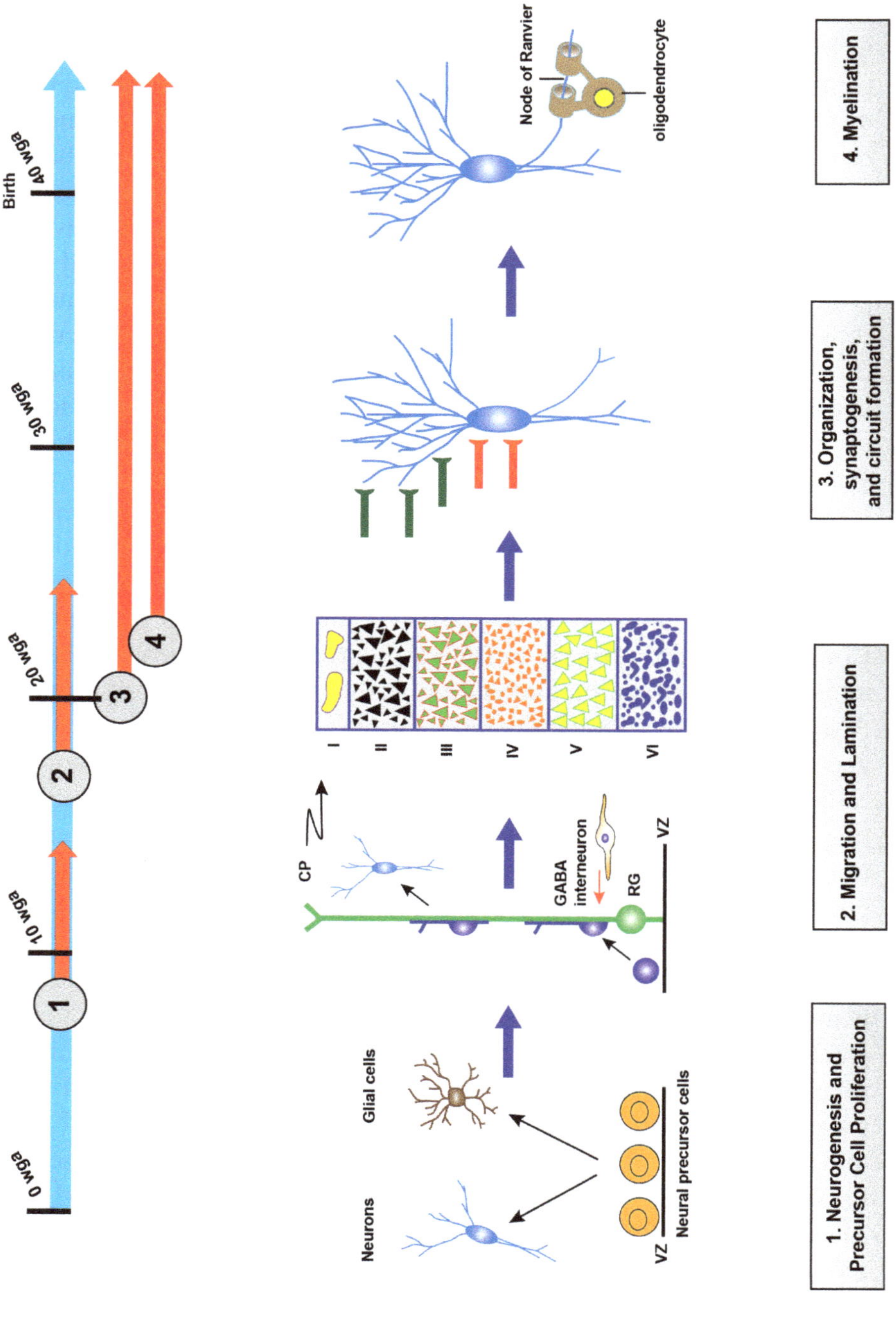
0 wga
10 wga
20 wga
30 wga
40 wga
Birth
1
2
3
4
Neurons
Glial cells
VZ
Neural precursor cells
CP
GABA
interneuron
RG
VZ
I
II
III
IV
V
VI
Node of Ranvier
oligodendrocyte
1. Neurogenesis and
Precursor Cell Proliferation
2. Migration and Lamination
3. Organization,
synaptogenesis,
and circuit formation
4. Myelination

disorders including schizophrenia and autism [Schmidt and Mirnics, 2015]. Relevant to this chapter, abnormal migration often results in abnormal circuit connectivity, comprising foci for seizure generation (discussed further in Section 4.2).

1.2.3 *Cortical organization and synaptogenesis*

Once neurons are in place in the cortex, and even while they are *en route* to their ultimate destinations, a period of growth and elongation of axons and dendrites occurs. This cortical organization begins in mid gestation, prior to synaptogenesis (the process of synapse formation), and extends into early childhood. The timing and extent of the growth and maturation of these processes varies substantially in different cortical layers and brain regions. Proper growth and guidance of axons and dendrites is crucial not only for inter-neuronal connectivity and synaptogenesis, but also for the ontogeny of the intrinsic electrical properties and ion conductances of neurons.

Figure 1.2. Sequence of human neuronal development on a cellular basis. Time line at the top of the figure indicates weeks of gestation (wga) from conception (0 wga) to birth (40 wga). Numbers in gray circles correspond to the stages of brain development below. 1. Neural precursor cells proliferate at the ventricular zone (VZ) and form either neurons or glial cells. 2. Neurons migrate from the VZ to the cortical plate (CP) in a radial fashion along radial glia (RG) cells. Neurons arrive at the CP and establish their final cortical location in an "inside-out" fashion — layer VI neurons are born and arrive first, and layer I cells are last-born and bypass all other layers to migrate to their final destination. Inset: GABA interneurons arrive at the CP via tangential migration rather than radial migration, from their site of origin in the forebrain medial and lateral ganglionic eminences. The third panel shows the mature pattern of the cortical plate consisting of six layers, I–VI. 3. During migration and after having arrived at the CP, neurons elaborate processes including axons and dendrites, and form synapses with other neurons. Shown here are three excitatory synapses (green) onto the distal dendritic tree of the neuron, and two perisomatic inhibitory synapses (red). 4. During the third trimester and after birth, axons are myelinated by oligodendrocytes, which extend multiple processes to envelop axons of multiple neurons. Nodes of Ranvier are axonal regions not covered by myelin; the velocity of neural activity is increased by impulses transmitted down axons in a saltatory (jumping) fashion.

All of the above events follow a developmental sequence. In the earliest neurons, calcium channels are expressed first and become functional prior to potassium channels, favoring increased excitability that is enhanced further when sodium channels are expressed [Moody and Bosma, 2005]. Early action potentials have smaller amplitudes and broader durations than later in development. The earliest synchronized activity of developing neurons is mediated through electrical synapses and calcium currents via a variety of oscillatory waves at different time points and regions. Closer to term, larger scale synaptically-driven networks are activated (e.g., giant depolarizing potentials or GDPs — see Section 3.2 for more details) [Dehorter *et al.*, 2012; Egorov and Draguhn, 2013]. Various types of spontaneous activity are transient and specific for certain periods of development, but at all phases of development network oscillations affect cellular connectivity and function [Kirischuk *et al.*, 2017].

Synaptogenesis begins in the cervical spinal cord around wga 6, whereas the earliest synapses in the cortex form around wga 18. Dendritic spines typically start to appear on mature neocortical neurons first and on interneurons later, between wga 24 and 27, after the massive ingrowth of thalamocortical axons into the cortical plate that starts around wga 21–22. It is thought that many of these early prenatal synapses and circuits are transient, with overproduction of synapses occurring and continuing during the first few postnatal years. Their elimination by activity-dependent pruning enables consolidation of the pathways. That is, synaptic connections are strengthened by neural activity; pathways that do not fire consistently will be pruned.

As is true for the temporal development of ion channel expression, there is also a developmental sequence to the maturation of synaptic function. Excitatory synapses, with glutamate as the primary transmitter, develop prior to inhibitory synapses that utilize GABA as the transmitter. Importantly, GABA is depolarizing rather than hyperpolarizing through most of prenatal life [Ben-Ari, 2002]. Gradually, beginning in late gestation or early in postnatal life in humans, GABA's action transitions from depolarizing (usually but not always excitatory — see Section 3.2) to hyperpolarizing (inhibitory).

This topic is discussed in detail in Section 3.2 and in Chapter 2. Glutamate receptor subunits also mature sequentially, with the earliest receptor subunit isoforms favoring greater excitation. These physiological adaptations are important early in development for neuronal plasticity, trophic function, and connectivity.

It is estimated that a newborn's brain weighs about one-quarter of its weight in early adulthood [Dekaban, 1978]. By birth, the human brain's morphology grossly resembles that of the adult, and the types and arrangement of neurons in the neocortex is largely similar. However, neurogenesis continues in many brain regions throughout infancy and early childhood. After birth, synaptogenesis and the massive growth of dendrites and axons continue, along with glial proliferation and myelination. The fastest rate of brain growth occurs during the first three years of life, demarcating a period of critical neuronal plasticity that can be influenced by multiple pathological processes, including seizures [Isaeva *et al.*, 2013].

1.2.4 *Myelination*

The myelination of central axons by oligodendrocytes represents a critical developmental step necessary for rapid ("saltatory") axonal transmission [Bergles and Richardson, 2016]. Myelination begins in the second trimester but becomes most prominent and rapid in the third trimester and for several years after birth. The various tracts and regions of the CNS myelinate at different rates and at different times, usually progressing from caudal to rostral, dorsal to ventral, and central to peripheral. This pattern of myelination corresponds to attainment of developmental milestones involving visual, sensorimotor, and cognitive function. The degree of myelination will govern the rate of seizure propagation within the brain and peripherally.

1.2.5 *Peripheral nervous system development*

The PNS derives from neural crest cells and placodes. After the neural tube closes, neural crest cells proliferate and migrate to peripheral destinations, and differentiate into a wide spectrum of structures comprising the PNS (Figure 1.1A, bottom). Neural crest gives rise to dorsal root ganglia, autonomic ganglia and Schwann cells. Spinal nerves are comprised of a mixture of sensory and motor axons. The motor manifestations of a seizure require a sufficiently intact and myelinated PNS to allow the excessive neuronal firing to propagate and manifest as observable clinical signs.

1.3 Increased seizure susceptibility of the developing brain

Seizure incidence is highest in childhood, especially in the first year of life. Numerous physiologic factors (Table 1.2) contribute to the increased susceptibility of the developing brain to seizures [Wong, 2005; Ben-Ari and Holmes, 2006; Silverstein and Jensen, 2007; Stafstrom, 2007a; Dulac *et al.*, 2013; Nardou *et al.*, 2013; Miller *et al.*, 2017; Stafstrom and Rho, 2017]. Animal models have provided important insights into the mechanisms of heightened neuronal excitability and seizures (see Chapters 8, 9). Understanding seizure susceptibility as a developmental sequence requires the comparison of nervous system development in humans and rodents (the most commonly used animal model). Such comparisons are approximate since the timing and ultimate completion of various aspects of brain development differ between species, as well as between sexes, brain regions, and neuron types [Katsarou *et al.*, 2017]. However, some informative comparisons can be made, since the exact timing of developmental milestones differs among species, but the sequence of when each milestone occurs is similar across species. The P1–10 rat is roughly equivalent to the third trimester and early postnatal life in humans, with P8–10 rats considered to be similar to full term newborn in humans with respect to brain growth, neurochemical maturation, oligodendrocyte formation, myelination, and other factors [Clancy *et al.*, 2007; Molnar and Clowry, 2012; Semple *et al.*, 2013]. In rodents, during the second postnatal week there is a consistently lower threshold to a wide variety of seizure inducers. This window of hyperexcitability in animal models corresponds approximately to the first year of life in the human infant [Dobbing and Sands, 1973;

Table 1.2. Factors promoting increased seizure susceptibility in the developing brain.

Factor	Consequence
Higher input resistance and shorter membrane time constant in immature neurons	Amplifies synaptic inputs, longer lasting voltage changes
Earlier maturation of sodium and calcium channels, later maturation of potassium channels	Longer action potentials, shorter refractory periods, increased neuron firing
Electrical synapses; more common early in development	Enhanced synchrony of neuronal networks
Excitatory synapses develop before inhibitory synapses	Relative predominance of excitation over inhibition early in development
Overexpression of excitatory synapses during critical period	Window of heightened seizure susceptibility
Increased ratio of NMDA subunits (NR2B/NR2A) favors prolonged depolarizing responses; NR2D relative overexpression reduces Mg^{2+} block	Favors hyperexcitability
Late appearance of inhibitory synapses	Less functional inhibition contributes to neuronal excitatory drive
Excitatory effect of GABA	GABA is depolarizing (and usually excitatory) early in life
Developmental changes in $GABA_A$ receptor subunits	Developmental differences in inhibitory effectiveness and benzodiazepine responsiveness
Immature $GABA_A$ binding pattern in substantia nigra	Proconvulsant effect
Immature homeostatic mechanisms: Na^+,K^+-ATPase, glial K^+ regulation, K^+-Cl^- cotransporters	Prolonged exposure to elevated extracellular K^+ leads to further neuronal depolarization

GABA, gamma-aminobutyric acid; NR, N-methyl-d-aspartate (NMDA) receptor; Mg, magnesium.

Romijn *et al.*, 1991; Clancy *et al.*, 2007], the peak of seizure incidence.

Any physiological factor that alters the brain's excitatory/inhibitory balance in favor of enhanced excitation will favor seizure susceptibility.

Some of these factors have already been mentioned, including ion channels and transmembrane gradients, neurotransmitters and their receptors, and structural and connectivity changes in the developing brain (Table 1.2). Seizure propensity in the very young involves a complex interplay between the timing of cellular and molecular changes [Rakhade and Jensen, 2009]. The various adaptations that make the immature brain especially vulnerable to hyperexcitability and seizure generation, and their specific timing, also provide the opportunity to develop novel, age-specific therapies (see Chapter 4).

1.3.1 *Development of membrane properties and ionic channels*

Intrinsic membrane properties include membrane resistance R_N (defined as voltage change V divided by current I, V/I) and time constant τ_m, a measure of how quickly a neuron's voltage returns to baseline after a signal ($\tau_m = C_m \cdot R_N$, where C_m is membrane capacitance). These passive membrane properties act in concert with ionic conductances to determine a neuron's response to synaptic input. Early in development, neurons have a relatively higher membrane resistance and a shorter time constant, so a depolarizing or hyperpolarizing current of a given amplitude and duration will cause a greater voltage change in an immature neuron than in a mature one [Zhang, 2004]. Therefore, immature neurons are more efficient in converting excitatory synaptic potentials into action potentials.

The relative timing of ion channel development plays a major role in the enhanced excitability of the immature brain [Moody and Bosma, 2005; Spitzer, 2006]. Calcium ion channels, which mediate neuronal excitation and a variety of subcellular signaling functions, develop earliest, followed by potassium and sodium channels. Action potentials are longer early in development, permitting enhanced calcium influx, particularly at the presynaptic terminal, thereby enhancing excitability by increasing the probability of neurotransmitter release. However, the brain must achieve a critical balance between activity-driven calcium channel activation that is necessary for normal developmental processes such as cellular differentiation, migration, and synaptogenesis, and excessive depolarizing currents can that may lead to seizures and neuronal damage [Spitzer *et al.*, 2002].

1.3.2 *Development of neurotransmitters, receptors, and transporters*

Intercellular communication via gap junctions plays a pivotal role in neuronal development [Belousov and Fontes, 2013; Connors, 2017]. Gap junctions mediate electrical synaptic transmission especially in the developing brain prior to chemical synapse formation. Electrical synapses have been reported in several brain regions, including neonatal neocortex and hippocampus. Fast-acting electrical transmission can facilitate rapid synchrony of the neuronal network and precipitate seizures [Velazquez and Carlen, 2000]. In addition to rapid electrical communication, gap junctions also mediate the transmission of small molecules such as second messengers and ions between neurons as well as between neurons and other cell types such as glia. Electrical synapses also participate in the adhesion between migrating neurons and radial glia. The ontogeny of gap junction subunit expression underlies diverse roles for these junctions. For example, excitatory and inhibitory neurons differ in their gap junction expression over time, leading to a dynamic interplay between excitation and inhibition. Electrical synapses are essential for correlated electrical activity and metabolic synchronization [Niculescu and Lohmann, 2014]. It can be hypothesized that the profusion of electrical synapses in prenatal and early postnatal development can facilitate various oscillatory activities, both normal and pathological, contributing to the hyperexcitability and seizure predisposition of the immature brain [Egorov and Draguhn, 2013; Scemes and Velíšková, 2017].

Excitatory chemical synapses form before inhibitory chemical synapses. Each glutamate receptor type, and each glutamate receptor subunit, possesses a distinct maturational profile. For example, excitatory N-methyl-D-aspartate (NMDA)-type glutamate receptors are present (and transiently overexpressed) as early as the second trimester of gestation, when they modulate progenitor cell proliferation and cell fate determination [Simeone *et al.*, 2004;

Bagasrawala *et al.*, 2017; Ewald and Cline, 2009]. The early developmental stoichiometry of NMDA receptor subunits favors prolonged depolarizing responses. In the first postnatal week in rodents, NMDA receptor subunits GluN1 and GluN2B are relatively elevated and GluN2A expression is low; physiologically, this subunit combination confers decreased sensitivity to blockade by magnesium ions and enhanced calcium influx, adaptations that favor depolarization, seizures, and excitotoxicity. Similarly, α-amino-3-hydroxy-5-methyl-4-isoxazoleproprionic acid (AMPA)-type glutamate receptors have a developmental profile, with GluA2 subunits developing later than GluA1 and GluA3 subunits. GluA2 subunits restrict calcium influx, so their relative lack early in development favors enhanced calcium entry and greater excitability. Likewise, the developmental time course of metabotropic (G-protein coupled) glutamate receptors also favors heightened excitability [Avallone *et al.*, 2006; Ngomba *et al.*, 2011; Nardou *et al.*, 2013].

The GABA system follows a maturational trend as well, with different expression of $GABA_A$ receptor subunits expressed at different developmental stages [Brooks-Kayal, 2005; Huang, 2009]. As mentioned, GABA's physiologic action varies over development. The early GABA depolarizing action occurs because of the distribution of chloride ions [Staley, 2006] (Figure 1.3). In the developing brain (up to a few months of age in humans), the intracellular chloride concentration is much higher than in mature neurons. Chloride ion distribution is regulated by membrane pumps. The sodium, potassium, chloride co-transporter 1 (NKCC1) actively influxes chloride ions, utilizing the energy stored in the transmembrane sodium gradient to import a potassium ion, along with one sodium ion and two chloride ions. NKCC1's activity results in an intracellular chloride concentration about 3–4 times greater than that found in mature neurons. Thus, when $GABA_A$ receptors are activated by GABA released from interneurons, postsynaptic chloride-permeable channels open and chloride effluxes out of the neuron down its electrochemical gradient. This chloride efflux results in a depolarizing current; the membrane potential deviates toward the chloride equilibrium potential, which is several tens of millivolts less negative than resting potential

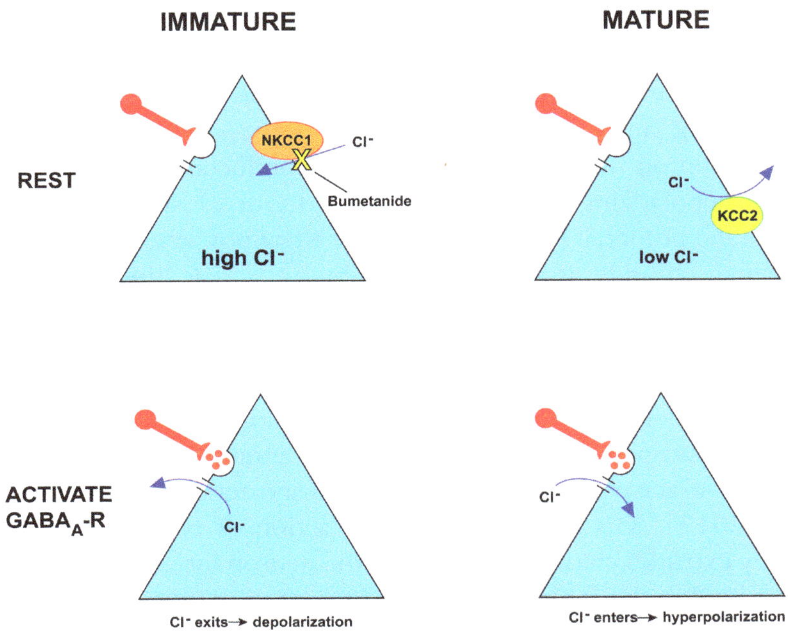

Figure 1.3. GABA responses as a function of age.

Depicted are neurons (blue triangles) illustrating the role of intracellular chloride concentration as a function of age on neuronal responses to GABA (red dots). At early developmental stages (left), intracellular chloride concentration is high due to the activity of a membrane transporter (NKCC1, orange oval) that imports chloride; activation of GABA$_A$ receptors at this age (lower left) causes chloride efflux and depolarization. In the mature brain (right), NKCC1 expression is much reduced, but another chloride transporter (KCC2, green oval) is highly expressed and extrudes chloride, keeping the intracellular chloride concentration relatively low. Therefore, in the mature brain, activation of GABA$_A$ receptors (lower right) results in chloride influx and hyperpolarization of the neuron. The relative intracellular chloride concentrations at the two ages are indicated by the sizes of the Cl^- lettering. Bumetanide (upper left) blocks NKCC1 action and may protect against neonatal seizures by reducing the depolarizing action of GABA at immature ages. GABA$_A$-R, gamma-aminobutyric acid type A receptor; KCC2, potassium-chloride co-transporter 2; NKCC1, sodium-potassium-chloride co-transporter 1.

(i.e., depolarizing). The resulting depolarization may reach the threshold for action potential generation. Glutamatergic excitation provides stronger depolarization than does excitatory GABA, but GABA-mediated depolarization is sufficient to activate NMDA receptors and subthreshold ion currents such as the persistent sodium current [Stafstrom, 2007b], and thus potentiate excitation.

It is important to note that even during the phase when GABA is depolarizing, another mechanism — shunting — can effectively produce inhibition by increasing membrane conductance. Shunting dissipates depolarizing synaptic currents without causing a change in membrane potential [Isaev *et al.*, 2007; Khazipov *et al.*, 2015]. That is, when chloride is passively distributed across the membrane, increasing chloride conductance will not generate transmembrane chloride current. Therefore, GABA can produce some inhibition in the neonatal brain, even in the face of its depolarizing action.

As development proceeds, the expression and activity of the NKCC1 transporter declines and that of another membrane pump increases — the potassium chloride co-transporter 2 (KCC2) [Ben-Ari *et al.*, 2012]. KCC2 has the opposite action of NKCC1 — KCC2 actively extrudes chloride from inside the neuron into the extracellular space, leaving the intracellular compartment with a lower basal chloride concentration (Figure 1.3). Binding of GABA to the $GABA_A$ receptor of a mature neuron with KCC2 present will cause chloride channel opening and influx of chloride into the neuron, down its concentration gradient. This increases intracellular negative charge, hyperpolarizing the neuron and keeping its membrane potential further from the threshold for action potential firing.

The transition from GABAergic depolarization/excitation to inhibition is a critical physiological milestone. As glutamatergic synapses develop and continue to mediate their powerful excitatory action, GABA switches to its mature inhibitory action. While the developmental change in expression of the chloride transporters described above partly explains the depolarizing-to-hyperpolarizing GABA transition, the situation is probably more complex. The early excitatory action of GABA may also be related to the specific distribution of impermeant anions in immature neurons, rather than just transporter expression, as elaborated in Chapter 2 [Glykys *et al.*, 2014]. This transition time point also corresponds to other developmental milestones, namely, the appearance of $GABA_B$–mediated inhibitory responses and disappearance of large oscillatory currents known as giant depolarizing potentials (GDPs) [Mohajerani and Cherubini, 2006]. GDPs are seen only at early ages (e.g., P4–8 in rodents or mid-to-late 3rd trimester in humans), are predominantly dependent upon depolarizing GABA action, and facilitate the formation of synapses and neuronal circuits [Allène *et al.*, 2008]. Seizure susceptibility peaks during this transition, when GABA is still excitatory, excitation via glutamate receptors is still maturing, and $GABA_B$-receptor-mediated inhibition is not yet complete; this window of increased seizure susceptibility occurs around postnatal (P) day 10–14 in rats, corresponding to approximately term in humans, when neonatal seizures are common [Khazipov *et al.*, 2015].

Phenobarbital, which enhances GABAergic inhibition by increasing postsynaptic chloride channel open time, is typically used to suppress seizures in the neonatal period, but its efficacy against neonatal seizures is limited [Painter *et al.*, 1999]. Relevant to neonatal seizure treatment, $GABA_A$ receptor sensitivity to benzodiazepines also varies over development [Haas *et al.*, 2013]. Novel approaches to the management of neonatal seizures are needed [El-Dib and Soul, 2017]. In this regard, bumetanide is a diuretic similar to furosemide that blocks NKCC1 (Figure 1.3) and suppresses epileptic activity in brain slices and animal models [Dzhala *et al.*, 2005], an effect that is enhanced with concomitant phenobarbital use [Dzhala *et al.*, 2008].

1.3.3 *Regulation of the ionic environment*

The development of several ion transport mechanisms favors excitability early in development. Expression of the chloride gradient depends on the development of the NKCC1 and KCC2 transporters, which partially determine whether GABA mediates depolarization or hyperpolarization. Expression of the sodium-potassium ion pump (Na^+, K^+-ATPase) follows a developmental pattern as well [Benarroch, 2011]. Extracellular accumulation of potassium after excessive neuronal activity (e.g., a seizure) can further depolarize the neuronal membrane, exacerbating or prolonging ictal activity. The ability of glial cells to clear extracellular potassium improves with age.

1.3.4 *Structural maturation of the brain and seizure susceptibility*

In the developing brain, synaptic connections are formed and pruned as a function of neuronal activity. Thus, neuronal activity determines which connections remain stable and which are lost. Such changes are referred to as plasticity, a general phenomenon that likely influences the brain's capacity to learn and respond to the environment [Ismail *et al.*, 2017]. The same properties that govern plasticity may also contribute to the tendency of neural networks to synchronize in association with brain pathology or injury. For example, during the second week of life in the rat, the hippocampal CA3 region is characterized by an exuberance of excitatory connections between pyramidal cells, endowing the region with heightened excitability [Casanova *et al.*, 2014]. These connections are later pruned, with stabilization of the excessive excitation seen during this developmental window.

1.4 Disorders of brain development with relevance to seizures and epilepsy

This section provides a few examples of epilepsy according to the stages of brain development outlined in this chapter.

1.4.1 *Disorders of neural tube closure*

Closure of the anterior and posterior neural pores occurs at the end of the 4th wga. At this early stage of brain development, seizures are unlikely, as the processes of neuronal migration, synaptogenesis, and circuit formation have not yet occurred. Postnatal disorders most closely associated with neural tube closure are encephaloceles and myelomeningoceles (spina bifida) when the anterior and posterior neural pores, respectively, fail to close normally. In severe brain malformations resulting from such early developmental pathology, subsequent developmental steps are often clearly altered as well. The increased incidence of epilepsy in children with spina bifida is thought to be due to secondary or additional developmental insults such as migration anomalies rather than to neural tube closure impairment itself [Talwar *et al.*, 1995].

1.4.2 *Disorders of neuronal migration*

It has become increasingly recognized that defects in neuronal migration can give rise to malformations of cortical development and epilepsy, due to either localized (focal) cortical dysplasia or to widespread migration abnormalities [Desikan and Barkovich, 2016]. In children with malformations of cortical development, seizures are very common and can begin in infancy or after several years of life. This topic is covered in detail in Chapter 11, but is discussed briefly below.

A wide spectrum of disorders of neuronal migration is associated with seizures, ranging from an excessive number of small, thin gyri (polymicrogyria), to a reduced number of thick gyri (pachygyria), to an almost completely smooth cortex without many gyri or sulci at all (lissencephaly) (Table 1.1) [Wynshaw-Boris *et al.*, 2010]. Other abnormalities of neuronal migration occurring slightly later in gestation include schizencephaly (wide cleft) or dysgenesis of the corpus callosum. Arrested migration can result in heterotopias, which are collections of neurons with normal or abnormal morphology that have failed to reach their targets in the cortical plate. The resultant abnormal neural circuits may cause focal or multifocal epilepsy.

Mutations in genes regulating numerous aspects of neuronal migration have been implicated in epilepsy. Two examples of abnormal migration due to genetic mutations, one affecting excitatory pyramidal neurons and one affecting inhibitory interneurons, illustrate the wide spectrum of developmental epilepsies. *LIS1* is a gene that regulates migration of neurons from the VZ to the CP. Mutations in *LIS1* are responsible for a number of human disorders, particularly Miller-Dieker syndrome [Parrini *et al.*, 2016]. Affected children have characteristic facial dysmorphic features and congenitally lissencephalic brains with minimal if any cortical gyri and sulci, leaving the cortex with a smooth appearance and neurons with disordered lamination. Nearly all children have seizures, presumably due to abnormal circuit formation between disordered neurons [Hippenmeyer, 2013].

ARX is a homeobox gene that regulates the tangential migration of GABAergic inhibitory interneurons from the ganglionic eminences [Parrini *et al.*, 2016; Katsarou *et al.*, 2017]. Mutations of *ARX* lead to a deficiency of cortical interneurons and decreased inhibitory tone and results in several epilepsy syndromes including infantile spasms. These examples, discussed in more detail in subsequent chapters (see Chapters 3, 8, 11), illustrate the importance of appropriate migration of excitatory and inhibitory neurons for the proper functioning of the cerebral cortex and how mutations in genes regulating either migration pathway can generate an epileptic phenotype.

1.4.3 *Disorders of cortical organization and synaptogenesis*

Once neurons have migrated to their respective locations, they need to further differentiate, express ion channels, elaborate dendritic arbors, specify and guide axons, and form synapses. Disorders, either acquired or genetic, can affect any of these processes and result in hyperexcitable circuits that predispose to seizure generation. Mutations in any of multiple genes that modulate cortical organization and synapse formation can alter the excitability of the developing brain and engender epilepsy, with the mutations exerting different effects at different developmental stages [Reid *et al.*, 2018].

In terms of ion channels, numerous gene mutations predispose to epilepsy. For example, loss-of-function mutations of the $\alpha 1$ subunit of the sodium channel gene (*SCN1A*) are responsible for a spectrum of developmental epilepsies, including genetic epilepsy with febrile seizures plus and Dravet syndrome (severe myoclonic epilepsy of infancy) (see Chapter 3) [Meisler and Kearney, 2005; Harkin *et al.*, 2007; Stafstrom, 2009; Steinlein, 2014]. Children with Dravet syndrome initially have typical development, but then develop medication-refractory seizures of several types along with developmental and cognitive regression; they also have an increased predisposition to sudden death in epilepsy (SUDEP) [Steinlein, 2014].

Similarly, potassium channel mutations can engender epileptic encephalopathies [Villa and Combi, 2016]. A large family of potassium channels mediates outward currents that counter depolarizing influences and stabilize membrane excitability. One example is the *KCNQ2* and *KCNQ3* genes that modulate subthreshold excitability via a muscarine-mediated current ("M-current") [Hille *et al.*, 2014]. Mutations in either gene can cause a spectrum of epilepsy from a benign familial neonatal syndrome to a severe epileptic encephalopathy [Maljevic and Lerche, 2014]. Thus, dysfunction of genes mediating ion fluxes during a window of early development can lead to benign or severe epilepsy.

Regarding synaptogenesis, multiple genetic mutations affecting synapse structure and function result in epilepsy as well as other neurodevelopmental disorders such as autism and schizophrenia. There is an intimate association between autism spectrum disorder (ASD) and epilepsy, with up to 30% of individuals with ASD having comorbid seizures, and the incidence of epilepsy in ASDs with a defined genetic basis is even higher [Strasser *et al.*, 2017]. These disorders likely share neurobiological mechanisms; abnormalities of synapse function and synaptogenesis are especially prevalent in both disorders [Stafstrom and Benke, 2015; Keller *et al.*, 2017]. Affected synaptic proteins in ASD and epilepsy include those that anchor synaptic machinery for vesicle fusion and neurotransmitter release (*SHANK3*, *STXBP1*), modulate subcellular signaling pathways (mTOR, *PTEN*), and regulate GTPase and thus NMDA- and AMPA-receptor function (*SYNGAP1*) [Peça and Feng, 2012]. Therefore, deficiencies in synapse formation and function, driven by mutations in genes coding for synaptic proteins, can create a substrate for developmental epilepsy and ASD [Huguet *et al.*, 2013].

1.4.4 *Disorders of myelination*

Central myelin is formed by oligodendrocytes beginning in the mid-second trimester through several years of life and even into late adolescence. The brain is sparsely myelinated at birth with the most rapid increase in central and peripheral myelin occurring during the first two postnatal years. The dearth of myelination prenatally and shortly after birth accounts in part for the multifocal nature of neonatal seizures and their slow propagation. Primary disorders affecting myelination can certainly be associated with seizures, but these disorders more commonly manifest with dysfunction of cognitive and motor skills.

The leukodystrophies are disorders of CNS white matter due to glial cell or myelin dysfunction and represent a classic example of disorders called dysmyelination [Tonduti and Vanderver, 2018]. Seizures frequently accompany the leukodystrophies but such seizures typically occur late in the disease course [Tonduti and Vanderver, 2018]. An exception is Alexander disease, caused by a gain-of-function mutation in the gene that encodes glial fibrillary acidic protein (GFAP), an astrocytic intermediate filament. While Alexander disease is a disease of astrocyte dysfunction (rather than a primary demyelinating disorder) demyelination is an inevitable consequence. Epilepsy in Alexander's disease appears early in the disease course, often as the presenting sign [Prust *et al.*, 2011].

1.4.5 *Epileptogenesis in the developing brain*

The preceding discussion emphasizes the mechanisms by which the immature brain is susceptible to seizures, or ictogenesis [Rakhade and Jensen, 2009; Nardou *et al.*, 2013]. The developing brain is also prone to the development of epilepsy, the condition of unprovoked, recurrent seizures. The process by which a normal brain becomes epileptic is called epileptogenesis. While there is some overlap between mechanisms of ictogenesis and epileptogenesis, the latter term refers to the development of spontaneous recurrent seizures, either following a brain injury or due to a genetic predisposition. Intensive investigation is now focusing on ways in which the developing brain becomes epileptic, and importantly, on interventions to retard or prevent epileptogenesis.

Numerous factors likely play a role in epileptogenesis, and these are best considered according to a temporal sequence [Bender and Baram, 2007; Pitkanen and Lukasiuk, 2009; Rakhade and Jensen, 2009; Wasterlain *et al.*, 2013; Katsarou *et al.*, 2018; Wasterlain *et al.*,

2013]. In the first hours to days following a precipitating brain injury or severe seizure, immediate early genes are activated that lead to transcription of proteins that alter subsequent excitability. In addition, after a seizure, many receptors and other proteins involved in excitability are phosphorylated, including potassium channels and $GABA_A$, AMPA, and NMDA receptors. Later, in the time frame of days to weeks, inflammation occurs, with elevations of cytokines and other inflammatory compounds, neurotrophic factors, ion channels, and neurotransmitter receptors (see Chapter 10). These changes underlie chronic epileptogenesis that occurs weeks, months to years later, including altered neurogenesis and gliosis, along with the emergence of cognitive and behavioral abnormalities (see Chapter 13). Therefore, the epileptogenic cascade progresses from changes at the gene level to changes at the structural level; these multifactorial processes may provide biomarkers to identify which individuals are at most risk for the development of epilepsy and optimal ways to intervene in the process [Sankar and Rho, 2007]. With accumulating evidence that antiepileptic drugs can cause apoptosis in the developing brain, there is an urgent need for alternative treatments [Wasterlain *et al.*, 2013; Kaushal *et al.*, 2016].

1.5 Conclusion

This chapter has reviewed normal brain development and has provided examples of the rich diversity of mechanisms and pathologies that can give rise to developmental epilepsy. Many of these disorders are considered in greater detail in subsequent chapters. Knowledge of normal and abnormal brain development is providing invaluable information about developmental epilepsy and revealing opportunities to intervene so as to avert the epileptic consequences and associated comorbidities.

References

Allène, C., Cattani, A., Ackman, J.B., Bonifazi, P., Aniksztejn, P., Ben-Ari, Y., and Cossart, R. (2008). Sequential generation of two distinct synapse-driven network patterns in developing neocortex, *J. Neurosci.*, 28, 12851–12863.

Avallone, J., Gashi, E., Magrys, E., and Friedman, L.K. (2006). Distinct regulation of metabotropic glutamate receptor (mGluR1 alpha) in the developing limbic system following multiple early-life seizures, *Exp. Neurol.*, 202, 100–111.

Back, S.A. (2014). Cerebral white and gray matter injury in newborns: new insights into pathophysiology and management, *Clin. Perinatol.*, 41, 1–24.

Bagasrawala, I., Memi, F., Radonjic, N.V., and Zecevic, N. (2017). N-methyl-D-aspartate receptor expression patterns in the human fetal cerebral cortex, *Cereb. Cortex*, 27, 5041–5053.

Belousov, A.B. and Fontes, J.D. (2013). Neuronal gap junctions: making and breaking connections during development and injury, *Trends Neurosci.*, 36, 227–236.

Ben-Ari, Y. (2002). Excitatory actions of GABA during development: the nature of the nurture, *Nat. Rev. Neurosci.*, 3, 728–739.

Ben-Ari, Y. and Holmes, G.L. (2006). Effects of seizures on developmental processes in the immature brain, *Lancet Neurol.*, 5, 1055–1063.

Ben-Ari, Y., Khalilov, I., Kahle, K.T., and Cherubini, E. (2012). The GABA excitatory/inhibitory shift in brain maturation and neurological disorders, *Neuroscientist*, 18, 467–486.

Benarroch, E.E. (2011). Na+, K+-ATPase: functions in the nervous system and involvement in neurologic disease, *Neurology*, 76, 287–293.

Bender, R.A. and Baram, T.Z. (2007). Epileptogenesis in the developing brain: what can we learn from animal models?, *Epilepsia*, 48(Suppl 5), 2–6.

Bergles, D.E. and Richardson, W.D. (2016). Oligodendrocyte development and plasticity, *Cold Spring Harb. Perspect. Biol.*, 8, a020453.

Blanquie, O., Kilb, W., Sinning, A., and Luhmann, H.J. (2017). Homeostatic interplay between electrical activity and neuronal apoptosis in the developing neocortex, *Neuroscience*, 358, 190–200.

Brooks-Kayal, A.R. (2005). Rearranging receptors. *Epilepsia*, 46(Suppl 7), 29–38.

Casanova, J.R., Nishimura, M., and Swann, J.W. (2014). The effects of early-life seizures on hippocampal dendrite development and later-life learning and memory, *Brain Res. Bull.*, 103, 39–48.

Chu, J. and Anderson, S.A. (2015). Development of cortical interneurons, *Neuropsychopharm. Rev.*, 40, 16–23.

Clancy, B., Finlay, B.L., Darlington, R.B., and Anand, K.J. (2007). Extrapolating brain development from experimental species to humans, *Neurotoxicology*, 28, 931–937.

Connors, B.W. (2017). Synchrony and so much more: Diverse roles for electrical synapses in neural circuits, *Dev. Neurobiol.*, 77, 610–624.

DeFelipe, J., López-Cruz, P.L., Benavides-Piccione, R., Bielza, C., Larrañaga, P., Anderson, P., Burkhalter, A., Cauli, B., Fairén, A., Feldmeyer, D., Fishell, G., Fitzpatrick, D., Freund, T.F., González-Burgos, G., Hestrin, S., Hill, S., Hof, P.R., Huang, J., Jones, E.G., Kawaguchi, Y., Kisvárday, Z., Kubota, Y., Lewis, D.A., Marín, O., Markram, H., McBain, C.J., Meyer, H.S., Monyer, H., Nelson, S.B., Rockland, K., Rossier, J., Rubenstein, J.L., Rudy, B., Scanziani, M., Shepherd, G.M., Sherwood, C.C., Staiger, J.F., Tamás, G., Thomson, A., Wang, Y., Yuste, R., and Ascoli, G.A. (2013). New insights into the classification and nomenclature of cortical GABAergic interneurons, *Nat. Rev. Neurosci.,* 14, 202–216.

Dehorter, N., Vinay, L., Hammond, C., and Ben-Ari, Y. (2012). Timing of developmental sequences in different brain structures: physiological and pathological implications, *Eur. J. Neurosci.,* 35, 1846–1856.

Dekaban, A.S. (1978). Changes in brain weights during the span of human life: relation of brain weights to body heights and body weights. *Ann. Neurol.*, 4, 345–356.

Desikan, R.S. and Barkovich, A.J. (2016). Malformations of cortical development, *Ann. Neurol.*, 80, 797–810.

Dobbing, J. and Sands, J. (1973). Quantitative growth and development of the human brain, *Arch. Dis. Child.*, 48, 757–767.

Dulac, O., Milh, M., and Holmes, G.L. (2013). Brain maturation and epilepsy, *Handb. Clin. Neurol.*, 111, 441–446.

Dzhala, V.I., Brumback, A.C., and Staley, K.J. (2008). Bumetanide enhances phenobarbital efficacy in a neonatal seizure model, *Ann. Neurol.*, 63, 222–235.

Dzhala, V.I., Talos, D.M., Sdrulla, D.A., Brumback, A.C., Mathews, G.C., Benke, T.A., Delpire, E., Jensen, F.E., and Staley, K.J. (2005). NKCC1 transporter facilitates seizures in the developing brain, *Nat. Med.*, 11, 1205–1213.

Egorov, A.V. and Draguhn, A. (2013). Development of coherent neuronal activity patterns in mammalian cortical networks: common principles and local hetereogeneity, *Mech. Dev.*, 130, 412–423.

El-Dib, M. and Soul, J.S. (2017). The use of phenobarbital and other anti-seizure drugs in newborns, *Semin. Fetal Neonatal Med.*, 22, 321–327.

Ewald, R.C. and Cline, H.T. (2009). *Biology of the NMDA Receptor*, ed. Van Dongen, A. M., "NMDA receptors and brain development," (CRC Press/Taylor & Francis, Boca Raton FL), https://www.ncbi.nlm.nih.gov/books/NBK5287/.

Glykys, J., Dzhala, V., Egawa, K., Balena, T., Saponjian, Y., Kuchibhotla, K.V., Bacskai, B.J., Kahle, K.T., Zeuthen, T., and Staley, K.J. (2014). Local impermeant anions establish the neuronal chloride concentration, *Science*, 343, 670–675.

Haas, M., Qu, Z., Kim, T.H., Vargas, E., Campbell, K., Petrou, S., Tan, S.S., Reid, C.A., and Heng, J. (2013). Perturbations in cortical development and neuronal network excitability arising from prenatal exposure to benzodiazepines in mice, *Eur. J. Neurosci.*, 37, 1584–1593.

Harkin, L.A., McMahon, J.M., Iona, X., Dibbens, L., Pelekanos, J.T., Zuberi, S.M., Sadleir, L.G., Andermann, E., Gill, D., Farrell, K., Connolly, M., Stanley, T., Harbord, M., Andermann, F., Wang, J., Batish, S.D., Jones, J.G., Seltzer, W.K., Gardner, A.; Infantile Epileptic Encephalopthy Referral Consortium, G. Sutherland, S.F. Berkovic, J.C. Mulley and I.E. Scheffer (2007). The spectrum of *SCN1A*-related infantile epileptic encephalopathies, *Brain*, 130(Part 3), 843–852.

Hille, B., Dickson, E., Kruse, M., and Falkenburger, B. (2014). Dynamic metabolic control of an ion channel. *Prog. Mol. Biol. Transl. Sci.*, 123, 219–247.

Hippenmeyer, S. (2013). Molecular pathways controlling the sequential steps of cortical projection neuron migration, *Adv. Exp. Med. Biol.*, 800, 1–24.

Huang, Z.J. (2009). Activity-dependent development of inhibitory synapses and innervation pattern: role of GABA signalling and beyond, *J. Physiol.*, 587(Pt 9), 1881–1888.

Huguet, G., Ey, E., and Bourgeron, T. (2013). The genetic landscapes of autism spectrum disorders, *Annu. Rev. Genomics Hum. Genet.*, 14, 191–213.

Isaev, D., Isaeva, E., Khazipov, R., and Holmes, G.L. (2007). Shunting and hyperpolarizing GABAergic inhibition in the high-potassium model of ictogenesis in the developing rat hippocampus, *Hippocampus*, 17, 210–219.

Isaeva, E., Isaev, D., and Holmes, G.L. (2013). Alteration of synaptic plasticity by neonatal seizures in rat somatosensory cortex, *Epilepsy Res.*, 106, 280–283.

Ismail, F.Y., Fatemi, A., and Johnston, M.V. (2017). Cerebral plasticity: Windows of opportunity in the developing brain, *Eur. J. Paediatr. Neurol.*, 21, 23–48.

Jiang, X. and Nardelli, J. (2016). Cellular and molecular introduction to brain development. *Neurobiol. Dis.*, 92, 3–17.

Katsarou, A.M., Galanopoulou, A.S., and Moshé, S.L. (2017). Interneuronopathies and their role in early life epilepsies and neurodevelopmental disorders, *Epilepsia Open*, 2, 284–306.

Katsarou, A.M., Galanopoulou, A.S., and Moshé, S. L. (2018). Epileptogenesis in neonatal brain, *Semin. Fetal Neonatal Med.*, 23, 159–167.

Kaushal, S., Tamer, Z., Opoku, F., and Forcelli, P.A. (2016). Anticonvulsant drug-induced cell death in the developing white matter of the rodent brain, *Epilepsia*, 57, 727–734.

Keller, R., Basta, R., Salerno, L., and Elia, M. (2017). Autism, epilepsy, and synaptopathies: a not rare association, *Neurol. Sci.*, 38, 1353–1361.

Khazipov, R., Valeeva, G., and Khalilov, I. (2015). Depolarizing GABA and developmental epilepsies, *CNS Neurosci. Ther.*, 21, 83–91.

Kirischuk, S., Sinning, A., Blanquie, O., Yang, J.W., Luhmann, H.J., and Kilb, W. (2017). Modulation of neocortical development by early neuronal activity: Physiology and pathophysiology, *Front. Cell. Neurosci.*, 11, 379, doi:10.3389/fncel.2017.00379.

Luhmann, H.J., Fukuda, A., and Kilb, W. (2015). Control of cortical neuronal migration by glutamate and GABA, *Front. Cell. Neurosci.*, 9, 4, doi:10.3389/fncel.2015.00004.

Luhmann, H.J., Kirischuk, S., Sinning, A., and Kilb, W. (2014). Early GABAergic circuitry in the cerebral cortex, *Curr. Opin. Neurobiol.*, 26, 72–78.

Lui, J.H., Hansen, D.V., and Kriegstein, A.R. (2011). Development and evolution of the human neocortex, *Cell*, 146, 18–36.

Maljevic, S. and Lerche, H. (2014). Potassium channel genes and benign familial neonatal epilepsy, *Prog. Brain Res.*, 213, 17–53.

Meisler, M.H. and Kearney, J.A. (2005). Sodium channel mutations in epilepsy and other neurological disorders, *J. Clin. Invest.*, 115, 2010–2017.

Miller, S.M., Goasdoue, K., and Björkman, S.T. (2017). Neonatal seizures and disruption to neurotransmitter systems, *Neural Regen. Res.*, 12, 216–217.

Mohajerani, M.H. and Cherubini, E. (2006). Role of giant depolarizing potentials in shaping synaptic currents in the developing hippocampus, *Crit. Rev. Neurobiol.*, 18, 12–23.

Molnar, Z. and Clowry, G. (2012). Cerebral cortical development in rodents and primates, *Prog. Brain Res.*, 195, 45–70.

Moody, W.J. and Bosma, M.M. (2005). Ion channel development, spontaneous activity, and activity-dependent development in nerve and muscle cells, *Physiol. Rev.*, 85, 883–941.

Nardou, R., Ferrari, D.C., and Ben-Ari, Y. (2013). Mechanisms and effects of seizures in the immature brain, *Semin. Fetal Neonatal Med.*, 18, 175–184.

Ngomba, R.T., Santolini, I., Salt, T.E., Ferraguti, F., Battaglia, G., Nicoletti, F., and van Luijtelaar, G. (2011). Metabotropic glutamate receptors in the thalamocortical network: strategic targets for the treatment of absence epilepsy, *Epilepsia*, 52, 1211–1222.

Niculescu, D. and Lohmann, C. (2014). Gap junctions in developing thalamic and neocortical neuronal networks, *Cereb. Cortex*, 24, 3097–3106.

Ortega, J.A., Memi, F., Radonjic, N., Filipovic, R., Bagasrawala, I., Zecevic, N., and Jakovcevski, I. (2018). The subventricular zone: a key player in human neocortical development, *Neuroscientist*, 24, 156–170.

Painter, M.J., Scher, M.S., Stein, A.D., Armatti, S., Wang, Z., Gardner, J.C., Paneth, N., Minnigh, B., and Alvin, J. (1999). Phenobarbital compared with phenytoin for the treatment of neonatal seizures, *N. Engl. J. Med.*, 341, 485–489.

Parrini, E., Conti, V., Dobyns, W.B., and Guerrini, R. (2016). Genetic basis of brain malformations, *Mol. Syndromol.*, 7, 220–233.

Peça, J. and Feng, G. (2012). Cellular and synaptic network defects in autism, *Curr. Opin. Neurobiol.*, 22, 866–872.

Pitkanen, A. and Lukasiuk, K. (2009). Molecular and cellular basis of epileptogenesis in symptomatic epilepsy, *Epilepsy Behav.*, 14, 16–25.

Prust, M., Wang, J., Morizono, H., Messing, A., Brenner, M., Gordon, E., Hartka, T., Sokohl, A., Schiffmann, R., Gordish-Dressman, H., Albin, R., Amartino, H., Brockman, K., Dinopoulos, A., Dotti, M.T., Fain, D., Fernandez, R., Ferreira, J., Fleming, J., Gill, D., Griebel, M., Heilstedt, H., Kaplan, P., Lewis, D., Nakagawa, M., Pedersen, R., Reddy, A., Sawaishi, Y., Schneider, M., Sherr, E., Takiyama, Y., Wakabayashi, K., Gorospe, J.R., and Vanderver, A. (2011). GFAP mutations, age at onset, and clinical subtypes in Alexander disease, *Neurology*, 77, 1287–1294.

Rakhade, S.N. and Jensen, F.E. (2009). Epileptogenesis in the immature brain: emerging mechanisms, *Nat. Rev. Neurol.*, 5, 380–391.

Rakic, S. and Zecevic, N. (2003). Emerging complexity of layer I in human cerebral cortex, *Cereb. Cortex*, 13, 1072–1083.

Reid, C.A., Rollo, B., Petrou, S., and Berkovic, S.F. (2018). Can mutation-mediated effects occurring early in development cause long-term seizure susceptibility in genetic generalized epilepsies?, *Epilepsia*, 59, 915–922.

Romijn, H.J., Hofman, M.A., and Gransberger, A. (1991). At what age is the developing cerebral cortex of the rat comparable to that of the full term newborn baby?, *Early Hum. Dev.*, 26, 61–67.

Sankar, R. and Rho, J.M. (2007). Do seizures affect the developing brain? Lessons from the laboratory, *J. Child Neurol.*, 22(5 Suppl), 21S–29S.

Scemes, E. and Velíšková, J. (2017). Exciting and not so exciting roles of pannexins, *Neurosci. Lett.*, pii: S0304-3940(17)30220-3. doi: 10.1016/j.neulet.2017.03.010. [Epub ahead of print]

Schmidt, M.J. and Mirnics, K. (2015). Neurodevelopment, GABA system dysfunction, and schizophrenia, *Neuropsychopharmacology*, 40, 190–206.

Semple, B.D., Blomgren, K., Gimlin, K., Ferriero, D.M., and Noble-Haeusslein, L.J. (2013). Brain development in rodents and humans: Identifying benchmarks of maturation and vulnerability to injury across species, *Prog. Neurobiol.*, 106–107, 1–16.

Silbereis, J.C., Pochareddy, S., Zhu, Y., Li, M., and Sestan, N. (2016). The cellular and molecular landscapes of the developing human central nervous system, *Neuron*, 89, 248–268.

Silverstein, F.S. and Jensen, F.E. (2007). Neonatal seizures. *Ann. Neurol.*, 62, 112–120.

Simeone, T.A., Sanchez, R.M., and Rho, J.M. (2004). Molecular biology and ontogeny of glutamate receptors in the mammalian central nervous system, *J. Child Neurol.*, 19, 343–360.

Spitzer, N.C. (2006). Electrical activity in early neuronal development, *Nature*, 444, 707–712.

Spitzer, N.C., Kingston, P.A., Manning, T.J., and Conklin, M.W. (2002). Outside and in: development of neuronal excitability, *Curr. Opin. Neurobiol.*, 12, 315–323.

Stafstrom, C.E. (2007a). Neurobiological mechanisms of developmental epilepsy: translating experimental findings into clinical application, *Semin. Pediatr. Neurol.*, 14, 164–172.

Stafstrom, C.E. (2007b). Persistent sodium current and its role in epilepsy, *Epilepsy Curr.*, 7, 15–22.

Stafstrom, C.E. (2009). Severe epilepsy syndromes of early childhood: the link between genetics and pathophysiology with a focus on *SCN1A* mutations, *J. Child Neurol.*, 24(8 Suppl), 15S–23S.

Stafstrom, C.E. and Benke, T.A. (2015). Autism and epilepsy: exploring the relationship using experimental models, *Epilepsy Curr.*, 15, 206–210.

Stafstrom, C.E. and Rho, J.M. (2017). *Swaiman's Pediatric Neurology: Principles and Practice*, 6th edition, eds. Swaiman, K., Ashwal, S., Ferriero, D. M., Schor, N. F., Finkel, R. S., Gropman, A. L., Pearl, P. L., and Shevell, M. I., Chapter 63 "Neurophysiology of seizures and epilepsy," (Elsevier, Amsterdam), pp. 506–512.

Staley, K. (2006). Wrong-way chloride transport: is it a treatable cause of some intractable seizures?, *Epilepsy Curr.*, 6, 124–127.

Steinlein, O.K. (2014). Mechanisms underlying epilepsies associated with sodium channel mutations, *Prog. Brain Res.*, 213, 97–111.

Stiles, J. and Jernigan, T.L. (2010). The basics of brain development, *Neuropsychol. Rev.*, 20, 327–348.

Strasser, L., Downes, M., Kung, J., Cross, J.H., and De Haan, M. (2017). Prevalence and risk factors for autism spectrum disorder in epilepsy: a systematic review and meta-analysis, *Dev. Med. Child Neurol.*, 60, 19–29.

Talwar, D., Baldwin, M.A., and Horbatt, C.L. (1995). Epilepsy in children with meningomyelocele, *Pediatr. Neurol.*, 13, 29–32.

Tonduti, D. and Vanderver, A. (2018). *Inherited Metabolic Epilepsies*, ed. Pearl, P. L., Chapter 37 "Leukodystrophies and epilepsy." (Demos, New York) pp. 483–487.

Velazquez, J.P. and Carlen, P. (2000). Gap junctions, synchrony, and seizures, *Trends Neurosci.*, 23, 68–74.

Villa, C. and Combi, R. (2016). Potassium channels and human epileptic phenotypes: an updated overview, *Front. Cell. Neurosci.*, 10, 81, doi:10.3389/fncel.2016.00081.

Wasterlain, C.G., Gloss, D.S., Niquet, J., and Wasterlain, A.S. (2013). Epileptogenesis in the developing brain, *Handb. Clin. Neurol.*, 3, 427–439.

Wichterle, H., Garcia-Verdugo, J.M., Herrera, D.G., and Alvarez-Buylla, A. (1999). Young neurons from medial ganglionic eminence disperse in adult and embryonic brain, *Nat. Neurosci.*, 2, 461–466.

Wong, M. (2005). Advances in the pathophysiology of developmental epilepsies, *Semin. Pediatr. Neurol.*, 12, 72–87.

Wu, Q., Liu, J., Fang, A., Li, R., Bai, Y., Kriegstein, A.R., and Wang, X. (2014). The dynamics of neuronal migration, *Adv. Exp. Med. Biol.*, 800, 25–36.

Wynshaw-Boris, A., Pramparo, T., Youn, Y.H., and Hirotsune, S. (2010). Lissencephaly: mechanistic insights from animal models and potential therapeutic strategies, *Semin. Cell Dev. Biol.*, 21, 823–830.

Zhang, Z.W. (2004). Maturation of layer V pyramidal neurons in the rat prefrontal cortex: intrinsic properties and synaptic function, *J. Neurophysiol.*, 91, 1171–1182.

Chapter 2
Physiology and Pathophysiology of Seizures in the Developing Brain

Lila T. Worden,* MD
Kevin J. Staley,† MD

**Division of Neurology, Children's Hospital of Philadelphia, Philadelphia, PA, USA*
†Department of Neurology, Massachusetts General Hospital, Boston, MA, USA

2.1 Introduction

Seizures are the abnormal, hypersynchronous firing of neurons that disrupt normal brain functioning. An imbalance of excitation and inhibition, either from an overstimulation of excitatory conductances [Walther *et al.*, 1986] or by blocking inhibitory conductances [Matusmoto and Ajmonemarsan, 1964; Prince and Wilder, 1967], is commonly cited as a fundamental ictogenic mechanism, but might be more accurately described as a commonly-used experimental condition to induce epileptiform activity in normal brain tissue [Staley, 2015].

Genetic studies have highlighted the heterogeneity of conditions that may lead to epilepsy. Many early onset epilepsies are due to mutations that could engender hyperexcitability, such as increased excitation via gain of function mutation in *SCN8A* [Wagnon *et al.*, 2016], or decreased inhibition via loss of function mutations in $GABA_A$ receptors

[Macdonald and Kang, 2012] or *KCNQ2* potassium channels [Singh *et al.*, 1998]. However, an equal number of mutations underlying seizures *enhance* inhibition (e.g., gain of function mutations in *KCNT1* [Barcia *et al.*, 2012]) or *decrease* excitation (e.g., loss of function mutation in *SCN1A* [Yu *et al.*, 2006; Carvill *et al.*, 2014]). Additionally, many gene mutations underlying epilepsy do not affect the balance of excitatory and inhibitory forces [Ran *et al.*, 2015].

The genetic heterogeneity underlying epilepsies makes them inadequate models for understanding seizure pathophysiology. As such, we will defer a review of the genetics of developmental epilepsies to other chapters. To understand seizure physiology in the developing brain, we will focus on neonatal seizures, as this population has unique susceptibilities to seizures and more homogenous pathology than those with genetic epilepsies, and as such serves as a useful model for understanding seizure pathophysiology.

2.1.1 *Seizures in the neonatal period*

The neonatal period is one of the highest risk intervals for the onset of seizures and epilepsy throughout the lifespan (Figure 2.1). The incidence falls dramatically after the first year of life and does not reach similar levels again until the 8th decade [Olafsson *et al.*, 2005].

In neonates, the incidence of seizure is 1–3.5 per 1000 live births [Ronen *et al.*, 1999; Wirrell, 2005; Glass *et al.*, 2009; Vasudevan and

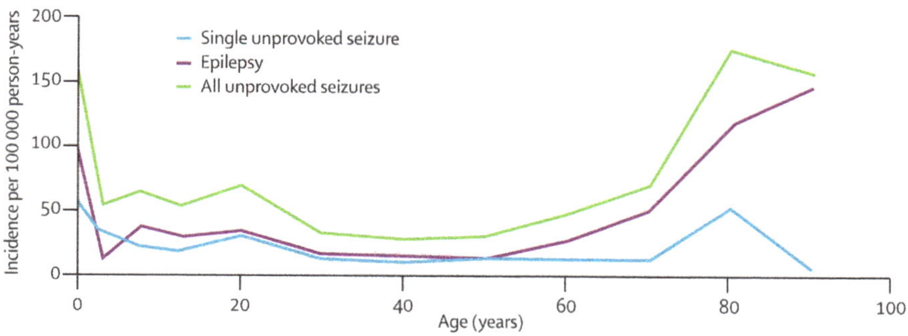

Figure 2.1. Incidence of seizures and epilepsy throughout the lifespan. Reprinted from Olafsson *et al.*, 2005.

Levene, 2013]. Postnatal day 7–14 (P7–P14) mice are at approximately the same stage of brain development as human infants between term birth and the first year of life [Semple *et al.*, 2013]. A variety of experimentally-induced seizures in these animals confirms the unique susceptibility to seizure at this developmental stage: kindling [Moshé, 1981], hypoxia [Jensen *et al.*, 1991], kainic acid [Tremblay *et al.*, 1984; Stafstrom, Thompson and Holmes, 1992], or $GABA_B$ receptor antagonism [Velíšková *et al.*, 1996].

Increased seizure incidence during this period is due to both intrinsic factors and external factors, such as complications of birth. The most common cause of seizure in this group is hypoxic-ischemic injury [Glass *et al.*, 2016], accounting for over 1/3 of all neonatal seizures. The birth process is also associated with an increased incidence of intracranial hemorrhage, stroke, and meningitis (Table 2.1). Additionally, neonates with severe congenital brain malformations such as hemimegalencephaly or lissencephaly, and those with certain metabolic conditions, like nonketotic hyperglycinemia, frequently present with seizures in the newborn period.

We will first review the physiology of normal neuronal signaling, including ion channels, membrane potentials and synaptic transmission. We will then discuss changes in early brain development that underlie the enhanced vulnerability to seizures. Lastly, we will

Table 2.1. Seizure etiology in term neonates. Adapted from Glass *et al.*, 2016.

Hypoxic-ischemic encephalopathy	38%
Ischemic stroke	18%
Intracranial hemorrhage	12%
Genetic epilepsy	6%
Intracranial infection	4%
Brain malformation	4%
Transient metabolic disturbance	4%
Inborn error of metabolism	3%
Benign familial neonatal epilepsy	1%
Other/unknown	9%

explore seizure pathophysiology after brain injury, and a model for the repetitive seizures of epilepsy.

2.2 Normal physiology: Ion channels, neurotransmitters, and action potentials

2.2.1 *Ion channel overview*

Ion channels are transmembrane proteins that allow passive movement of ions down their electrochemical gradient. While some channels are open at rest and help to maintain the resting membrane potential, many are gated. Gated ion channels are activated or opened based on a particular state. For example, ligand-gated channels require the presence of a molecule such as a neurotransmitter to open, while voltage-gated channels are activated by a threshold membrane depolarization or hyperpolarization. Other channels are pH- or mechanically-gated, responding to pressure or stretch. In general, voltage-gated ion channels are involved in modulation of the membrane potential and electrical signal transmission via action potentials, whereas ligand-gated ion channels are involved in signal transmission across synapses.

Ion channels are involved in fast transmission of neuronal signals. A single channel opening allows passive diffusion of many ions along their electrochemical gradient. This contrasts with pumps, which are active transporters that move ions *against* their electrochemical gradients and require ATP to function. Pumps act slowly because a protein conformational change occurs with ion each transport cycle. Comparatively, the movement of ions is 100 to 100,000 times slower than through channels [Kandel *et al.*, 2013]; however, pumps play an essential role in maintaining the electrochemical gradient. Secondary ion transporters drive movement of one ion *against* its electrochemical gradient by using energy derived from moving another, co-transported ion moving *down* its electrochemical gradient. The distribution of ion channels is not uniform throughout a neuron and varies according to local function. For example, the initial segment of the axon has a very high density of voltage-gated Na channels, leading to easy generation of action potentials [Kandel *et al.*, 2013].

2.2.2 *Resting membrane potential*

To understand the movement of ions into and out of cells that underlies neuronal signaling, it is first necessary to understand the neuronal membrane at homeostasis, or rest.

The neuron cell membrane is made up of a lipid bilayer which is impermeable to the free diffusion of ions and water, enabling a separation of charge across the membrane based on the relative concentrations and charges of ions in the intracellular and extracellular spaces. This electrical potential difference across the membrane is called the membrane potential. At rest, there is a net negative charge inside the cell relative to the external milieu. By convention, the electrical potential outside the cell is defined as zero; consequently, the resting membrane potential is –60 to –70 mV in most neurons.

The resting potential is influenced by the permeability of the membrane to each ion. The main ions contributing to the membrane potential are sodium (Na^+), potassium (K^+), chloride (Cl^-), and organic anions; while there are other charged ions such as hydrogen, calcium and bicarbonate, their significantly lower concentrations make their impact much less. The neuronal membrane is most permeable to potassium and chloride, and significantly less to sodium; in contrast, the organic anions are fixed intracellularly and do not have the potential to diffuse, and so can contribute to the creation of electrical and osmotic gradients across the membrane. The concentrations of permeant ions that contribute to the resting membrane potential are maintained via active transport to regain baseline charge separation, otherwise over time the ionic gradients would dissipate. The Na-K-ATPase pump is the most well-known primary ion transporter, moving 3 Na^+ ions out for every 2 K^+ in, and while there are other primary ion transporters, Na-K-ATPase is responsible for the majority of primary active neuronal membrane ion transport at rest.

On the extracellular side, there is a high concentration of sodium and chloride. The main intracellular ions are potassium and organic anions. The intracellular organic anions are formed by structural proteins and amino acids. Ribosomes, the proteins involved in RNA translation and protein synthesis, have a large negative charge, as do

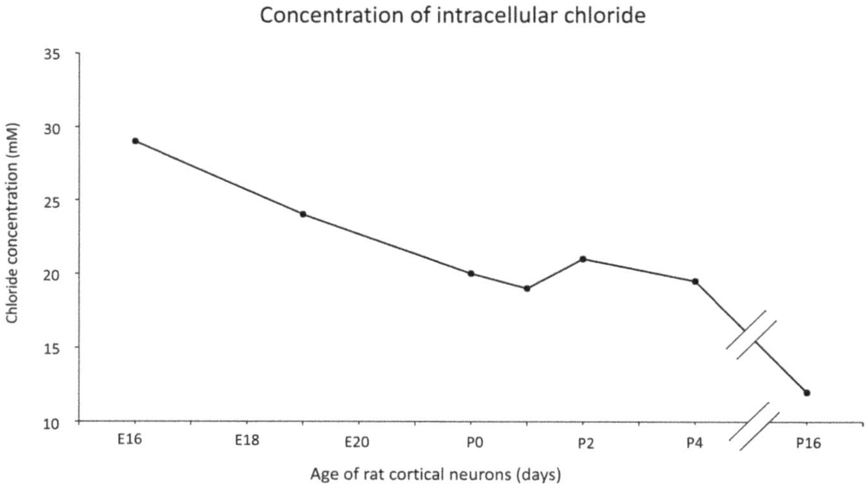

Figure 2.2. Developmental decrease of intracellular chloride in rat neurons. VZ = Ventricular zone. Adapted from Owens *et al.*, 1996.

nucleic acids due to the phosphate groups that provide the backbone structure of DNA [Baker *et al.*, 2001]. The cytoskeleton, which maintains the cell structure and is essential for axonal transport and cell trafficking, also has a large negative charge due its major component — microtubules, whose negative charge facilitates interactions with microtubule-associated proteins [Baker *et al.*, 2001; Sanabria *et al.*, 2006].

Chloride is a relatively minor intracellular anion, but it plays a critical role by virtue of its high permeability through ligand-gated $GABA_A$ receptor channels. The chloride concentration varies notably through early development (Figure 2.2). In immature neurons, chloride is high intracellularly and drops to very low concentrations over time [Owens *et al.*, 1996; Ben-Ari, 2002]. Chloride concentration is important in regulating the susceptibility to seizures, so we explore this in more detail.

2.2.2.1 *Chloride concentration is determined by impermeable anions*

In the 1990s, the identification of the electroneutral cation-chloride cotransporters NKCC1 and KCC2 provided a mechanism for pumping chloride across the cell membrane against its equilibrium potential using secondary active transport. NKCC1 is a Na^+–K^+–$2Cl^-$ cotransporter that imports 2 Cl^- into neurons accompanied by 1 Na^+ and 1 K^+. NKCC1-mediated transport is driven largely by the energy of the Na^+ gradient that is generated by the Na-K-ATPase pump. KCC2 is a K^+–Cl^- cotransporter that exports 1 Cl^- and 1 K^+ out of neurons by using the energy of the K^+ gradient [Delpire, 2000; Ben-Ari, 2002; Blaesse *et al.*, 2009; Kahle *et al.*, 2015].

The change in intracellular chloride from high to low in early development was initially thought due to differential developmental expression of NKCC1 and KCC2, with earlier expression of NKCC1 [Plotkin *et al.*, 1997; Dzhala *et al.*, 2005; Kahle *et al.*, 2008] than KCC2 [Lu *et al.*, 1999; Rivera *et al.*, 1999; Stein *et al.*, 2004; Dzhala *et al.*, 2005] resulting in a higher intracellular chloride concentration early in development. More recent studies have shown that both NKCC1 and KCC2 are expressed outside of these developmental windows [Sedmak *et al.*, 2016]. Furthermore, there are neurons with high intracellular chloride that do not express NKCC1 [Balakrishnan *et al.*, 2003; Nickell *et al.*, 2006; Zhang *et al.*, 2007] and neurons with low intracellular chloride that do not express KCC2 or the related potassium-chloride cotransporter KCC3 [Kahle *et al.*, 2015]. These cotransporters are equilibrative, meaning they transport ions in whichever direction the concentration gradients dictate [Delpire and Staley, 2014]. Thus NKCC1 and KCC2 can engage in bidirectional transport under the right conditions [Glykys *et al.*, 2014]. While the cation-chloride cotransporters are *not* the main determinants of chloride concentration as previously thought, they are important in returning chloride to homeostatic levels after chloride shifts from ion channel openings.

Instead, the current evidence supports that chloride concentration is regulated by the quantity of impermeable anions, both intracellular and extracellular [Glykys *et al.*, 2014]. Intracellular and extracellular impermeable anions displace chloride and account for changes in the local chloride concentration. New study techniques have shown that chloride does *not* decrease uniformly in all neurons at the same point in development [Tyzio *et al.*, 2008; Glykys *et al.*, 2009; Glykys and Staley, 2015] and additionally, different areas of the same neuron can have differing chloride concentrations [Duebel *et al.*, 2006; Glykys *et al.*, 2014]. In early life, cytoplasmic chloride concentration is initially high due to a relatively lower density of intracellular anions [Audebert *et al.*, 1994; McClatchy *et al.*, 2007]. Extracellular chloride concentrations may also change with development as a consequence of changes in the concentration and sulfation of the glycosaminoglycan moieties of extracellular and membrane-bound glycoproteins [Miyata *et al.*, 2012]. With development, chloride near the neuronal membrane may decrease due to displacement by these extracellular impermeant organic anions [Glykys *et al.*, 2017].

2.2.3 *Equilibrium potentials and membrane conductances*

Each ion has an equilibrium potential, which is the membrane potential at which the electric driving force from electromagnetic charge equals the chemical driving force from the concentration gradient. At the equilibrium potential there is no net flux of the ion across the cell membrane; it is also known as the reversal potential as it is the membrane potential at which the ion flow through an open channel will reverse direction. The equilibrium potential for an ion can be calculated using the Nernst equation:

$$E_{rev} = RT/ZF \times \ln\left([\text{ion}]_{outside}/[\text{ion}]_{inside}\right) \qquad (2.1)$$

where R is the ideal gas constant, T is the temperature, Z is the valence of the ion (e.g., −1 for chloride), and F is the Faraday constant. For any permeant anion, if the equilibrium potential is more negative than the resting membrane potential, then free flow across an ion channel will lead to an inward current. In this condition, anions move out of the neuron and depolarize the membrane. The opposite is true if the equilibrium potential is greater (less negative) than the resting membrane potential — the anion will move inwards (by convention, this is called an outward current) and hyperpolarize the membrane.

Depolarizing or hyperpolarizing conductances are defined by their effects on the membrane potential. Depolarizing conductances

Table 2.2. The idealized distribution of major ions across the cell membrane at rest in a mature neuron. Adapted from Hammond, 2015; Lodish *et al.*, 2000.

	Intracellular concentration (mM)	**Extracellular concentration (mM)**	**Equilibrium potential (mV)**
Na^+	14	140	+60
K^-	140	3	−88
Cl^-	14	146	−61
Ca^+	0.0001	1.5	+125
Anions (−)	138	9	None

decrease the voltage difference across the membrane whereas hyperpolarizing currents make the voltage across the membrane more negative. Channels are permeable to a single or limited number of ions. Under most circumstances, sodium and calcium are considered depolarizing or excitatory currents due to their influx when channels are open, whereas potassium and chloride are thought of as hyperpolarizing or inhibitory currents due potassium efflux and influx of chloride. However, since flow across open ion channels is passive, the direction of ion flow is dependent on the equilibrium potential for each ion and can be reversed depending on the membrane potential and the concentrations of ions on either side of the membrane.

2.2.4 *Electrical signaling and action potentials*

Electrical signaling in the neuron involves brief changes in the resting membrane potential due to currents across the membrane. Temporary depolarizations of the post-synaptic membrane by excitatory currents caused by opening of ligand-gated channels are called excitatory post-synaptic potentials (EPSP). Temporary hyperpolarizations caused by the opening of ligand-gated channels are called inhibitory post-synaptic potentials (IPSP).

When the depolarizing potential crosses a critical level or threshold, typically −40 to −50 mV, an action potential occurs, which is an

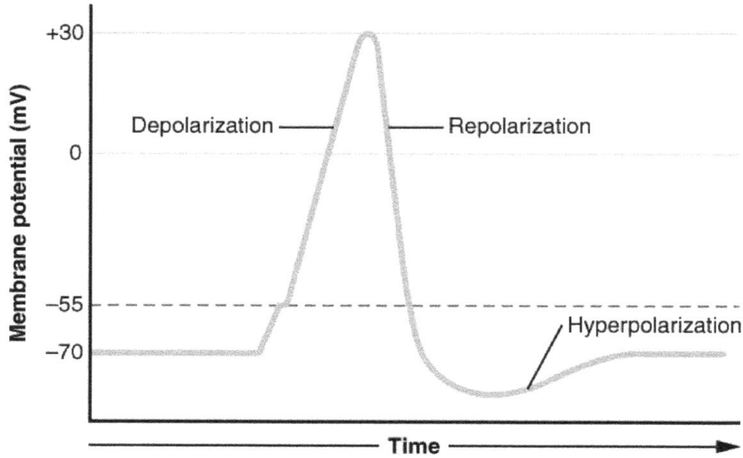

Figure 2.3. Phases of an action potential; adapted with Creative Commons license.

all-or-none phenomenon that spurs the opening of voltage-gated sodium channels, leading to a cascade of events resulting in propagation of an electrical impulse down the axon.

An action potential can be separated into multiple phases: depolarization, repolarization, and hyperpolarization (See Figure 2.3).

(1) Depolarization: a sharp rise in membrane conductance is due the positive-feedback of rapidly activated voltage-gated sodium channels that drives the membrane potential towards the equilibrium potential of sodium (+60 mV), though this potential is rarely reached due to the rapid inactivation of Na^+ channels and slow opening of repolarizing K^+ channels. Voltage-gated calcium channels also contribute to membrane depolarization during action potentials.
(2) Repolarization: at the peak of the action potential (+30 mV), the Na^+ channels are completely inactivated and voltage-gated K^+ channels are fully activated, leading to K efflux and membrane repolarization.
(3) Afterhyperpolarization: Voltage- and calcium-gated potassium channels inactivate more slowly than the membrane potential returns to rest, resulting in an afterhyperpolarization or undershoot of the membrane potential below resting membrane potential.

Lastly, the absolute refractory period is a period during which it is impossible to evoke another action potential due Na^+ channel inactivation. This is followed by a relative refractory period when an action potential *could* be elicited but requires a much stronger stimulus than usual, as Na^+ channels are recovered from inactivation but some K^+ channels remain open.

2.3 Neurotransmission at the synapse

Glutamate and γ-aminobutyric acid (GABA) are the main neurotransmitters involved in fast synaptic signaling.

2.3.1 *Glutamate*

Glutamate is the main excitatory neurotransmitter of the brain. Glutamate is a non-essential amino acid that does not cross the blood-brain barrier, requiring local synthesis from a precursor (primarily glutamine). Glutamate synapses are critical for learning and plasticity.

Glutamate receptors are divided into metabotropic and ionotropic subtypes. Metabotropic glutamate receptors are G-protein-coupled receptors that have many downstream effects. This is a large family ($mGlu_{1-8}$) of receptors that transmit signals through second messenger pathways such as mitogen-activated protein (MAP) kinase phosphorylation and formation of cyclic adenosine monophosphate (cAMP), and play a role in synaptic modulation, including indirect gating of ion channels [Fagni and Pin, 2015].

Ionotropic glutamate receptors are direct, ligand-gated ion channels. Ionotropic glutamate receptors are separated into *N*-methyl-D-aspartate (NMDA) and non-NMDA subtypes.

2.3.1.1 *Non-NMDA receptors*

Non-NMDA ionotropic receptors open channels permeable to Na^+ with more limited permeability to K^+ and Ca^{2+}. There are 2 types of non-NMDA glutamate receptors: α-amino-3-hydroxy-5-methyl-4-isoxazoleprpionic acid (AMPA) and kainate receptors. AMPA plays the main role in fast excitatory synaptic transmission by causing rapid EPSPs. AMPA receptors are heteromeric, made up of 4 subunits: GluR1, 2, 3, 4 in combination. GluR2 is not expressed until 3rd week of life rats or late in the 1st year of life in humans [Talos *et al.*, 2006ab]; glutamate receptors that do not contain GluR2 subunits are more permeable to calcium [Sanchez *et al.*, 2001; Kumar *et al.*, 2002].

2.3.1.2 *NMDA receptors*

NMDA receptors are so named because of the selective binding of NMDA to this glutamate receptor. Activation of NMDA receptors opens a channel permeable to multiple cations, resulting in K^+ efflux, as well as Na^+ and Ca^{2+} influx.

NMDA receptors are unique in being both voltage-gated as well as ligand-gated. NMDA receptors have several binding sites: in addition to glutamate, the NMDA receptor has binding sites for glycine, zinc, PCP, MK801, protons (H^+), and magnesium, which all modulate the functioning of the channel. Magnesium regulates NMDA receptor function in a voltage-dependent way: at rest, magnesium is bound tightly within the channel pore and acts as an extrinsic plug. During depolarization the magnesium block is removed, allowing the flow of ions. Due to the voltage-gated magnesium block, NMDA activation leads to slow but prolonged EPSPs and substantial Ca^{2+} influx.

NMDA receptors are heterotetramers containing two obligatory GluN1 (=GRIN1) subunits in combination with two other subunits (GluN2 and/or GluN3). The combination of the subunits changes throughout development which contributes to differing sensitivity to activation.

2.3.2 *GABA*

GABA is the main inhibitory neurotransmitter in the brain. It is synthesized from glutamate via glutamic acid decarboxylase. There are 2 types of GABA receptors: $GABA_A$ and $GABA_B$.

The $GABA_A$ receptor is a ligand-gated receptor composed of 5 homologous subunits surrounding a central channel permeable to chloride and bicarbonate, though the electrochemical driving force and permeability for chloride significantly surpasses bicarbonate and makes chloride the dominant ion under most circumstances. Each receptor is composed of two α subunits, two β subunits, and either one γ or one δ subunit; there are multiple isoforms of each subunit which modulates receptor characteristics such as binding affinity and sensitivity. $GABA_A$ receptors have two endogenous modulators, neurosteroids and endocannabinoids, and multiple binding sites activated by exogenous molecules, including benzodiazepines, barbiturates, ethanol, the anesthetic drug etomidate, as well as pharmacological reagents such as the competitive antagonist bicuculline and the non-competitive channel blocker picrotoxin.

$GABA_B$ receptors are metabotropic receptors located pre- and post-synaptically. They act through GTP-binding proteins to mediate slow, long lasting IPSPs on dendrites and presynaptic terminals; the latter receptors ultimately decrease the amount of GABA released. $GABA_B$ receptor activation also modulates inhibitory conductances, and can stimulate the opening of potassium channels, or decrease the conductance to calcium.

The excitatory or inhibitory effect of GABA depends on the flow of chloride across the channel. The chloride driving force is small and can be readily reversed with small changes in intracellular concentration. Opening of $GABA_A$ channels can lead to either inward or outward currents of chloride depending on local conditions. In mature neurons, opening $GABA_A$ causes an influx of chloride, further hyperpolarizing the cell and generating a fast-inhibitory post-synaptic potential. In immature neurons, intracellular chloride concentration is higher, resulting in reversal of the electrochemical gradient, so $GABA_A$ activation causes chloride efflux and depolarization, resulting in an excitatory post-synaptic potential.

Even without flow of chloride ions across the membrane, $GABA_A$ activation can still be inhibitory through a phenomenon called "shunting inhibition." If the equilibrium potential of chloride is near the resting membrane potential, opening of chloride channels may not lead to flow of anions. Shunting does not change the membrane potential of the cell, but it reduces the amplitude of any coincident

EPSP by reducing electrical resistance of the local cell membrane and holding the cell membrane close to the chloride equilibrium potential, thus dampening the depolarizing impact of the EPSP [Paulus and Rothwell, 2016].

2.4 Transition from normal signaling to synchronized hyperexcitability

How does the neuron go from an action potential to seizure? A seizure results from the abnormal, hypersynchronous firing of neurons. Seizure activity is characterized by high-frequency bursts of action potentials that occur during paroxysmal depolarizing shifts (PDS) in the membrane potential, and synchronization of these PDS across a network of neurons.

The PDS is an intracellular depolarization that is sudden, large, and long-lasting, and triggers a train of action potentials at its onset. The PDS is the single-cell correlate of a focal interictal epileptiform discharge on surface EEG recording [Ayala *et al.*, 1973] (Figure 2.4).

The synergistic action of AMPA and NMDA glutamate receptors is thought to initiate a PDS. AMPA receptor activation induces a fast

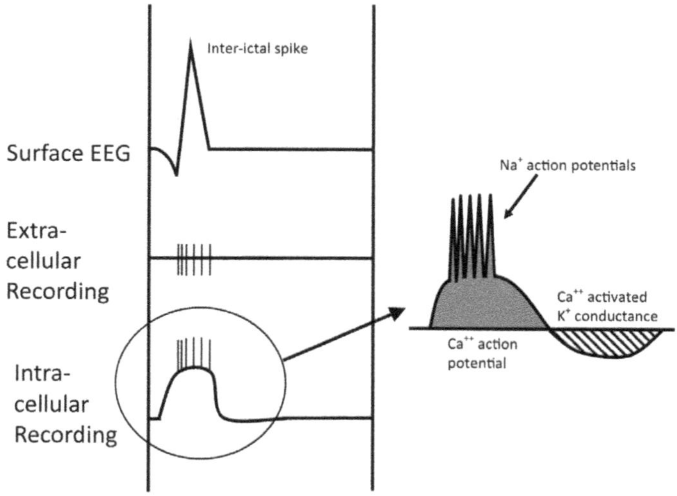

Figure 2.4. Paroxysmal depolarizing shift. Adapted from Ayala *et al.*, 1973.

EPSP, causing adequate depolarization to relieve the magnesium blocking of the NMDA channels and allows for subsequent activation of NMDA receptors. Longer NMDA receptor activation sustains the prolonged depolarization of the PDS and permits influx of extracellular calcium, as well as the opening of voltage-gated sodium channels and the repetitive generation of action potentials over a few hundred milliseconds. Similar to a single action potential, the PDS is followed by an afterhyperpolarization that temporally stabilizes the neuron's resting membrane potential; however failure of these mechanisms can cause the depolarization to spread [Stafstrom and Rho, 2017].

Synchronization of neurons is the second requirement for aberrant firing to become a seizure. Spread of an excitatory burst is typically prevented by surround inhibition, a local inhibitory environment driven by inhibitory interneurons. When a neuron is sufficiently active, surround inhibition is lost, which facilitates the spread of the excitatory burst [Prince and Wilder, 1967] and propagation of a seizure. Prolonged depolarizations lead to sustained opening of calcium- and voltage dependent potassium channels, causing accumulation of extracellular K^+, which shifts the potassium equilibrium potential in a direction that blunts the hyperpolarizing effect of potassium channel opening. Calcium also accumulates in pre-synaptic terminals which increases the probability of neurotransmitter release.

2.5 Intrinsic susceptibilities to seizures in the developing brain

Immature neurons are intrinsically more susceptible to seizures due to differences in brain development. These changes are noted at all levels of the brain, from ion channels to synapses to neural networks.

2.5.1 *Synapse formation*

Excitatory synapses predominate during early development. Synaptic density peaks within a few months of birth [Huttenlocher and de Courten, 1987], and synaptogenesis is dependent on activity

[Rakhade and Jensen, 2009]. Although GABAergic synapses form before glutamatergic synapses [McLean *et al.*, 1996; Khazipov *et al.*, 2001; Ben-Ari, 2002], the effect of GABA is excitatory at the early developmental stages which correlates with dendritic aborization [Tyzio *et al.*, 1999; Khazipov *et al.*, 2001; Ben-Ari, 2007]. While this excess of excitation is critical for normal development due to its role in synaptic plasticity, it leads to globally heightened excitability [Insel *et al.*, 1990]. The overexpression of excitatory synapses during the critical period corresponds to window of heightened seizure susceptibility [Casanova *et al.*, 2014].

Additionally, the most rapid method of synaptic transmission — gap junctions that transmit signals via direct electrical coupling — are increased in the developing brain [Brooks-Kayal, 2005; Casanova *et al.*, 2014]. This allows for extremely rapid transmission of signals through neural networks and enhancement of neural synchronization [Talhouk *et al.*, 2008] in the developing brain.

2.5.2 *Conductances and ion channels*

Voltage-gated sodium and calcium channels develop earlier relative to potassium channels [Stafstrom and Rho, 2017]. Additionally, early developmental action potentials are longer and allow for more calcium entry intracellularly, which increases neurotransmitter release and activates second messenger pathways. This is important for normal neuronal development as excitatory synapses and calcium-dependent processes are needed for normal differentiation, migration, and synapse formation; however, there is a developmental period when hyperpolarizing and inhibitory inputs are not yet active. Consequently, there are more frequent and longer action potentials, and a decreased refractory period [Moody, 1998; Bender *et al.*, 2001; Jensen, 2009].

Potassium currents are similarly biased toward excitation early in development; HCN (or h-channels) are less selective K^+ channels that reverse at membrane potentials that are positive to the pure potassium reversal potential. HCN channels are active at or below membrane potential. They function to temper dendritic excitability [Poolos *et al.*,

2002]. Immature neurons have decreased levels of HCN1, which increases dendritic excitability [Pape, 1996; Bender *et al.*, 2001].

Additionally, there is a high level of intracellular chloride in immature neurons. This decreases over time due to increasing concentrations of large, impermeant anions in the cytoplasm and extracellular matrix. The net effect is that GABA activation is excitatory in early development due to a reversed electrochemical gradient compared to mature neurons, causing ligand-gated chloride efflux and membrane depolarization. The depolarizing effect of GABA is seen up to about P14 in rats, corresponding to mid-to-late preterm gestation in primates [Ben-Ari *et al.*, 1989, 2007; Khazipov *et al.*, 2001; Ben-Ari, 2002].

Immature neurons have higher membrane resistances due to delayed maturation of inward rectifying K^+ currents [Mongiat *et al.*, 2009], and shorter time constants due to reduced Na^+ channel opening and inactivation times [Huguenard *et al.*, 1988]. They additionally have lower thresholds for the activation of action potentials than mature neurons [Mongiat *et al.*, 2009]. The result is that young neurons are very efficient at translating an EPSP into an action potential, so that an EPSP of a certain magnitude has a larger effect on immature neurons than on a mature neuron and contributes to the excitatory skew in the developing brain.

Together, the prolonged depolarizing currents of early $GABA_A$ and NMDA receptor activation can form oscillations that facilitate synaptic network development. Giant depolarizing potentials (GDPs) are large oscillatory currents of recurrent membrane depolarizations with superimposed fast action potentials separated by quiescent intervals. These oscillations help to facilitate synaptic network formation and synchronization, are seen maximally at P8 [Ben-Ari *et al.*, 1989], corresponding to a near-term infant and the critical period for synapse development.

2.5.3 *Neurotransmitter receptor composition*

The receptor subunit composition of both GABA and glutamate changes throughout development, and early patterns of expression additionally favor excitatory responses.

Glutamate NMDA receptor NR2 subunits are predominantly NR2B in the immature brain compared with NR2A in the mature brain; this alteration of the NR2B/NR2A ratio results in prolonged current decay and favors prolonged EPSPs [Dunah *et al.*, 1996]. Additionally, there is relative overexpression of the NR2C, NR2D, and NR3A subunits in the critical period up to P14 in rodents; this configuration lowers the sensitivity to magnesium ions, thereby decreasing the voltage-gated magnesium block [Hollmann and Heinemann, 1994; Dunah *et al.*, 1996; Wong *et al.*, 2002]. AMPA receptors also lack GluR2 expression until late in the first year of life in humans; this configuration allows for additional calcium permeability of the AMPA receptor and increased activation of second messenger pathways via the resultant calcium influx [Sanchez *et al.*, 2001; Kumar *et al.*, 2002].

GABA receptors also display differences in subunit composition early in development. $GABA_A$ receptors have overexpression of α-2 and α-4 subunits compared to α-1, which results in decreased sensitivity to benzodiazepines [Kapur and Macdonald, 1999; Brooks-Kayal, 2005]. $GABA_B$ also shows delayed maturation [Gaiarsa *et al.*, 1995], furthering the lack of early inhibitory signals.

2.5.4 *Immature glia*

While immature neurons are less prone to glutamate-induced excitotoxicity than mature neurons [Liu *et al.*, 1996], there is decreased glutamate clearance from extracellular spaces. Clearance of excess glutamate in the synapses is normally accomplished by glutamate transporters (GLT1 and GLAST1) found on astrocytes but these transporters are not present on immature glia [Nardou *et al.*, 2013]. Excessive extracellular glutamate enhances firing of adjacent neurons and increases neuronal synchronization.

2.6 Pathophysiology of seizures after brain injury

While neonatal brains are uniquely susceptible to seizures due to inherent differences in physiology compared to the mature brain, they are also at increased risk due to potential for brain injury around birth. Indeed, the most common causes of seizures in the neonatal period — hypoxic-ischemic encephalopathy, stroke, and intracranial hemorrhage — are all related to acute brain injury [Glass *et al.*, 2016]. Exploration of the timing and trends of seizures after acute brain injury provides insights into the underlying pathophysiology.

2.6.1 *Clues to seizure pathophysiology*

After an hypoxic-ischemic insult, seizure onset is delayed by 6–12 hours and reaches peak burden at 23 hours after birth in neonates [Lynch *et al.*, 2012]. The seizure burden then wanes over the subsequent 1–2 days. In the era of therapeutic hypothermia, a neuroprotective strategy for neonates born with suspected hypoxic-ischemic insult, the time to seizure has shifted. Wusthoff and colleagues [2011] found that the peak time to seizure onset in these infants is delayed to 35 hours, with broader variability in start time, though there is no difference in seizure incidence compared to uncooled neonates.

Seizure frequency is correlated with other indicators of brain injury. A brain MRI scan within 5–7 days after an ischemic insult will show decreases in the apparent diffusion coefficient (ADC) signal signifying restricted water diffusion secondary to cytotoxic edema and neuronal injury [Triulzi *et al.*, 2006; Bednarek *et al.*, 2012]. Worsening MRI measures of ADC have been shown to correlate with seizure frequency [McKinstry *et al.*, 2002]. In the traumatic brain injury literature, it is known that seizure frequency trends with increases in intracranial pressure and reductions in cerebral perfusion pressure [Levene *et al.*, 1987]. Both delay in seizures after hypoxic ischemic insult and the correlation between cell swelling and seizure burden suggest an association between cytotoxic edema and development of seizures.

2.6.2 *Chloride, impermeable anions, and seizures*

The equilibrium potential is not static and can be altered by changing the ion concentration. The equilibrium potential of chloride (–61 mV)

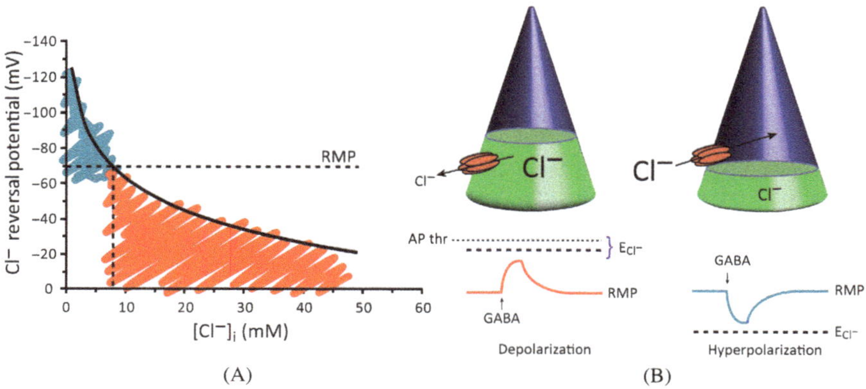

Figure 2.5. Direction of chloride flow based on equilibrium potential. (A) No chloride flows through GABA receptors at the intracellular concentration (vertical line) that crosses the resting membrane potential (RMP, horizontal line) but a few millimolar shift in concentration can lead to outward (blue) or inward (red) flow. (B) Neurons with varying intracellular chloride concentrations (green) are variably depolarized or hyperpolarized. Reprinted from Glykys *et al.*, 2017.

is near the resting membrane potential (–70 mV), and as a consequence, a few millimolar change in the chloride concentration can change the equilibrium potential enough to reverse the direction of Cl^- flow (Figure 2.5).

Chloride concentration is regulated by large, immobile anions [Glykys *et al.*, 2014]. Intracellularly, these are proteins and amino acids, including ribosomes, nucleic acids, actin and tubulin of the ubiquitous cytoskeleton as discussed previously. However, there are also *extracellular* fixed anions — the extracellular matrix. The extracellular matrix is primarily made up of glycoproteins, which is a class of molecules containing one or more glycosaminoglycan covalently linked to a core protein. Each glycosaminoglycan unit is composed of a disaccharide pair containing between 0 and 4 sulfate groups. Sulfates are trivalent anions, so the extracellular matrix has the capacity for a large amount of negative charge and consequent displacement of extracellular chloride. Chloride distribution and concentration is thus determined in local environments by the presence of these impermeant anions that displace chloride.

2.6.2.1 *Depolymerizaton of anionic macromolecules occurs in the setting of brain injury*

What happens to these intracellular anionic macromolecules in the setting of brain injury? In the setting of traumatic injury, there is an increase in the calcium-sensitive phosphatase calcineurin, which changes neuronal function. In a rat model of trauma, Campbell and colleagues [2012] showed that increase in calcineurin levels leads to dendritic spine loss through degradation of the actin-rich cytoskeleton. This leads to degeneration of post-synaptic neuronal dendrites and dendritic beading, secondary to a disruption in osmotic equilibrium. Neuronal injury can also lead to cytoskeleton degradation more proximally at the initial axon segment, even in the absence of axonal loss [Schafer *et al.*, 2009].

Hypoxic-ischemic injury also leads to breakdown of anionic macromolecules. Ischemia disrupts the neuronal cytoskeleton by changing phosphorylation of the microtubule-associated protein, tau [Kitagawa *et al.*, 1989; Shackelford and Nelson, 1996; Burkhart *et al.*, 1998; Li *et al.*, 1998; Shackelford and Yeh, 1998]. Both dephosphorylation and hyperphosphorylation occur, leading to destabilization of the microtubule [Psilodimitrakopoulos *et al.*, 2013]. Changes in cytoskeleton secondary to an hypoxic insult have been observed in neocortical cells [Friedman *et al.*, 1998] as well as in the brainstem [Mironov and Richter, 1999].

Lastly, recurrent or prolonged seizures directly cause calcineurin-mediated breakdown of actin [Halpain *et al.*, 1998; Ouyang *et al.*, 2007; Kurz *et al.*, 2008] and remodeling of dendritic spines, even in the absence of cell death or changes in oxygen levels [Zeng *et al.*, 2007].

2.6.2.2 *Extracellular biopolymers are released in the setting of trauma*

Externally, the extracellular matrix also mobilizes its impermeable anions in the setting of acute brain injury by releasing matrix metalloproteinases (MMP) from neurons and glia. MMPs are zinc- and calcium-dependent endopeptidases that are released into the interstitial space and hydrolyze glycosaminoglycans, thereby releasing the negatively charged sulfate groups. MMP-2 and MMP-9 are known to be overexpressed following traumatic brain injury [Zhang *et al.*, 2016], and MMP-9 knockout mice show reduced lesion volumes and have less motor deficits after stroke [Wang *et al.*, 2000]. In seizure models, MMP increases after administration of kainate [Gasche *et al.*, 2006] and in pilocarpine-induced status epilepticus [Rankin-Gee *et al.*, 2015]. In non-human primate models of ischemia, different subtypes were found to be overexpressed both acutely (MMP9) and chronically (MMP2 and MMP7) [Anthony *et al.*, 1997; Clark *et al.*, 1997; Morita-Fujimura *et al.*, 2000; Gasche *et al.*, 2001].

MMPs additionally increase the permeability of the blood brain barrier, which, in addition to clearance of the glycosoaminoglycans through leukocyte and cytokine activation, allows for replacement of the lost negative glycosaminoglycan charge with chloride from the intravascular space [Syková and Nicholson, 2008]. The increase in extracellular chloride concentration leads to a subsequent increase in intracellular chloride through the actions of the equilibrative NKCC1 cation-chloride cotransporter due to chemical driving forces.

Damage to the intracellular and extracellular anionic macromolecules will disrupt the local chloride concentrations and distort $GABA_A$ receptor-mediated signaling, which is likely to contribute to seizure activity. Movement of chloride intracellularly is also accompanied by movements of water and cations through NKCC1. Neurons are impermeable to water and lack aquaporins so the water that is transported with cations across the membrane results in cell swelling and may be a key mechanism of cytotoxic edema [Glykys *et al.*, 2017].

2.6.2.3 *Intracellular chloride increases after brain injury*

Chloride accumulates intracellularly after injury to the brain and is observed in diverse mechanisms of brain injury. In models of trauma [Dzhala *et al.*, 2012; Glykys and Staley, 2016], increases in intracellular chloride is seen not just in those neurons with transected axons but also in neurons with active synapses, which could potentially have network-wide effects. Increases in intracellular chloride have also been seen in hypoxic-ischemic conditions [Inglefield and Schwartz-Bloom, 1998; Galeffi *et al.*, 2004; Pond *et al.*, 2006] and status epilepticus [Khalilov *et al.*, 2003; Dzhala *et al.*, 2010; Lillis *et al.*, 2012].

While there are multiple potential channels for chloride entry into cells after injury, including ligand-gated $GABA_A$ anion channels [van den Pol *et al.*, 996; Hasbani *et al.*, 1998] and volume sensitive chloride channels [Inoue and Okada, 2007], there is evidence that membrane chloride transporters are principally responsible for the increase in intracellular chloride. After a traumatic injury to the brain, there is a significant transient upregulation of NKCC1 protein [Hasbargen *et al.*, 2010], and blocking these cotransporters mitigates some of the malignant changes. The FDA-approved diuretic bumetanide is a highly-specific NKCC1 antagonist [Isenring *et al.*, 1998; Hannaert *et al.*, 2002]. Blocking NKCC1 reduces intracellular chloride across multiple types of acute brain injury, including hypoxia, seizures, and trauma [Pond *et al.*, 2006; Dzhala *et al.*, 2010, 2012]. NKCC1 also mediates flux of chloride from the blood to the brain across the blood-brain barrier [O'Donnell *et al.*, 2004] so bumetanide may also function to reduce chloride flux into the brain after injury, and thereby stabilize GABA signaling.

A novel anti-seizure strategy, currently under investigation, involves inhibition of cation-chloride cotransporters to slow the accumulation of chloride. In pre-clinical trials, addition of bumetanide to the $GABA_A$ agonist phenobarbital has been shown to reduce seizure activity in the hippocampus and neocortex [Dzhala *et al.*, 2008; Glykys *et al.*, 2009; Dzhala and Staley, 2015; Sivakumaran and Maguire, 2016]. Clinical trials are ongoing to address the question of whether bumetanide can potentiate the inhibitory effects of GABA. While conclusions have been mixed, data show that bumetanide was effective. In a pharmacokinetic study by Pressler and colleagues [2015], bumetanide as an add-on medication to phenobarbital did not improve seizure control; however, over 1/3 of subjects did not have seizures during the baseline period [Thoresen and Sabir, 2015]. Examination of those who did have seizures and received bumetanide suggests that bumetanide was effective in reducing the seizure burden [Pressler *et al.*, 2015]. An additional randomized, placebo-controlled trial (NCT00830531) of bumetanide administered along with escalating doses of phenobarbital has recently closed and may help to further clarify the potential benefit of bumetanide in neonatal seizure control.

Additional avenues to reduce intracellular chloride may have benefit as novel anti-seizure strategies, including modulation of KCC2 and KCC3 [Lee *et al.*, 2007; Kahle and Delpire, 2016], volume regulation via mannitol [Glykys *et al.*, 2018, under review], and stabilization of the extracellular matrix.

2.7 Neonatal onset epilepsy

While the model of imbalance between excitatory and inhibitory conductances works reasonably well to understand a single seizure, it fails when applied to the condition of epilepsy, a state defined by predisposition to recurrent, spontaneous seizures. Nonetheless, patients who have recurrent seizures are not seizing the majority of the time, even those with status epilepticus [Moran *et al.*, 2004]. What dynamics allow for the transition from steady-state into a seizure in the first place and lead to the sustained high neuronal firing of a seizure?

Activity-dependent decreases in neuronal inhibition ("activity-dependent disinhibition") can account for networks in which rare events occur that can be maintained through self-reinforcing, positive feedback mechanisms. Each neural network has its own baseline level seizure probability based on intrinsic characteristics such as ionic gradients, connectivity, receptor sensitivity; this would differ in a network of immature versus mature neurons, or intact versus injured neurons. If a transient imbalance favoring excitation could lead to further disinhibition via positive-feedback, the ultimate result is propagation of further excitation into a seizure. Once established, the seizure itself provides the mechanism for maintaining further imbalance of excitation and inhibition, thereby providing some stability to the rare, hyperexcited state that prevents immediate return to the network's homeostatic levels. Activity-dependent disinhibition explains the abrupt state transitions that correspond to spontaneous seizures. There are several possible molecular mechanisms and we will touch on each below.

2.7.1 *Reduced GABA-mediated inhibition*

The first mechanism is a reduction in GABA-mediated inhibition. A reduction in GABA conductance could occur at the pre- or post-synaptic level by change in neurotransmitter release, or post-synaptic changes: neurotransmitter reuptake, receptor desensitization, receptor membrane trafficking, and post-translational modification of receptor subunits affecting transmitter affinity and gating. Reduction in GABA-mediated inhibition can also be due to a shift in the reversal potential of GABA, which can happen with relatively small changes in the intracellular chloride concentration as discussed earlier. Prolonged activation of the $GABA_A$ receptor leads to a large influx of chloride, which occurs rapidly through opening of ion channels. Conversely, the return of chloride to homeostatic levels and re-establishment of the chloride gradient is dependent upon chloride efflux through the cation-chloride cotransporter KCC2, which acts much more slowly since cotransporter shifts have sharply different requirements for protein conformational changes with ion pumping compared to channel-mediated ion flux, as discussed earlier. Thus, prolonged $GABA_A$ receptor activation can paradoxically be excitatory, arising from the bicarbonate co-conductance through the GABA channel [Staley *et al.*, 1995; Staley and Proctor, 1999; Doyon *et al.*, 2011, 2016; Jedlicka *et al.*, 2011; Lewin *et al.*, 2012] and the greater stability of bicarbonate compared to chloride concentrations. The bicarbonate concentration gradient is stabilized by active and passive pH buffering systems in concert with the action of carbonic anhydrase [Staley *et al.*, 1995].

2.7.1.1 *Anticonvulsant efficacy in neonatal seizures*

$GABA_A$ receptor activation thus may be excitatory due to both steady-state changes in intracellular chloride concentrations as well as activity-dependent shifts in the fluxes of chloride and bicarbonate through the open $GABA_A$ channel. Both of these effects will degrade the anticonvulsant efficacy of the anticonvulsants that are commonly used to treat neonatal seizures, because both benzodiazepines and barbiturates such as phenobarbital work by increasing the open probability of the $GABA_A$ receptor [Twyman *et al.*, 1989]. When currents flow in the wrong direction through these channels, increasing their open time will not diminish, and might exacerbate, seizure activity. Thus, an important strategy for improving neonatal seizure therapy is enhancement of ionic homeostasis in the injured and epileptic neonatal brain. Anticonvulsants that work through other mechanisms, such as phenytoin, have thus far not proven to be more effective [Painter *et al.*, 1999; Yau *et al.*, 2015], perhaps because their activity also depends on an intact system of GABA-mediated synaptic inhibition.

2.7.2 *Degradation in cationic homeostasis*

Local changes in ion concentrations of the intracellular and extracellular spaces can also mediate activity-dependent disinhibition. In chemical models of seizure, prolonged seizure activity increases the extracellular K^+ concentration to the point where it overwhelms the ability of the Na-K-ATPase to maintain cation gradients on which normal cellular function and other cotransporters like the KCC2 depend [Ransom *et al.*, 2000]. Failure of KCC2 further causes a cascade of other ion imbalances, as it plays an important role in regulation the chloride concentration across the membrane, and hence inhibitory currents [Viitanen *et al.*, 2010]. Loss of function Na-K-ATPase mutations can also lead to high extracellular K^+ and failure of the pump to maintain cation gradients [Heinzen *et al.*, 2014]. The high extracellular potassium concentration also shifts the equilibrium potential for K^+ so that it is a less effective repolarizing conductance.

Calcium homeostatic mechanisms similarly can be overwhelmed in the setting of excessive activity. Intracellular calcium concentration is typically very low. If large influxes of calcium through voltage and ligand-gated channels overwhelm the transporters that allow recovery of calcium homeostasis, the resultant shift in calcium changes the probability of calcium-dependent neurotransmitter release and changes the effect of calcium-dependent potassium conductances [Heinemann *et al.*, 1986; Kovács *et al.*, 2005]. Degradation in ionic homeostasis during periods of increased network activity is a key mechanism of ictogenesis.

2.7.3 *Glial dysfunction*

Glial dysfunction secondary to failure of ionic homeostasis is a third mechanism for achieving activity-dependent disinhibition. Glia provide significant modulation of the synaptic environment as one astrocyte may contact thousands of synapses. Glia are responsible for excessive glutamate and potassium uptake [Rothstein *et al.*, 1996] and glia dysfunction resulting in excess extracellular glutamate engenders seizure propagation and excitotoxicity via excessive calcium influx into neurons [Attwell *et al.*, 1993]. Furthermore, in anoxia there is a massive release of additional glutamate into the extracellular space from glia due to the reversal of the glutamate uptake carrier due to loss of the Na-K-ATPase-generated electrochemical gradient [Attwell *et al.*, 1993; Grewer and Rauen, 2005].

Glia also modulate synapses by affecting the synchrony of surrounding neurons. Astrocytes act as a calcium buffer. Astrocytes are triggered to fire by K^+ released from nearby neurons during action potentials, leading to changes in the astrocyte intracellular calcium concentration. In the setting of excessive extracellular K^+ or in conditions where there is high adjacent neuronal activity, excessive glial calcium transients lead to synchronization of a large network of synapses [Sasaki *et al.*, 2014] due to gap junction connections between glia.

2.8 Conclusions

Most neonatal seizures arise from acute brain injuries, but epilepsy may also manifest in the neonatal period (Table 2.1). In both cases, acute shifts in ionic balances play key roles in the onset of seizure activity. Understanding the pathophysiology of these ion shifts requires insights into physiological ion homeostasis as well as how ion balances are altered by injury and network activity. Accumulating evidence suggests that some of these ion shifts may be ameliorated, although there is still much to be discovered regarding the most effective and least toxic means by which this can be accomplished.

References

Anthony, D.C., Ferguson, B., Matyzak, M.K., *et al.* (1997). Differential matrix metalloproteinase expression in cases of multiple sclerosis and stroke, *Neuropathol. Appl. Neurobiol.*, 23, 406–415.

Attwell, D., Barbour, B., and Szatkowski, M. (1993). Nonvesicular release of neurotransmitter, *Neuron*, 11, 401–407.

Audebert, S. Koulakoff, A., Berwald-Netter, Y., *et al.* (1994). Developmental regulation of polyglutamylated alpha- and beta-tubulin in mouse brain neurons, *J. Cell Sci.*, 107, 231323–231322.

Ayala, G.F., Dichter, M., Gumnit, R.J., *et al.* (1973). Genesis of epileptic interictal spikes New knowledge of cortical feedback systems suggests a neurophysiological explanation of brief paroxysms, *Brain Res.*, 52, 1–17.

Baker, N.A., Sept, D., Joseph, S., *et al.* (2001). Electrostatics of nanosystems: application to microtubules and the ribosome, *Proc. Natl. Acad. Sci. USA*, 98, 10037–10041.

Balakrishnan, V., Becker, M., Löhrke, S., *et al.* (2003). Expression and function of chloride transporters during development of inhibitory neurotransmission in the auditory brainstem, *J. Neurosci.*, 23, 4134–4145.

Barcia, G., Fleming, M.R., Deligniere, A., *et al.* (2012). De novo gain-of-function KCNT1 channel mutations cause malignant migrating partial seizures of infancy, *Nat. Genet.*, 44, 1255–1259.

Bednarek, N., Mathur A., Inder, T., *et al.* (2012). Impact of therapeutic hypothermia on MRI diffusion changes in neonatal encephalopathy, *Neurology*, 78, 1420–1427.

Ben-Ari, Y., Cherubini, E., Corradetti, R., and Gaiarsa J.L. (1989). Giant synaptic potentials in immature rat CA3 hippocampal neurones, *J. Physiol.*, 416, 303–325.

Ben-Ari, Y. (2002). Excitatory actions of gaba during development: the nature of the nurture, *Nat. Rev. Neurosci.*, 3, 728–739.

Ben-Ari, Y., Gaiarsa, J.L., Tyzio, R., and Khazipov, R. (2007). GABA: a pioneer transmitter that excites immature neurons and generates primitive oscillations, *Physiol. Rev.*, 87, 1215–1284.

Ben-Ari, Y. (2007). GABA excites and sculpts immature neurons well before delivery: modulation by GABA of the development of ventricular progenitor cells, *Epilepsy Curr.*, 7, 167–169.

Bender, R.A., Brewster, A., Santoro, B., *et al.* (2001). Differential and age-dependent expression of hyperpolarization-activated, cyclic nucleotide-gated cation channel isoforms 1-4 suggests evolving roles in the developing rat hippocampus, *Neuroscience*, 106, 689–698.

Blaesse, P., Airaksinen, M.S., Rivera, C., and Kaila, K. (2009). Cation-chloride cotransporters and neuronal function, *Neuron*, 61, 820–838.

Brooks-Kayal, A.R. (2005). Rearranging receptors, *Epilepsia*, 46 Suppl 7, 29–38.

Burkhart, K.K., Beard, D.C., Lehman, R.A., and Billingsley, M.L. (1998). Alterations in tau phosphorylation in rat and human neocortical brain slices following hypoxia and glucose deprivation, *Exp. Neurol.*, 154(2), 464–472.

Campbell, J.N., Low B., Kurz, J.E., *et al.* (2012). Mechanisms of dendritic spine remodeling in a rat model of traumatic brain injury, *J. Neurotrauma*, 29, 218–234.

Carvill, G.L., Weckhuysen, S., McMahon, J.M., *et al.* (2014). GABRA1 and STXBP1: novel genetic causes of Dravet syndrome, *Neurology*, 82, 1245–53.

Casanova, J.R., Nishimura, M., and Swann, J.W. (2014). The effects of early-life seizures on hippocampal dendrite development and later-life learning and memory, *Brain Res. Bull.*, 103, 39–48.

Clark, A.W., Krekoski, C.A., Bou, S.S., Chapman, K.R., and Edwards, D.R. (1997). Increased gelatinase A (MMP-2) and gelatinase B (MMP-9) activities in human brain after focal ischemia, *Neurosci. Lett.*, 238, 53–56.

Delpire, E. (2000). Cation-chloride cotransporters in neuronal communication, *News Physiol. Sci.*, 15, 309–312.

Delpire, E. and Staley, K.J. (2014). Novel determinants of the neuronal Cl(-) concentration, *J. Physiol.*, 592, 4099–4114.

Doyon, N., Prescott, S.A., Castonguay, A., *et al.* (2011). Efficacy of synaptic inhibition depends on multiple, dynamically interacting mechanisms implicated in chloride homeostasis, *PLoS Comput. Biol.*, 7, e1002149.

Doyon, N., Vinay, L., Prescott, S.A., and De Koninck, Y. (2016). Chloride regulation: a dynamic equilibrium crucial for synaptic inhibition, *Neuron*, 89, 1157–1172.

Duebel, J., Haverkamp, S., Schleich, W., *et al.* (2006). Two-photon imaging reveals somatodendritic chloride gradient in retinal ON-type bipolar cells expressing the biosensor Clomeleon, *Neuron*, 49, 81–94.

Dunah, A.W., Yasuda, R.P., Wang, Y.H., *et al.* (1996). Regional and ontogenic expression of the NMDA receptor subunit NR2D protein in rat brain using a subunit-specific antibody, *J. Neurochem.*, 67, 2335–2345.

Dzhala, V., Valeeva, G., Glykys, J., Khazipov, R., and Staley, K. (2012). Traumatic alterations in GABA signaling disrupt hippocampal network activity in the developing brain, *J. Neurosci.*, 32, 4017–4031.

Dzhala, V.I., Talos, D.M., Sdrulla, D.A., *et al.* (2005). NKCC1 transporter facilitates seizures in the developing brain, *Nat. Med.* 11, 1205–1213.

Dzhala, V.I., Kuchibhotla, K.V., Glykys, J.C., *et al.* (2010). Progressive NKCC1-dependent neuronal chloride accumulation during neonatal seizures, *J. Neurosci.*, 30, 11745–11761.

Dzhala, V.I., Brumback, A.C., and Staley, K.J. (2008). Bumetanide enhances phenobarbital efficacy in a neonatal seizure model, *Ann. Neurol.*, 63, 222–235.

Dzhala, V. and Staley, K.J. (2015). Acute and chronic efficacy of bumetanide in an *in vitro* model of posttraumatic epileptogenesis, *CNS Neurosci. Ther.*, 21, 173–180.

Fagni, L. and Pin, J.-P. (2015). The metabotropic glutamate receptors A2, in Hammond, C. (ed.) *Cellular and Molecular Neurophysiology*, 4th edn. Boston: Academic Press, pp. 269–282.

Friedman, J.E., Chow, E.J., and Haddad, G.G. (1998). State of actin filaments is changed by anoxia in cultured rat neocortical neurons, *Neuroscience*, 82, 421–427.

Gaiarsa, J.L., Tseeb, V., and Ben-Ari, Y. (1995). Postnatal development of pre- and postsynaptic GABAB-mediated inhibitions in the CA3 hippocampal region of the rat, *J. Neurophysiol.*, 73, 246–255.

Galeffi, F., Sah, R., Pond, B.B., *et al.* (2004). Changes in intracellular chloride after oxygen-glucose deprivation of the adult hippocampal slice: effect of diazepam, *J. Neurosci.*, 24, 4478–4488.

Gasche, Y., Copin, J.C., Sugawara, T., *et al.* (2001). Matrix metalloproteinase inhibition prevents oxidative stress-associated blood-brain barrier disruption after transient focal cerebral ischemia, *J. Cereb. Blood Flow Metab.*, 21, 1393–400.

Gasche, Y., Soccal, P.M., Kanemitsu, M., and Copin, J. (2006). Matrix metalloproteinases and diseases of the central nervous system with a special emphasis on ischemic brain, *Front. Biosci.*, 11, 1289–301.

Glass, H.C., Pham, T.N., Danielsen, B., *et al.* (2009). Antenatal and intrapartum risk factors for seizures in term newborns: a population-based study, California 1998–2002, *J. Pediatr.*, 154, 24–28.e1.

Glass, H.C., Shellhaas, R.A., Wusthoff, C.J., *et al.* (2016). Contemporary profile of seizures in neonates: a prospective cohort study, *J. Pediatr.* 174, 98–103.e1.

Glykys, J., Dzhala, V.I., Kuchibhotla, K.V., *et al.* (2009). Differences in cortical versus subcortical GABAergic signaling: a candidate mechanism of electroclinical uncoupling of neonatal seizures, *Neuron.* 63, 657–672.

Glykys, J., Dzhala, V., Egawa, K., *et al.* (2014). Local impermeant anions establish the neuronal chloride concentration, *Science*, 343, 670–675.

Glykys, J., Dzhala, V., Egawa, K., *et al.* (2017). Chloride dysregulation, seizures, and cerebral edema: a relationship with therapeutic potential, *Trends Neurosci.*, 40, 276–294.

Glykys, J. *et al.* (2018). Mannitol decreases neocortical epileptiform activity during early brain development via cotransport of chloride and water, *Neurobiol. Dis.*, In review.

Glykys, J. and Staley, K.J. (2015). Diazepam effect during early neonatal development correlates with neuronal Cl(-), *Ann. Clin. Transl. Neurol.*, 2, 1055–1070.

Glykys, J. and Staley, K.J. (2016). Developmental decrease of neuronal chloride concentration is independent of trauma in thalamocortical brain slices, *PLoS One.* 11, e0158012.

Grewer, C. and Rauen, T. (2005). Electrogenic glutamate transporters in the CNS: molecular mechanism, pre-steady-state kinetics, and their impact on synaptic signaling, *J. Membr. Biol.*, 203, 1–20.

Halpain, S., Hipolito, A., and Saffer, L. (1998). Regulation of F-actin stability in dendritic spines by glutamate receptors and calcineurin, *J. Neurosci.*, 18, 9835–9844.

Hammond, C. (2015). Ionic gradients, membrane potential and ionic currents, in *Cellular and Molecular. Neurophysiology*, 4th edn. Boston: Elsevier, pp. 39–54.

Hannaert, P., Alvarez-Guerra, M., Pirot, D., Nazaret, C., and Garay, R.P. (2002). Rat NKCC2/NKCC1 cotransporter selectivity for loop diuretic drugs, *Naunyn. Schmiedebergs. Arch. Pharmacol.*, 365, 193–199.

Hasbani, M.J., Hyrc, K.L., Faddis, B.T., Romano, C., and Goldberg, M.P. (1998). Distinct roles for sodium, chloride, and calcium in excitotoxic dendritic injury and recovery, *Exp. Neurol.*, 154, 241–258.

Hasbargen, T., Ahmed, M.M., Miranpuri, G., Li, L., Kahle, K.T., Resnick, D., and Sun D. (2010). Role of NKCC1 and KCC2 in the development of chronic neuropathic pain following spinal cord injury, *Ann. N. Y. Acad. Sci.*, 1198, 168–172.

Heinemann, U., Konnerth, A., Pumain, R., and Wadman, W.J. (1986). Extracellular calcium and potassium concentration changes in chronic epileptic brain tissue, *Adv. Neurol.*, 44, 641–661.

Heinzen, E.L., Arzimanoglou, A., Brashear, A., *et al.* (2014). Distinct neurological disorders with ATP1A3 mutations, *Lancet. Neurol.*, 13, 503–514.

Hollmann, M. and Heinemann, S. (1994). Cloned glutamate receptors, *Annu. Rev. Neurosci.*, 17, 31–108.

Huguenard, J.R., Hamill, O.P., and Prince, D.A. (1988). Developmental changes in Na^+ conductances in rat neocortical neurons: appearance of a slowly inactivating component, *J. Neurophysiol.*, 59, 778–795.

Huttenlocher, P.R. and de Courten, C. (1987). The development of synapses in striate cortex of man, *Hum. Neurobiol.*, 6, 1–9.

Inglefield, J.R. and Schwartz-Bloom, R.D. (1998). Optical imaging of hippocampal neurons with a chloride-sensitive dye: early effects of in vitro ischemia, *J. Neurochem.*, 70, 2500–2509.

Inoue, H. and Okada, Y. (2007). Roles of volume-sensitive chloride channel in excitotoxic neuronal injury, *J. Neurosci.*, 27, 1445–1455.

Insel, T.R., Miller, L.P., and Gelhard, R.E. (1990). The ontogeny of excitatory amino acid receptors in rat forebrain — I N-methyl-D-aspartate and quisqualate receptors, *Neuroscience*, 35, 31–43.

Isenring, P., Jacoby, S.C., Payne, J.A., and Forbush, B, 3rd. (1998). Comparison of Na-K-Cl cotransporters NKCC1, NKCC2, and the HEK cell Na-L-Cl cotransporter, *J. Biol. Chem.*, 273, 11295–11301.

Jedlicka, P., Deller, T., Gutkin, B.S., and Backus, K.H. (2011). Activity-dependent intracellular chloride accumulation and diffusion controls GABA(A) receptor-mediated synaptic transmission, *Hippocampus*, 21, 885–898.

Jensen, F.E., Applegate, C.D., Holtzman, D., Belin, T.R., and Burchfiel, J.L. (1991). Epileptogenic effect of hypoxia in the immature rodent brain, *Ann. Neurol.*, 29, 629–637.

Jensen, F.E. (2009). Neonatal seizures: an update on mechanisms and management, *Clin. Perinatol.*, 36, 881–900.

Kahle, K.T., Staley, K.J., Nahed, B.V., *et al.* (2008). Roles of the cation-chloride cotransporters in neurological disease, *Nat. Clin. Pract. Neurol.* 4, 490–503.

Kahle, K.T., Khanna, A.R., Alper, S.L., *et al.* (2015). K-Cl cotransporters, cell volume homeostasis, and neurological disease, *Trends Mol. Med.*, 21, 513–523.

Kahle, K.T. and Delpire, E. (2016). Kinase-KCC2 coupling: Cl^- rheostasis, disease susceptibility, therapeutic target, *J. Neurophysiol.*, 115, 8–18.

Kandel, E.R. *et al.* (2013). Ion channels, in *Principles of. Neural Science*, 5th edn. New York: McGraw-Hill, Health Professions Division.

Kapur, J. and Macdonald, R.L. (1999). Postnatal development of hippocampal dentate granule cell gamma-aminobutyric acidA receptor pharmacological properties, *Mol. Pharmacol.*, 55, 444–452.

Khalilov, I., Holmes, G.L., and Ben-Ari, Y. (2003). *In vitro* formation of a secondary epileptogenic mirror focus by interhippocampal propagation of seizures, *Nat. Neurosci.*, 6, 1079–1085.

Khazipov, R., Esclapez, M., Caillard, O., *et al.* (2001). Early development of neuronal activity in the primate hippocampus in utero, *J. Neurosci.*, 21, 9770–9781.

Kitagawa, K., Matsumoto, M., Niinobe, M., *et al.* (1989). Microtubule-associated protein 2 as a sensitive marker for cerebral ischemic damage — immunohistochemical investigation of dendritic damage, *Neuroscience*, 31, 401–411.

Kovács, R. *et al.* (2005). Mitochondrial calcium ion and membrane potential transients follow the pattern of epileptiform discharges in hippocampal slice cultures, *J. Neurosci.*, 25, 4260–4269.

Kumar, S.S., Bacci, A., Kharazia, V., and Huguenard, J.R. (2002). A developmental switch of AMPA receptor subunits in neocortical pyramidal neurons, *J. Neurosci.* 22, 3005–3015.

Kurz, J.E., Moore, B.J., Henderson, S.C., Campbell, J.N., and Churn, S.B. (2008). A cellular mechanism for dendritic spine loss in the pilocarpine model of status epilepticus, *Epilepsia*, 49, 1696–1710.

Lee, H.H., Walker, J.A., Williams, J.R., *et al.* (2007). Direct protein kinase C-dependent phosphorylation regulates the cell surface stability and activity of the potassium chloride cotransporter KCC2, *J. Biol. Chem.*, 282, 29777–29784.

Levene, M.I., Evans, D.H., Forde, A., and Archer, L.N. (1987). Value of intracranial pressure monitoring of asphyxiated newborn infants, *Dev. Med. Child Neurol.*, 29, 311–319.

Lewin, N., Aksay, E., and Clancy, C.E. (2012). Computational modeling reveals dendritic origins of GABA(A)-mediated excitation in CA1 pyramidal neurons, *PLoS One*, 7, e47250.

Li, Y., Jiang, N., Powers, C., and Chopp, M. (1998). Neuronal damage and plasticity identified by microtubule-associated protein 2, growth-associated protein 43, and cyclin D1 immunoreactivity after focal cerebral ischemia in rats, *Stroke*, 29, 1972–1980.

Lillis, K.P., Kramer, M.A., Mertz, J., Staley, K.J., and White, J.A. (2012). Pyramidal cells accumulate chloride at seizure onset, *Neurobiol. Dis.*, 47, 358–366.

Liu, Z., Stafstrom, C.E., Sarkisian, M., *et al.* (1996). Age-dependent effects of glutamate toxicity in the hippocampus, *Brain Res. Dev. Brain Res.*, 97, 178–184.

Lodish, H., Berk, A., and Zipursky, S. (2000). Intracellular ion environment and membrane electric potential, in *Molecular and Cellular Biology*, 4th edn. New York, NY. Available from: https://www.ncbi.nlm.nih.gov/books/NBK21627/

Lu, J., Karadsheh, M., and Delpire, E. (1999). Developmental regulation of the neuronal-specific isoform of K-Cl cotransporter KCC2 in postnatal rat brains, *J. Neurobiol.* 39, 558–568.

Lynch, N.E., Stevenson, N.J., Livingstone, V., *et al.* (2012). The temporal evolution of electrographic seizure burden in neonatal hypoxic ischemic encephalopathy, *Epilepsia*, 53, 549–557.

Macdonald, R.L. and Kang, J.-Q. (2012). mRNA surveillance and endoplasmic reticulum quality control processes alter biogenesis of mutant GABAA receptor subunits associated with genetic epilepsies, *Epilepsia*, 53 Suppl 9, 59–70.

Matusmoto, H. and Marsan, C.A. (1964). Cellular mechanisms in experimental epileptic seizures, *Science*, 144, 193–194.

McClatchy, D.B., Liao, L., Park, S.K., *et al.* (2007). Quantification of the synaptosomal proteome of the rat cerebellum during post-natal development, *Genome Res.*, 17, 1378–1388.

McKinstry, R.C., Miller, J.H., Snyder, A.Z., *et al.* (2002). A prospective, longitudinal diffusion tensor imaging study of brain injury in newborns, *Neurology*, 59, 824–833.

McLean, H.A., Caillard, O., Khazipov, R., *et al.* (1996). Spontaneous release of GABA activates GABAB receptors and controls network activity in the neonatal rat hippocampus, *J. Neurophysiol.*, 76, 1036–1046.

Mironov, S.L. and Richter, D.W. (1999). Cytoskeleton mediates inhibition of the fast Na^+ current in respiratory brainstem neurons during hypoxia, *Eur. J. Neurosci.*, 11, 1831–1834.

Miyata, S., Komatsu, Y., Yoshimura, Y., *et al.* (2012). Persistent cortical plasticity by upregulation of chondroitin 6-sulfation, *Nat. Neurosci.*, 15, 414–422, S1-2.

Mongiat, L.A., Esposito, M.S., Lombardi, G., and Schinder, A.F. (2009). Reliable activation of immature neurons in the adult hippocampus, *PLoS One*, 4, e5320.

Moody, W.J. (1998). The development of voltage-gated ion channels and its relation to activity-dependent development events, *Curr. Top. Dev. Biol.*, 39, 159–185.

Moran, N., Poole, K., Bell, G., *et al.* (2004). Epilepsy in the United Kingdom: seizure frequency and severity, anti-epileptic drug utilization and impact on life in 1652 people with epilepsy, *Seizure*, 13, 425–433.

Morita-Fujimura, Y., Fujimura, M., Gasche, Y., Copin, J.C., and Chan, P.H. (2000). Overexpression of copper and zinc superoxide dismutase in transgenic mice prevents the induction and activation of matrix metalloproteinases after cold injury-induced brain trauma, *J. Cereb. Blood Flow Metab.*, 20, 130–138.

Moshé, S.L. (1981). The effects of age on the kindling phenomenon, *Dev. Psychobiol.*, 14, 75–81.

Nardou, R., Ferrari, D.C., and Ben-Ari, Y. (2013). Mechanisms and effects of seizures in the immature brain, *Semin. Fetal Neonatal Med.*, 18, 175–184.

Nickell, W.T., Kleene, N.K., Gesteland, R.C., and Kleene, S.J. (2006). Neuronal chloride accumulation in olfactory epithelium of mice lacking NKCC1, *J. Neurophysiol.*, 95, 2003–2006.

O'Donnell, M.E., Tran, L., Lam, T.I., *et al.* (2004). Bumetanide inhibition of the blood-brain barrier Na-K-Cl cotransporter reduces edema formation in the rat middle cerebral artery occlusion model of stroke, *J. Cereb. Blood Flow Metab.*, 24, 1046–1056.

Olafsson, E., Ludvigsson, P., Gudmundsson, G., *et al.* (2005). Incidence of unprovoked seizures and epilepsy in Iceland and assessment of the epilepsy syndrome classification: a prospective study, *Lancet. Neurol.*, 4, 627–634.

Ouyang, Y., Yang, X.F., Hu, X.Y., *et al.* (2007). Hippocampal seizures cause depolymerization of filamentous actin in neurons independent of acute morphological changes, *Brain Res.*, 1143, 238–246.

Owens, D. F., Boyce, L.H., Davis, M.B., and Kriegstein, A.R. (1996). Excitatory GABA responses in embryonic and neonatal cortical slices demonstrated by gramicidin perforated-patch recordings and calcium imaging, *J. Neurosci.*, 16, 6414–6423.

Painter, M.J., Scher, M.S., Stein, A.D., *et al.* (1999). Phenobarbital compared with phenytoin for the treatment of neonatal seizures, *N. Engl. J. Med.*, 341, 485–489.

Pape, H.C. (1996). Queer current and pacemaker: the hyperpolarization-activated cation current in neurons, *Annu. Rev. Physiol.*, 58, 299–327.

Paulus, W. and Rothwell, J.C. (2016). Membrane resistance and shunting inhibition: where biophysics meets state-dependent human neurophysiology, *J. Physiol.*, 594, 2719–2728.

Plotkin, M.D., Snyder, E.Y., Hebert, S.C., and Delpire, E. (1997). Expression of the Na-K-2Cl cotransporter is developmentally regulated in postnatal rat brains: a possible mechanism underlying GABA's excitatory role in immature brain, *J. Neurobiol.*, 33, 781–795.

van den Pol, A.N., Obrietan, K., and Chen, G. (1996). Excitatory actions of GABA after neuronal trauma, *J. Neurosci.*, 16, 4283–4292.

Pond, B. B., Berglund, K., Kuner, T., *et al.* (2006). The chloride transporter Na^+-K^+-Cl^- cotransporter isoform-1 contributes to intracellular chloride increases after in vitro ischemia, *J. Neurosci.*, 26, 1396–1406.

Poolos, N.P., Migliore, M., and Johnston, D. (2002). Pharmacological upregulation of h-channels reduces the excitability of pyramidal neuron dendrites, *Nat. Neurosci.*, 5, 767–774.

Pressler, R.M., Boylan, G.B., Marlow, N., *et al.* (2015). Bumetanide for neonatal seizures-back from the cotside, *Nat. Rev. Neurol.*, 11, 724, doi: 10.1038/nrneurol.2015.116.

Pressler, R.M., Boylan, G.B., Marlow, N., *et al.* (2015). Bumetanide for the treatment of seizures in newborn babies with hypoxic ischaemic encephalopathy (NEMO): an open-label, dose finding, and feasibility phase 1/2 trial, *Lancet Neurol.*, 14, 469–477.

Prince, D.A. and Wilder, B.J. (1967). Control mechanisms in cortical epileptogenic foci 'surround' inhibition, *Arch. Neurol.*, 16, 194–202.

Psilodimitrakopoulos, S., Petegnief, V., de Vera, N., *et al.* (2013). Quantitative imaging of microtubule alteration as an early marker of axonal degeneration after ischemia in neurons, *Biophys. J.*, 104, 968–975.

Rakhade, S.N. and Jensen, F.E. (2009). Epileptogenesis in the immature brain: emerging mechanisms, *Nat. Rev. Neurol.*, 5, 380–391.

Ran, X., Li, J., Shao, Q., *et al.* (2015). EpilepsyGene: a genetic resource for genes and mutations related to epilepsy, *Nucleic Acids Res.*, 43(Database issue), D893–9.

Rankin-Gee, E.K., McRae, P.A., Baranov, E., *et al.* (2015). Perineuronal net degradation in epilepsy, *Epilepsia*, 56, 1124–1133.

Ransom, C.B., Ransom, B.R., and Sontheimer, H. (2000). Activity-dependent extracellular K^+ accumulation in rat optic nerve: the role of glial and axonal Na^+ pumps, *J. Physiol.*, 522 Pt 3, 427–442.

Rivera, C., Voipio, J., Payne, J.A., *et al.* (1999). The K^+/Cl^- co-transporter KCC2 renders GABA hyperpolarizing during neuronal maturation, *Nature*, 397, 251–255.
Ronen, G.M., Penney, S., and Andrews, W. (1999). The epidemiology of clinical neonatal seizures in Newfoundland: a population-based study, *J. Pediatr.*, 134, 71–75.
Rothstein, J.D., Dykes-Hoberg, M., Pardo, C.A., *et al.* (1996). Knockout of glutamate transporters reveals a major role for astroglial transport in excitotoxicity and clearance of glutamate, *Neuron*, 16, 675–686.
Sanabria, H., Miller, J.H. Jr, Mershin, A., *et al.* (2006). Impedance spectroscopy of alpha-beta tubulin heterodimer suspensions, *Biophys. J.*, 90, 4644–4650.
Sanchez, R.M., Koh, S., Rio, C., *et al.* (2001). Decreased glutamate receptor 2 expression and enhanced epileptogenesis in immature rat hippocampus after perinatal hypoxia-induced seizures, *J. Neurosci.*, 21, 8154–8163.
Sasaki, T., Ishikawa, T., Abe, R., *et al.* (2014). Astrocyte calcium signalling orchestrates neuronal synchronization in organotypic hippocampal slices, *J. Physiol.*, 592, 2771–2783.
Schafer, D.P., Jha, S., Liu, F., *et al.* (2009). Disruption of the axon initial segment cytoskeleton is a new mechanism for neuronal injury, *J. Neurosci.*, 29, 13242–13254.
Sedmak, G., Jovanov-Milošević, N., Puskarjov, M., *et al.* (2016). Developmental expression patterns of KCC2 and functionally associated molecules in the human brain, *Cereb. Cortex*, 26, 4574–4589.
Semple, B.D., Blomgren K., Gimlin, K., *et al.* (2013). Brain development in rodents and humans: identifying benchmarks of maturation and vulnerability to injury across species, *Prog. Neurobiol.*, 106–107, 1–16.
Shackelford, D.A. and Nelson, K.E. (1996). Changes in phosphorylation of tau during ischemia and reperfusion in the rabbit spinal cord, *J. Neurochem.*, 66, 286–295.
Shackelford, D.A. and Yeh, R.Y. (1998). Dephosphorylation of tau during transient forebrain ischemia in the rat, *Mol. Chem. Neuropathol.*, 34, 103–120.
Singh, N.A., Charlier, C., Stauffer, D., *et al.* (1998). A novel potassium channel gene, KCNQ2, is mutated in an inherited epilepsy of newborns, *Nat. Genet.*, 18, 25–29.
Sivakumaran, S. and Maguire, J. (2016). Bumetanide reduces seizure progression and the development of pharmacoresistant status epilepticus, *Epilepsia*, 57, 222–232.

Stafstrom, C.E. and Rho, J.M. (2017). Swaiman's Pediatric Neurology, 6th edition, eds. Swaiman, K. F. *et al.*, Chapter 63 "Neurophysiology of seizures and epilepsy", (Elsevier, Amsterdam), 506–512.

Stafstrom, C.E., Thompson, J.L., and Holmes, G.L. (1992). Kainic acid seizures in the developing brain: status epilepticus and spontaneous recurrent seizures, *Brain Res. Dev. Brain Res.*, 65, 227–236.

Staley, K. (2015). Molecular mechanisms of epilepsy, *Nat. Neurosci.*, 18, 367–672.

Staley, K.J. and Proctor, W.R. (1999). Modulation of mammalian dendritic GABA(A) receptor function by the kinetics of Cl^- and $HCO3^-$ transport, *J. Physiol.*, 519 Pt 3, 693–712.

Staley, K.J., Soldo, B.L., and Proctor, W.R. (1995). Ionic mechanisms of neuronal excitation by inhibitory GABAA receptors, *Science*, 269, 977–981.

Stein, V., Hermans-Borgmeyer, I., Jentsch, T.J. and Hübner, C.A. (2004). Expression of the KCl cotransporter KCC2 parallels neuronal maturation and the emergence of low intracellular chloride, *J. Comp. Neurol.*, 468, 57–64.

Syková, E. and Nicholson, C. (2008). Diffusion in brain extracellular space, *Physiol. Rev.*, 88, 1277–1340.

Talhouk, R.S., Zeinieh, M.P., Mikati, M.A., and El-Sabban, M.E. (2008). Gap junctional intercellular communication in hypoxia-ischemia-induced neuronal injury, *Prog. Neurobiol.*, 84, 57–76.

Talos, D.M., Fishman, R.E., Park, H., *et al.* (2006). Developmental regulation of alpha-amino-3-hydroxy-5-methyl-4-isoxazole-propionic acid receptor subunit expression in forebrain and relationship to regional susceptibility to hypoxic/ischemic injury I. Rodent cerebral white matter and cortex, *J. Comp. Neurol.*, 497, 42–60.

Talos, D.M., Follett, P.L., Folkerth, R.D., *et al.* (2006). Developmental regulation of alpha-amino-3-hydroxy-5-methyl-4-isoxazole-propionic acid receptor subunit expression in forebrain and relationship to regional susceptibility to hypoxic/ischemic injury II. Human cerebral white matter and cortex, *J. Comp. Neurol.*, 497, 61–77.

Thoresen, M. and Sabir, H. (2015). Epilepsy: neonatal seizures still lack safe and effective treatment, *Nat. Rev. Neurol.*, 11, 311–312.

Tremblay, E., Nitecka, L., Berger, M.L., and Ben-Ari, Y. (1984). Maturation of kainic acid seizure-brain damage syndrome in the rat. I. Clinical, electrographic and metabolic observations, *Neuroscience*, 13, 1051–1072.

Triulzi, F., Parazzini, C., and Righini, A. (2006). Patterns of damage in the mature neonatal brain, *Pediatr. Radiol.*, 36, 608–620.

Twyman, R.E., Rogers, C.J., and Macdonald, R.L. (1989). Differential regulation of γ-aminobutyric acid receptor channels by diazepam and phenobarbital, *Ann. Neurol.*, 25, 213–220.

Tyzio, R., Represa, A., Jorquera, I., *et al.* (1999). The establishment of GABAergic and glutamatergic synapses on CA1 pyramidal neurons is sequential and correlates with the development of the apical dendrite, *J. Neurosci.*, 19, 10372–10382.

Tyzio, R., Minlebaev, M., Rheims, S., *et al.* (2008). Postnatal changes in somatic gamma-aminobutyric acid signalling in the rat hippocampus, *Eur. J. Neurosci.*, 27, 2515–2528.

Vasudevan, C. and Levene, M. (2013). Epidemiology and aetiology of neonatal seizures, *Semin. Fetal Neonatal Med.*, 18, 185–191.

Velíšková, J., Velíšek, L., and Moshé, S.L. (1996). Age-specific effects of baclofen on pentylenetetrazol-induced seizures in developing rats, *Epilepsia*, 37, 718–722.

Viitanen, T., Ruusuvuori, E., Kaila, K., and Voipio, J. (2010). The K^+-Cl^- cotransporter KCC2 promotes GABAergic excitation in the mature rat hippocampus, *J. Physiol.*, 588(Pt 9), 1527–1540.

Wagnon, J.L., Barker, B.S., Hounshell, J.A., *et al.* (2016). Pathogenic mechanism of recurrent mutations of SCN8A in epileptic encephalopathy, *Ann. Clin. Transl. Neurol.*, 3, 114–123.

Walther, H., Lambert, J.D., Jones, R.S., Heinemann, U., and Hamon, B. (1986). Epileptiform activity in combined slices of the hippocampus, subiculum and entorhinal cortex during perfusion with low magnesium medium, *Neurosci. Lett.*, 69, 156–161.

Wang, X., Jung, J., Asahi, M., *et al.* (2000). Effects of matrix metalloproteinase-9 gene knock-out on morphological and motor outcomes after traumatic brain injury, *J. Neurosci.*, 20, 7037–7042.

Wirrell, E.C. (2005). Neonatal seizures: to treat or not to treat?, *Semin. Pediatr. Neurol.*, 12, 97–105.

Wong, H.K., Liu, X.B., Matos, M.F., *et al.* (2002). Temporal and regional expression of NMDA receptor subunit NR3A in the mammalian brain, *J. Comp. Neurol.*, 450, 303–317.

Wusthoff, C.J., Dlugos, D.J., Guitierrez-Colina, A., *et al.* (2011). Electrographic seizures during therapeutic hypothermia for neonatal hypoxic-ischemic encephalopathy, *J. Child Neurol.*, 26, 724–728.

Yau, M. L.-Y., Fung, E.L.-W., and Ng, P.C. (2015). Response of levetiracetam in neonatal seizures, *World J. Clin. Pediatr.*, 4, 45–49.

Yu, F.H., Mantegazza, M., Westenbroek, R.E., *et al.* (2006). Reduced sodium current in GABAergic interneurons in a mouse model of severe myoclonic epilepsy in infancy, *Nat. Neurosci.*, 9, 1142–1149.

Zeng, L., Xu, L., Rensing, N.R., *et al.* (2007). Kainate seizures cause acute dendritic injury and actin depolymerization in vivo, *J. Neurosci.*, 27, 11604–11613.

Zhang, L.-L., Delpire, E., and Vardi, N. (2007). NKCC1 does not accumulate chloride in developing retinal neurons, *J. Neurophysiol.*, 98, 266–277.

Zhang, S., Kojic, L., Tsang, M., *et al.* (2016). Distinct roles for metalloproteinases during traumatic brain injury, *Neurochem. Int.*, 96, 46–55.

Chapter 3

Neonatal Genetic Epilepsies: Electroclinical Phenotypes and Basic Mechanisms

Maria-Roberta Cilio,*,† MD, PhD
Charbel El Kosseifi,* MD

**Pediatric Neurology Unit, Department of Pediatrics, Catholic University of Louvain, Brussels, Belgium*
†Pediatric Epilepsy Unit, Department of Neurology, University of California, San Francisco, USA

3.1 Introduction

While the majority of seizures in neonates are related to acute brain injury, a substantial minority represents the first symptom of a neonatal-onset epilepsy, often linked to a pathogenic genetic variant [Shellhaas *et al.*, 2017]. In addition to the concept of genetic epilepsy — directly resulting from a known or presumed genetic mutation in which seizures are a core symptom of the disorder — the last International League Against Epilepsy (ILAE) position paper on the classification of the epilepsies [Scheffer *et al.*, 2017] introduced the new concept of developmental encephalopathies. This concept is particularly relevant for genetic epilepsies that begin in the neonatal period. The concept of epileptic encephalopathy is that the epileptic activity itself contributes to the poor neurologic outcome above and beyond what might be expected from the underlying pathology alone. The implication is that amelioration of the epileptiform activity may improve the developmental consequences of the disorder. However, in some neonatal epilepsies, such as *KCNQ2* or *STXBP1* encephalopathy, the disease *per se* may directly lead to both severe epilepsy and profound intellectual disability as two independent dimensions of the phenotype. The developmental consequences may arise more from the direct effect of the genetic mutation than from the effect of the frequent epileptic activity on development. The relevance of these two components, the epileptic component and the developmental component, can vary in the course of neonatal-onset epilepsies. For instance, in some patients with *KCNQ2* or *STXBP1* encephalopathy, the epilepsy may settle down relatively early, but the developmental consequences remain profound. These concepts are crucial to understanding the disease processes for both families and clinicians [Scheffer *et al.*, 2017]. In this chapter, we review the most relevant monogenic neonatal-onset epilepsies, detail their underlying pathophysiologic mechanisms, and present their electro-clinical phenotypes.

3.2 Channelopathies

Signaling via changes in membrane potential and transmembrane ion fluxes is essential to life in all biological organisms, from bacteria to humans. Most cellular functions are properly executed only within a narrow range of intracellular and extracellular concentration for each ion species; thus, evolution has spent a tremendous effort in overcoming the thermodynamic cost required to translocate charges across low dielectric media such as the lipid membranes and selecting the appropriate means to perform such delicate regulation. Ion channel proteins, by allowing highly regulated ion fluxes across cellular compartments separated by a lipid membrane, provide a solution to this problem. Schematically speaking, two main properties characterize ion channel function: the first one is the gating mechanism, namely the ability to sense the appropriate stimulus; the other is selectivity, namely the capacity to discriminate the ion species allowed to permeate. These two properties, although conceptually separate, are clearly linked in the operation of ion channels, as the structural rearrangement accompanying gating are tightly coupled to ion permeation [Miceli *et al.*, 2011].

In voltage-gated ion channels, the gating mechanism is triggered by transmembrane voltage changes. Differences of only a few millivolts can dramatically modify the opening probability of voltage gated-ion channels, leading to the massive ion fluxes responsible for electrical signaling in excitable cells.

3.2.1 *KCNQ2 and KCNQ3-associated neonatal epilepsy*

KCNQ2 and *KCNQ3* genes encode the voltage-gated potassium channels, Kv7.2 and Kv7.3, respectively. These potassium channels underlie the muscarine-regulated M-current (I_M), a widely distributed slowly activating and non-activating current, which plays a dominant role in modulating neuronal excitability by causing spike-frequency adaptation and setting the subthreshold membrane potential [Shah *et al.*, 2008]. In 1998, *KCNQ2* and *KCNQ3* were the first epilepsy genes to be discovered, when mutations in those genes were identified as a cause of Benign Familial Neonatal Epilepsy (BFNE) [Singh *et al.*, 1998; Charlier *et al.*, 1998, Soldovieri *et al.*, 2007a].

In Kv7.2, most BFNS-causing mutations are localized either in the large C-terminal domain, a critical region for subunit assembly and channel regulation by intracellular molecules, and in the voltage-sensing domains. Functional analysis of Kv7 channel subunits carrying mutations causing BFNE has revealed several mechanisms by which these genetic alterations impair I_M function [Soldovieri *et al.*, 2007a].

Some mutations drastically decrease channel subunit expression, while others affect intracellular trafficking [Soldovieri *et al.*, 2007a]. A mild decrease of I_M function appears sufficient to cause BFNE, and haploinsufficiency seems to be the primary pathogenetic mechanism for both familial and sporadic forms of the disorder.

Other mutations, instead, alter the function of Kv7.2 subunits normally inserted into the plasma membrane; among these, changes in gating properties have been suggested to play a major role in

BFNE pathogenesis [Dedek *et al.*, 2001; Castaldo *et al.*, 2002; Soldovieri *et al.*, 2007b], a result consistent with these mutations affecting residues located within the voltage sensing domain.

The fact that I_M gating changes can be responsible for human epilepsies provides strong support for the hypothesis that this current is a crucial regulator of neuronal excitability in humans; to achieve such delicate functional role, a fine control of I_M gating properties within a precise range of membrane potential values is required. In general, small changes in the channels' voltage dependence, particularly at sub-threshold voltages (between –60 and –30 mV), can profoundly affect neuronal excitability.

BFNE arises from *KCNQ2/3* alleles causing haploinsufficiency (including deletion of the entire gene) and from missense variants that exhibit partial loss-of-function *in vitro* [Miceli *et al.*, 2010; Schroeder *et al.*, 1998]. More than 10 years later, *KCNQ2* surprisingly also linked to a severe epilepsy syndrome named *KCNQ2* encephalopathy [Weckhuysen *et al.*, 2012]. The fact that mutations in the same gene can give rise either to a self-limited epilepsy or a severe epileptic/developmental encephalopathy demonstrates the importance of *KCNQ2* in brain development and suggests that the resulting potassium currents may be differently affected in the two disorders. Interestingly, mutations at the same position in *KCNQ2* were found in children with BFNE (R213W) and in children with *KCNQ2*-encephalopathy (R213Q). A functional study comparing the impact of these mutations showed that more severe functional deficits are associated with more severe epilepsy phenotypes [Miceli *et al.*, 2013]. In order for the KCNQ channel to properly allow ion flow, all four gates of the tetramer must work in tandem. If one of the subunits has a mutation leading to electromechanical uncoupling or pore-blocking, the tetramer becomes non-conducting, despite 3 normal wild-type subunits. This dominant-negative effect is exhibited by many of the mutations leading to *KCNQ2* encephalopathy with a pronounced loss of the I_M in the severe phenotypes [Orhan *et al.*, 2014].

The severe phenotype seen in *KCNQ2* encephalopathy may be further explained by the separation of the mutated potassium channels from their usual axonal partner, the voltage-gated sodium channels. Ankyrin-G is a sub-membranous framework that binds potassium and sodium channels together in the axon initial segment. The failure of appropriate clustering of channels in the membrane can lead to abnormal excitability [Yue and Yaari, 2006; Shah *et al.*, 2008]. This theory provides further grounds for the development of pharmacologic interventions that could reconnect or bind the channels and prevent the excessive or sustained firing of action potentials seen with seizures.

Finally, recent work has revealed a previously unexplored level of complexity in pathogenic mechanisms underlying *KCNQ2* encephalopathy. Indeed, some of the mutations stabilized the activated state of the channel, thereby producing gain-of-function effects [Miceli *et al.*, 2015]. However, careful analysis of the early phenotype of these patients showed that instead of the typical neonatal epileptic encephalopathy, these neonates present with encephalopathy, a burst-suppression pattern on EEG and non-epileptic myoclonus, often misdiagnosed as seizure [Mulkey *et al.*, 2017]. This clinical presentation is distinct from the phenotype associated with loss-of-function variants, supporting the value of *in vitro* functional screening.

3.2.2 *Benign Familial Neonatal Epilepsy*

BFNE is associated, in over 80% of cases, with mutations or deletions in the potassium channel genes *KCNQ2* or less often *KCNQ3* [Sands *et al.*, 2016]. BFNE mostly occurs as an autosomal dominant disorder with incomplete penetrance, although cases of de novo germline mutations with a mild effect or a post-zygotic mosaicism for a more severe variant in *KCNQ2* gene have been described [Milh *et al.*, 2015]. Screening for mosaicism and accurate variant classification in individuals with de novo *KCNQ2* mutations has important implications for genetic counseling.

In a recent multicenter study, BFNE was responsible for about 3% of all neonatal seizures [Glass *et al.*, 2016]. Seizures occur within the first days of life and have a pathognomonic semiology, characterized by asymmetric tonic posturing, sometimes evolving to unilateral or asynchronous bilateral clonic movements, shifting laterality, accompanied in many cases by apnea and oxygen desaturation. Seizures last 1 to 2 minutes and can occur up to 30 times per day, sometimes leading to status epilepticus. On EEG, the interictal background activity is continuous and well organized without focal slowing or attenuation to suggest an underlying lesion. Bilateral independent epileptiform abnormalities, mainly over the central regions, can be present [Sands *et al.*, 2016]. A distinctive ictal pattern has been described on EEG consisting of a sudden rise of the lower and upper margin, followed by a marked depression of the EEG amplitude [Vilan *et al.*, 2017]. Neurodevelopmental outcome is generally good, although it has been reported that up to 25% of patients develop epilepsy later in life. The recurrence risk seems to correlate with seizure burden in the neonatal period [Grinton *et al.*, 2015]. In the context of a positive family history, recognition of the typical electro-clinical phenotype should allow rapid suspicion of BFNE, without the need for extensive ancillary testing [Sands *et al.*, 2016; Vilan *et al.*, 2017]. In a recent multicenter study of 19 patients, low dose oral carbamazepine (10 mg/kg/day) or oxcarbazepine were reported to be safe and rapidly effective, even in the context of status epilepticus, and were associated with shortened hospital stay [Sands *et al.*, 2016]. Carbamazepine is a sodium-channel blocker seldom used in the NICU [Singh *et al.*, 1996; Hoppen *et al.*, 2001; Sands and McDonough, 2016]. It has been used in children and adults for over 30 years to treat focal seizures with an excellent therapeutic and side effect profile. Interestingly, carbamazepine is effective in focal epilepsy involving the supplementary sensorimotor area that resembles seizures presenting in infants with *KCNQ2*-related epilepsy [Connolly *et al.*, 1995].

3.2.3 *KCNQ2 encephalopathy*

On the other end of the spectrum, *de novo KCNQ2* variants leading to loss-of-function are responsible for over 10% of severe early-onset epileptic encephalopathy [Weckhuysen *et al.*, 2013]. Nearly 90% of mutations leading to *KCNQ2* encephalopathy occur in 4 high-risk zones. This strongly supports dominant-negative suppression as the primary factor underlying severe phenotypes in a substantial majority of *KCNQ2* encephalopathy cases [Orhan *et al.*, 2014].

KCNQ2 encephalopathy is characterized by onset within the first week of life of focal tonic seizures, similar in semiology to the ones seen in BFNE [Numis *et al.*, 2014], associated with encephalopathy (hypotonia, paucity of spontaneous movements, no visual fixation and altered reactivity). The neonatal EEG background demonstrates multifocal epileptiform abnormalities with random attenuation or burst-suppression. The ictal EEG shows the onset of low voltage fast activity over a single hemisphere followed by focal spike and wave complexes. While seizure durations are quite short, the post ictal phase is typically characterized by marked and prolonged diffuse voltage attenuation. Seizure frequency is high with 10 or more seizures per day or even per hour. Seizures tend to remit in early childhood, though most children have severe intellectual disability [Weckhuysen *et al.*, 2013], exemplifying the concept of developmental encephalopathy. This observation highlights the need for therapeutic approaches that address the developmental outcome in addition to the seizures, by targeting the underlying pathophysiology directly. As in BFNE, sodium channel blockers such as carbamazepine and phenytoin have been particularly effective [Numis *et al.*, 2014; Pisano *et al.*, 2015] and are now considered an established precision medicine treatment for *KCNQ2*-related epilepsies [Reif *et al.*, 2017].

As highlighted above, gain-of-function variants (R201H and R201C) have also been reported to cause *KCNQ2* encephalopathy although they are associated with a different phenotype than the loss-of-function variants. In this case, while epileptic seizures are not seen in the neonatal period, the clinical presentation is characterized by encephalopathy from birth, irregular breathing patterns and prominent startle-like non-epileptic myoclonus, which can be triggered by sound or touch. The EEG in the neonatal period shows a burst-suppression pattern. Some neonates subsequently develop infantile spasms and all have profound developmental delay. Interestingly, one patient had a later onset, and sequencing indicated that a low abundance (~20%) R201C variant had arisen by postzygotic mosaicism [Mulkey *et al.*, 2017].

3.2.4 *KCNT1*-associated epilepsy

KCNT1 encodes a weakly voltage-dependent sodium-gated potassium channel subunit also known as SLACK (Sequence Like a Calcium-Activated K^+ channel). It is widely expressed in the nervous system and represents the largest known potassium channel subunit. Its activity contributes to the slow hyperpolarization that follows repetitive firing of action potentials [Kim *et al.*, 2014]. Functional studies show that *KCNT1* mutations causing Epilepsy of Infancy with Migrating Focal Seizure (EIMFS; also called malignant migrating focal seizures of infancy (MMFSI)) are associated with a gain-of-function phenotype *in vitro*, leading to increased current amplitude of the sodium-activated potassium channel [Barcia *et al.*, 2012; McTague *et al.*, 2018]. However, no correlation has been found between the magnitude of the impact on the protein and the phenotype.

The first disease-causing mutation in *KCNT1* was described in 2012 [Barcia *et al.*, 2012]. MMFSI was first described in 1995 by Coppola and Dulac [Coppola *et al.*, 1995], as a disorder characterized by nearly continuous multi-focal partial seizures arising independently and sequentially from both hemispheres, progression through a period of intractable seizures, subsequent neurologic deterioration or arrest with complete loss of both cognitive and motor abilities, and in most children, progressive microcephaly [Coppola *et al.*, 1995]. Although MMFSI was initially described in infants, many neonatal cases have been reported. The first seizures occur before 6 months of age (1 day to 6 months; mean 25 days) in previously normal infants. During the first phase of the disorder, focal seizures with a unilateral motor onset may be sporadic and alternate from one side of the body to the other with lateral deviation of head and eyes, limb myoclonic jerks and increase tone in one or both limbs. In half of patients, seizures are associated autonomic symptoms, such as apnea and desaturation, and are sometimes misdiagnosed as gastro-esophageal reflux. Electrical seizures without clinical correlates have also been reported. EEG background may initially be normal or show diffuse slowing but soon becomes abnormal with lack of organization, and frequent seizures with shifting laterality between recordings. Electrographic seizures are monomorphic in each patient, consisting of focal rhythmic alpha or theta beginning in one region and progressively involving adjacent areas. The ictal onset locations vary. During the second phase, which may already start in the first month of life, seizures become very frequent, occurring in clusters of 5 to 30 seizures during drowsiness and awakening several times a day or being almost continuous for days or weeks. During clusters, between seizures, infants are often hypotonic and somnolent. They may partially recover between clusters. However, with the next cluster, infants regress. Over time, seizures tend to generalize more often. EEG shows multifocal paroxysmal abnormalities affecting alternately both hemispheres with migrating features characterized by multiple independent prolonged seizures evolving simultaneously from different regions of the brain. Seizures tend to be highly refractory to both conventional antiepileptic drugs (AEDs) and corticosteroids. However, some response has been reported with potassium bromide [Okuda *et al.*, 2000; Caraballo *et al.*, 2014] and levetiracetam [Hmaimess *et al.*, 2006; Cilio *et al.*, 2009]. About 25% of patients die within a year of onset. After 1 to 5 years, seizures may become less frequent, but severe developmental disability remains [Coppola *et al.*, 1995; Cilio *et al.*, 2007].

While the *KCNT1* mutation in itself could account for the increased excitability and seizure phenotype, the severity of the developmental delay in children with EIMFS suggests an independent developmental role for this gene. In addition to regulating ion flux, a number of channels have non-conducting functions that regulate biochemical activities independent of ion flux [Fleming and Kaczmarek, 2009]. This is likely to be the case for the KCNT1 channel, which, at its C-terminal domain, interacts with protein networks including fragile-X mental retardation protein (FMRP). *KCNT1* mutations may alter the conformation of the C-terminal region of the protein, impairing not only the gating of the channel but also its ability to interact with developmentally relevant proteins such as FMRP, accounting for the severe developmental delay [Barcia *et al.*, 2012].

KCNT1 mutations have also been associated with other types of epilepsies occurring later in life such as Autosomal Dominant Nocturnal Frontal Lobe Epilepsy (ADNFLE). In some families, the same mutation can lead to both EIMFS and ADNFLE, illustrating the phenomenon of phenotypic heterogeneity.

Quinidine, a class I antiarrhythmic drug, was found to reverse *in vitro* the increased conductance of *KCNT1* [Milligan *et al.*, 2014], and the first use of quinidine in a patient with EIMFS paved the way as a future cornerstone in precision medicine [Bearden *et al.*, 2014]. Subsequently, trials of quinidine in patients with *KCNT1* mutations have shown mixed results [Bearden *et al.*, 2014; Mikati *et al.*, 2015; Chong *et al.*, 2016; Abdelnour *et al.*, 2017; Fukuoka *et al.*, 2017; Mullen *et al.*, 2017; McTague *et al.*, 2018]. Initially it was hypothesized that one reason for lack of effect of quinidine in patients was the fact that quinidine was trialed late in the disease course in many patients. However, recent data do not support 'age at quinidine initiation' as a variable that can modify overall outcome [Abdelnour *et al.*, 2017; Numis *et al.*, 2018, in press].

A recent study suggested that this apparent mismatch between *in vitro* and *in vivo* responses to quinidine therapy may be explained by target-specific tissue concentrations. A better understanding of exposure and necessary receptor occupancy may tailor future *in vitro* assays to assess the efficacy of novel therapeutics at lower concentration ranges and predict clinical efficacy in patients with KCNT1 variants [Numis *et al.*, 2018, in press]. While targeting the KCNT1 channel with quinidine in EIMFS did not provide universal benefit, genomic-guided therapy with potassium bromide showed reductions in seizure frequency and severity [Okuda *et al.*, 2000; Caraballo *et al.*, 2014, Numis *et al.*, 2018, in press].

3.2.5 *SCN2A-associated neonatal epilepsy*

SCN2A pathogenic variants are also responsible for a channelopathy associated with a wide phenotypic spectrum including neonatal forms and later-onset disease including epilepsy, developmental delay and autism spectrum disorders.

SCN2A encodes $Na_v1.2$, a major voltage gated sodium channel in the central nervous system early in development. $Na_v1.2$ is supplanted over time, to some extent, by $Na_v1.6$ (SCN8A), which may account for the limited temporal expression of *SCN2A*-associated epilepsy [Liao *et al.*, 2010]. A recent large study reported on the genotype-phenotype presentation of 201 patients with *SCN2A* mutations half of whom had seizure onset before 3 months of life. Interestingly, patients with early seizure onset (<3 mo) presented with missense mutations resulting in a gain-of-function of the sodium channel, whereas patients with later onset often had loss-of-function mutations. The severity of the gain-of-function mutations correlated with the severity of the clinical phenotype [Wolff *et al.*, 2017], and dynamic action potential clamp can predict functional separation in mild familial and severe *de novo* forms of SCN2A epilepsy [Berecki *et al.*, 2018].

One of the typical presentations of *SCN2A* mutations is the Benign Familial Neonatal-Infantile epilepsy (BFNIE). In patients with BFNIE, seizure onset is between 2 days and 3 to 6 months of life. Although half of the patients present in the neonatal period, there is heterogeneity within the same family and different members with the same mutation may have a different age at onset (phenotype heterogeneity). Seizures tend to occur in clusters and are predominantly focal tonic and focal clonic. The interictal EEG is normal or shows occasional focal spikes. Seizures abate within the first two years of life with low recurrence risk and good neurodevelopmental outcome although cases of episodic ataxia later in life have been reported with two specific mutations (A263V and R1882G) [Berkovic *et al.*, 2004; Wolff *et al.*, 2017].

On the other end of the spectrum, *de novo* missense variants in *SCN2A* can be associated with refractory epilepsy presenting either in the neonatal period (neonatal-onset) or in the infantile period (late-onset). The predominant seizure types in the neonatal form are focal seizures with tonic components and apnea. The initial EEG is abnormal with a burst suppression pattern or multi-focal spikes. In the late-onset form, patients typically present with epileptic spasms. Patients have severe intellectual disabilities, axial hypotonia and microcephaly, sometimes accompanied by a movement disorder [Wolff *et al.*, 2017].

Analogous to the situation with *KCNQ2*, potential benefit of sodium channel blockers, such as carbamazepine and phenytoin, has been suggested [Dilena *et al.*, 2017; Berecki *et al.*, 2018]. It seems that sodium channel blockers, by counteracting the increased conductance through the mutant sodium channels, decrease the effect of the gain-of-function mutation.

3.3 Disorders of cell signaling

3.3.1 *CDKL5 encephalopathy*

The *CDKL5* (cyclin-dependent kinase-like 5) gene is located on the short arm of chromosome X (Xp22) and plays a crucial role in brain development. Dominantly acting loss-of-function variants are responsible for this early onset epilepsy associated with encephalopathy, affecting mainly girls. Pathogenic *CDKL5* variants are found across the majority of the coding regions of the gene but missense variants clearly cluster in the N-terminal catalytic domain, suggesting that the kinase function of *CDKL5* is particularly important for brain function. Genotype-phenotype correlation studies have found that mutations in the N-terminal kinase domain are often associated with more severe clinical symptoms than mutations in the C terminus [Fehr *et al.*, 2016; Hector *et al.*, 2017]. However, patients harboring the same mutation have varied severity of the epileptic encephalopathy. This could be due to X-chromosome random inactivation, with the same genetic mutation having different mosaic expression patterns of *CDKL5*, resulting in a spectrum of phenotypes [Bahi-Buisson *et al.*, 2008; Hector *et al.*, 2017].

In *CDKL5* encephalopathy, seizure onset is around 3–6 weeks of life. At onset, seizures are brief but frequent and often intractable. During this early stage, the interictal EEG may remain normal. Some of these infants experience successful seizure control after several weeks to months. Subsequently, the EEG background deteriorates, and the developmental delays, including hypotonia, lack of head control, and poor eye contact become evident. Seizures often display a distinctive "hypermotor-tonic-spasms" sequence [Klein *et al.*, 2011]. Interestingly, epileptic spasms can be present with or without hypsarrhythmia. Later, there is evolution to multifocal and myoclonic epilepsy [Bahi-Buisson *et al.*, 2008; Melani *et al.*, 2011; Auvin *et al.*, 2015]. Marked motor and cognitive impairment associated with feeding and sleep difficulties are typical [Mangatt *et al.*, 2016]. In addition, many patients show a deceleration of head growth and hand stereotypies similar to those seen in girls with Rett syndrome. Some boys have been reported with very severe early-onset phenotype or mosaicism for the pathogenic variant [Nemos *et al.*, 2009; Stosser *et al.*, 2017].

The mechanism by which a mutation in the *CDKL5* gene leads to such a severe and early-onset epileptic encephalopathy is not yet fully understood. One of the functions of the CDKL5 protein is to phosphorylate other proteins, and one of its major targets is *MECP2*, known to be involved in neuronal function and synapse maintenance. *MECP2* mutations are associated with Rett syndrome, a disease that shares some similarities with *CDKL5* encephalopathy. Two *CDKL5* knockout mouse models have been described [Wang *et al.*, 2012; Amendola *et al.*, 2014]. Behavioral analysis reveals that the knockout models reproduce key features of the human disorder, including limb clasping, hypo-activity, and abnormal eye tracking. Investigations of these mouse models have uncovered potential substrates for the *CDKL5*-associated encephalopathy, including reduced dendritic arborization of cortical neurons, decreased visual evoked responses, and alterations in Akt/rpS6 signaling pathways. Particularly interesting is the dissociation of behavioral phenotypes resulting from a conditional knockout of *CDKL5* in glutamatergic cortical neurons and GABAergic forebrain neurons, respectively. These findings suggest that the behavioral phenotype (motor hypoactivity) observed in *CDKL5* encephalopathy derives from the localized absence of CDKL5 in GABAergic forebrain neurons, and that the limb control and eye tracking phenotypes depend on glutamatergic neuron function. However, these mouse models lack spontaneous seizures or epileptiform activity, which are key features of *CDKL5* encephalopathy.

3.3.2 *BRAT1-associated lethal neonatal rigidity and multifocal seizures*

Mutations in the *BRAT1* gene have been associated with Lethal Neonatal Rigidity and Multifocal Seizures (LNRMFS) syndrome. This condition was first described in 2012 in a study using genetic mapping and exome sequencing to identify variant associated with diseases in an Amish population [Puffenberger *et al.*, 2012]. Subsequently, 10 additional patients with LNRMFS have been reported. Little is known about the neonatal electro-clinical phenotype of *BRAT1* related conditions. Neonates present with diffuse hypertonia, microcephaly, multifocal myoclonic jerks with and without EEG correlates, and multifocal refractory seizures leading to early death often in a context of refractory apnea and bradycardia [Saitsu *et al.*, 2014; Van De Pol *et al.*, 2015; Straussberg *et al.*, 2015; Saunders *et al.*, 2015; Horn *et al.*, 2016].

More recently, mutations in *BRAT1* were also associated with a milder presentation characterized by either later-onset epilepsy and survival past infancy or intellectual disability, ataxia/dyspraxia, and cerebellar atrophy with or without epilepsy [Srivastava *et al.*, 2016; Fernández-Jaén *et al.*, 2016; Mundy *et al.*, 2016]. Phenotypic variability has been reported within the same family with siblings presenting with forms of variable severity [Smith *et al.*, 2016]. Early genetic testing helps to prevent unnecessary procedures and futile treatments. Genetic counseling is critical as familial recurrence is common in this autosomal recessive condition. Families with two or more siblings affected by LNRMFS have been described.

BRAT1 encodes a protein that interacts with the tumor suppressor BRCA1 and binds to ATM-1. It is involved in cell-cycle signaling pathways required for cellular responses to DNA damage. Knockdown models of *BRAT1* results in p53-mediated apoptosis [Aglipay *et al.*, 2006]. Autopsy findings in one patient showed progressive atrophy and neuronal cell loss in the cerebrum and cerebellum leading to the assumption that disturbed apoptosis may be caused by *BRAT1* mutations [Saitsu *et al.*, 2014]. Recent studies also showed that loss of *BRAT1* suppresses growth signaling, increases apoptosis, and induces mitochondrial dysfunction, which is associated with mitochondria-dependent intrinsic apoptosis [So and Ouchi, 2014].

3.4 Disorders of synaptic transmission

3.4.1 *STXBP1 encephalopathy*

De novo mutations in *STXBP1* (syntaxin-binding protein 1) gene are one of the major causes of neonatal-onset developmental encephalopathy associated with epilepsy most often presenting as Ohtahara syndrome (OS) [Stamberger *et al.*, 2016].

The *STXBP1* gene, also known as *MUNC18-1*, is predominantly expressed in the brain. It encodes a membrane trafficking protein, which plays an important role in synaptic vesicle docking and fusion, necessary for neurotransmitter secretion. Through interaction with both vesicle-associated (synaptobrevin 2) and target-associated (syntaxin-1) soluble N-ethylmaleimide-sensitive factor attachment protein receptors (SNARE) proteins, *STXBP1* modulates the presynaptic vesicular fusion reaction. Syntaxin-1 includes both an N-terminal peptide (N-peptide) and a large conserved Habc-domain that binds to *STXBP1*. While the N-peptide is essential for vesicle fusion as such, the Habc-domain regulates the fusion, in part by forming the closed syntaxin-1 conformation. Hence the complex structure of *STXBP1* is required for its multifaceted role in different types of synaptic vesicle fusion [Zhou *et al.*, 2013].

An *STXBP1* knockout mouse model showed that total disruption of *STXBP1* leads to a complete loss of neurotransmitter secretion from synaptic vesicles. *STXBP1* knockout mice further showed neurodegeneration after an initially normal brain assembly, indicating that neurotransmitter secretion, and thus functional *STXBP1*, is important for the maintenance of neuronal synapses. Reduced *STXBP1* expression was further shown to increase synaptic depression at both GABAergic and glutamatergic synapses with a greater impact on GABAergic interneurons. This might result in net hyperexcitability and epileptic activity in case of *STXBP1* haploinsufficiency [Toonen *et al.*, 2006; Stamberger *et al.*, 2016]. These studies shed light on the pathophysiology of OS, which, in the setting of normal brain architecture, could be related to altered neurotransmission.

STXBP1 mutations were initially described in patients diagnosed with OS [Saitsu *et al.*, 2008]. Later, *STXBP1* was also associated with unclassified early-onset epileptic encephalopathy, and a variety of phenotypes including West syndrome, Dravet syndrome, non-syndromic epilepsy and intellectual disability, and autism [Stamberger *et al.*, 2016].

Ninety-five percent of patients with *STXBP1* mutations have epilepsy. In patients with *STXBP1* encephalopathy, seizures tend to occur early in life, often in the neonatal period (median onset age: 6 weeks). Neonates tend to present with epileptic spasms, often associated with refractory focal seizures. EEG at onset is markedly abnormal, usually showing a burst suppression pattern, sometimes multi-focal abnormalities. Half of the patients evolve to West syndrome. They have moderate to severe cognitive impairment and a normal head circumference [Di Meglio *et al.*, 2015; Stamberger *et al.*, 2016]. Epilepsy may settle down relatively early in the child's course, but the developmental consequences often remain profound. Affected infants also tend to develop an ataxic gait and paroxysmal non-epileptic movements later in childhood [Milh *et al.*, 2011; Di Meglio *et al.*, 2015].

Recently, 3 cases of focal cortical dysplasia (FCD) associated with *STXBP1* mutations raised the possibility of a causal relationship between neuronal expression of *STXBP1* mutations and FCD. One patient with a *STXBP1* mutation, early infantile epileptic encephalopathy, developmental delays and autism spectrum disorder achieved complete seizure remission following resection of dysplastic brain tissue. Examination of excised brain tissue identified mosaicism for *STXBP1*, providing evidence for a somatic mechanism [Uddin *et al.*, 2017]. This finding, although preliminary, also highlights the link between genetic and structural epilepsies.

3.5 Conclusions

Advances in our understanding of the genetic basis of neonatal epilepsies have opened the way for precision medicine approaches. It is well known that any effective cure will benefit from an early diagnosis. However, many neonates with genetic epilepsies remain undiagnosed until later in life, without an opportunity for early intervention. We believe that early recognition of the electro-clinical phenotype specific to each condition is essential for early diagnosis and potential targeted treatment. For example, *KCNQ2*- and *KCNQ3*-related epilepsies have been demonstrated to respond selectively to sodium channel blocking agents (carbamazepine, phenytoin).

Precision medicine in the neonatal intensive care nursery offers a unique opportunity to embrace therapeutic approaches stratified on the basis of etiology. Translational studies demonstrate that distinct pathophysiological mechanisms can be associated with different mutations and are reflected in different phenotypes. Novel therapeutic approaches for neonatal epilepsies have been either the result of attentive clinical observation (carbamazepine in *KCNQ2*-related epilepsies), or rationally directed therapies with *in vitro* validation (quinidine in EIMFS associated with *KCNT1* mutations).

Knowledge of the molecular mechanisms of epileptogenesis and developmental impairment is the basis of our advances in precision medicine in neonates with specific genetic defects. There is an urgent clinical need to clarify these mechanisms for the development of therapies effective against the common denominator causing both seizures and cognitive impairment.

Acknowledgments

Charbel El Kosseifi received a scholarship from Université catholique de Louvain, Cliniques universitaires aint-Luc, Service de Neurologie Pédiatrique.

References

Abdelnour, E., Gallentine, W., McDonald, M., *et al.* (2017). Does age affect response to quinidine in patients with KCNT1 mutations? Report of three new cases and review of the literature, *Seizure*, 55, 1–3.

Aglipay, J.A., Martin, S.A., Tawara, H., *et al.* (2006). ATM activation by ionizing radiation requires BRCA1-associated BAAT1. *J. Biol. Chem.*, 281, 9710–9718.

Amendola, E., Zhan, Y., Mattucci, C., *et al.* (2014). Mapping pathological phenotypes in a mouse model of CDKL5 disorder, *PLoS ONE*, 9, e91613.

Auvin, S., Cilio, M.R., and Vezzani, A. (2015). Current understanding and neurobiology of epileptic encephalopathies, *Neurobiol. Dis.*, 92 (Part A), 72–89.

Bahi-Buisson, N., Kaminska, A., Boddaert, N., *et al.* (2008). The three stages of epilepsy in patients with CDKL5 mutations, *Epilepsia*, 49, 1027–1037.

Barcia, G., Fleming, M.R., Deligniere, A., *et al.* (2012). De novo gain-of-function KCNT1 channel mutations cause malignant migrating partial seizures of infancy, *Nat. Gen.*, 44, 1255–1259.

Bearden, D., Strong, A., Ehnot, J., *et al.* (2014). Targeted treatment of migrating partial seizures of infancy with quinidine, *Ann. Neurol.*, 76, 457–461.

Berecki, G., Howell, K.B., Deerasooriya, Y.H., *et al.* (2018). Dynamic action potential clamp predicts functional separation in mild familial and severe de novo forms of SCN2A epilepsy, *Proc. Natl. Acad. Sci. USA*, 115, E5516–E5525.

Berkovic, S.F., Heron, S.E., Giordano, L., *et al.* (2004). Benign familial neonatal-infantile seizures: characterization of a new sodium channelopathy, *Ann. Neurol.*, 55, 550–557.

Caraballo, R., Pasteris, M.C., Fortini, P.S., *et al.* (2014). Epilepsy of infancy with migrating focal seizures: six patients treated with bromide, *Seizure*, 23, 899–902.

Castaldo, P., del Giudice, E.M., Coppola, G., *et al.* (2002). Benign familial neonatal convulsions caused by altered gating of KCNQ2/KCNQ3 potassium channels, *J. Neurosci.*, 22, RC199.

Charlier, C., Singh, N.A., Ryan, S.G., *et al.* (1998). A pore mutation in a novel KQT-like potassium channel gene in an idiopathic epilepsy family, *Nat. Gen.*, 18, 53–55.

Chong, P.F., Nakamura, R., Saitsu, H., *et al.* (2016). Ineffective quinidine therapy in early onset epileptic encephalopathy with KCNT1 mutation, *Ann. Neurol.*, 79, 502–503.

Chung, H.J., Jan, Y.N., and Jan, L.Y. (2006). Polarized axonal surface expression of neuronal KCNQ channels is mediated by multiple signals in the KCNQ2 and KCNQ3 C-terminal domains, *Proc. Natl. Acad. Sci. USA*, 103, 8870–8875.

Cilio, M.R., Bianchi, R., Balestri, M., *et al.* (2009). Intravenous levetiracetam terminates refractory status epilepticus in two patients with migrating partial seizures in infancy, *Epilepsy Res.*, 86, 66–71.

Cilio, M.R., Dulac, O., Guerrini, R., *et al.* (2007). "Migrating partial seizures in infancy." In Engel Jr., J. and Pedley, T.A. (eds.) *Epilepsy; A comprehensive textbook*, Vol. 3, 2nd ed,. pp. 2323–2328.

Connolly, M.B., Langill, L., Wong, P.K.H., *et al.* (1995). Seizures involving the supplementary sensorimotor area in children: a video-EEG analysis, *Epilepsia*, 36, 1025–1032.

Coppola, G., Plouin, P., Chiron, C., *et al.* (1995). Migrating partial seizures in infancy: a malignant disorder with developmental arrest, *Epilepsia*, 36, 1017–1024.

Dedek, K., Kunath, B., Kananura, C., *et al.* (2001). Neonatal epilepsy caused by a mutation in the voltage sensor of the KCNQ2 K channel, *Proc. Natl. Acad. Sci. USA*, 98, 12272–12277.

Di Meglio, C., Lesca, G., Villeneuve, N., *et al.* (2015). Epileptic patients with de novo STXBP1 mutations: Key clinical features based on 24 cases, *Epilepsia*, 56, 1931–1940.

Dilena, R., Striano, P., Gennaro, E., *et al.* (2017). Efficacy of sodium channel blockers in SCN2A early infantile epileptic encephalopathy, *Brain Dev.*, 39, 345–348.

Fehr, S., Wong, K., Chin, R., *et al.* (2016). Seizure variables and their relationship to genotype and functional abilities in the CDKL5 disorder, *Neurology*, 87, 2206–2213.

Fernández-Jaén, A., Álvarez, S., Young So, E., *et al.* (2016). Mutations in BRAT1 cause autosomal recessive progressive encephalopathy: Report of a Spanish patient, *Eur. J. Paediatr. Neurol.*, 20, 421–425.

Fleming, M.R. and Kaczmarek, L.K. (2009). Use of optical biosensors to detect modulation of Slack potassium channels by G protein-coupled receptors, *J. Recep. Sig. Transduc.*, 29, 173–181.

Fukuoka, M., Kuki, I., Kawawaki, H., *et al.* (2017). Quinidine therapy for West syndrome with KCNTI mutation: a case report, *Brain Dev.*, 39, 80–83.

Glass, H.C., Shellhaas, R.A.R.A., Wusthoff, C.J., *et al.* (2016). Contemporary profile of seizures in neonates: a prospective cohort study, *J. Pediatr.*, 174, 98–103.e1.

Grinton, B.E., Heron, S.E., Pelekanos, J.T., *et al.* (2015). Familial neonatal seizures in 36 families: clinical and genetic features correlate with outcome, *Epilepsia*, 56, 1071–1080.

Hector, R.D., Kalscheuer, V.M., Hennig, F., *et al.* (2017). CDKL5 variants: improving our understanding of a rare neurologic disorder, *Neurol. Gen.*, 3, e200.

Hmaimess, G., Kadhim, H., Nassogne, M.-C., *et al.* (2006). Levetiracetam in a neonate with malignant migrating partial seizures, *Pediatr. Neurol.*, 34, 55–59.

Hoppen, T., Elger, C.E., and Bartmann, P. (2001). Carbamazepine in phenobarbital-nonresponders: experience with ten preterm infants, *Eur. J. Pediatr.*, 160, 444–447.

Horn, D., Weschke, B., Knierim, E., *et al.* (2016). BRAT1 mutations are associated with infantile epileptic encephalopathy, mitochondrial dysfunction, and survival into childhood, *Am. J. Med. Gen. Part A*, 170, 2274–2281.

Kim, G.E., Kronengold, J., Barcia, G., *et al.* (2014). Human slack potassium channel mutations increase positive cooperativity between individual channels, *Cell Rep.*, 9, 1661–1673.

Klein, K.M., Yendle, S.C., Harvey, A.S., *et al.* (2011). A distinctive seizure type in patients with CDKL5 mutations: hypermotor-tonic-spasms sequence, *Neurology*, 76, 1436–1438.

Liao, Y., Deprez, L., Maljevic, S., *et al.* (2010). Molecular correlates of age-dependent seizures in an inherited neonatal-infantile epilepsy, *Brain*, 133, 1403–1414.

Mangatt, M., Wong, K., Anderson, B., *et al.* (2016). Prevalence and onset of comorbidities in the CDKL5 disorder differ from Rett syndrome, *Orphanet J. Rare Dis.*, 11, 39.

McTague, A., Nair, U., Malhotra, S., *et al.* (2018). Clinical and molecular characterization of KCNT1-related severe early-onset epilepsy, *Neurology*, 90, e55–e66.

Melani, F., Mei, D., Pisano, T., *et al.* (2011). CDKL5 gene-related epileptic encephalopathy: electroclinical findings in the first year of life, *Dev. Med. Child Neurol.*, 53, 354–360.

Miceli, F., Soldovieri, M.V., Ambrosino, P., *et al.* (2013). Genotype-phenotype correlations in neonatal epilepsies caused by mutations in the voltage sensor of Kv7.2 potassium channel subunits, *Proc. Natl. Acad. Sci. USA*, 110, 4386–4391.

Miceli, F., Soldovieri, M.V., Ambrosino, P., *et al.* (2015). Early-onset epileptic encephalopathy caused by gain-of-function mutations in the voltage sensor of Kv7.2 and Kv7.3 potassium channel subunits, *J. Neurosci.*, 35, 3782–3793.

Miceli, F., Soldovieri M.V., Iannotti, F.A., *et al.* (2011). The voltage-sensing domain of K(v)7.2 channels as a molecular target for epilepsy-causing mutations and anticonvulsants, *Front Pharmacol.*, 2, 2.

Miceli, F., Soldovieri, M.V., Joshi, N., *et al.* (2010). KCNQ2-Related Disorders. In: Pagon, R.A., Adam, M.P., Ardinger, H.H., *et al.*, eds., Seattle (WA): University of Washington, Seattle; 2010. [[Updated 2016 Mar 31]], pp. 1993–2016.

Mikati, M.A., Jiang, Y.-H., Carboni, M., *et al.* (2015). Quinidine in the treatment of KCNT1-positive epilepsies, *Ann. Neurol.*, 78, 995–999.

Milh, M., Lacoste, C., Cacciagli, P., *et al.* (2015). Variable clinical expression in patients with mosaicism for KCNQ2 mutations, *Am. J. Med. Gen. Part A*, 167, 2314–2318.

Milh, M., Villeneuve, N., Chouchane, M., *et al.* (2011). Epileptic and non-epileptic features in patients with early onset epileptic encephalopathy and STXBP1 mutations, *Epilepsia*, 52, 1828–1834.

Milligan, C.J., Li, M., Gazina, E.V., *et al.* (2014). KCNT1 gain of function in 2 epilepsy phenotypes is reversed by quinidine, *Ann. Neurol.*, 75, 581–590.

Mulkey, S., Ben-Zeev, B., Nicolai, J., *et al.* (2017). Neonatal nonepileptic myoclonus is a prominent clinical feature of KCNQ2 gain-of-function variants R201C and R201H, *Epilepsia*, 58, 436–445.

Mullen, S.A., Carney, P.W., Roten, A., *et al.* (2017). Precision therapy for epilepsy due to KCNT1 mutations: A randomized trial of oral quinidine, *Neurology*, 90, e67–e72.

Mundy, S.A., Krock, B.L., Mao, R., *et al.* (2016). BRAT1-related disease-identification of a patient without early lethality, *Am. J. Med. Gen. Part A*, 170, 699–702.

Nemos, C., Lambert, L., Giuliano, F., *et al.* (2009). Mutational spectrum of CDKL5 in early-onset encephalopathies: a study of a large collection of French patients and review of the literature, *Clin. Gen.*, 76, 357–371.

Numis, A.L., Angriman, M., Sullivan, J.E., *et al.* (2014). KCNQ2 encephalopathy: Delineation of the electroclinical phenotype and treatment response, *Neurology*, 82, 368–370.

Numis, A.L., Nair, U., Datta, A., *et al.* (2018). Lack of response to quinidine in KCNT1-related neonatal epilepsy, *Epilepsia*, in press, doi: 10.1111/epi.14551.

Okuda, K., Yasuhara, A., Kamei, A., *et al.* (2000). Successful control with bromide of two patients with malignant migrating partial seizures in infancy, *Brain Dev.*, 22, 56–59.

Orhan, G., Bock, M., Schepers, D., *et al.* (2014). Dominant-negative effects of KCNQ2 mutations are associated with epileptic encephalopathy, *Ann. Neurol.*, 75, 382–394.

Pisano, T., Numis, A.L., Heavin, S.B., *et al.* (2015). Early and effective treatment of KCNQ2 encephalopathy, *Epilepsia*, 56, 685–691.

Puffenberger, E.G., Jinks, R.N., Sougnez, C., *et al.* (2012). Genetic mapping and exome sequencing identify variants associated with five novel diseases, *PLoS ONE*, 7, 1.

Reif, P.S., Tsai, M.-H.H., Helbig, I., *et al.* (2017). Precision medicine in genetic epilepsies: break of dawn?, *Exp. Rev. Neurotherap.*, 17, 381–392.

Saitsu, H., Kato, M., Mizuguchi, T., *et al.* (2008). De novo mutations in the gene encoding STXBP1 (MUNC18-1) cause early infantile epileptic encephalopathy, *Nat. Gen.*, 40, 782–788.

Saitsu, H., Yamashita, S., Tanaka, Y., *et al.* (2014). Compound heterozygous BRAT1 mutations cause familial Ohtahara syndrome with hypertonia and microcephaly, *J. Hum. Gen.*, 59, 687–690.

Sands, T.T., Balestri, M., Bellini, G., *et al.* (2016). Rapid and safe response to low-dose carbamazepine in neonatal epilepsy, *Epilepsia*, 57, 2019–2030.

Sands, T.T. and McDonough, T.L. (2016). Recent advances in neonatal seizures, *Curr. Neurol. Neurosci. Rep.*, 16, 1–10.

Saunders, C.J., Miller, N.A., Soden, S.E., *et al.* (2015). Rapid whole-genome sequencing for genetic diseases in neonatal care units, *Sci. Transl. Med.*, 4, 154.

Scheffer, I.E., Berkovic, S., Capovilla, G., *et al.* (2017). ILAE classification of the epilepsies: position paper of the ILAE Commission for Classification and Terminology, *Epilepsia*, 58, 512–521.

Schroeder, B.C., Kubisch, C., Stein, V., and Jentsch, T.J. (1998). Moderate loss of function of cyclic-AMP-modulated KCNQ2/KCNQ3 K+ channels causes epilepsy, *Nature*, 396, 687–690.

Shah, M.M., Migliore, M., Valencia, I., *et al.* (2008). Functional significance of axonal Kv7 channels in hippocampal pyramidal neurons, *Proc. Natl. Acad. Sci. USA*, 105, 7869–7874.

Shellhaas, R.A., Wusthoff, C.J., Tsuchida, T.N., *et al.* (2017). Profile of neonatal epilepsies: characteristics of a prospective US cohort, *Neurology*, 89, 893–899.

Singh, B., Singh, P., Hifzi, I., *et al.* (1996). Treatment of neonatal seizures with carbamazepine, *J. Child Neurol.*, 11, 378–382.

Singh, N.A., Charlier, C., Stauffer, D., *et al.* (1998). A novel potassium channel gene, KCNQ2, is mutated in an inherited epilepsy of newborns, *Nat. Gen.*, 18, 25–29.

Smith, N.J., Lipsett, J., Dibbens, L.M., *et al.* (2016). BRAT1-associated neurodegeneration: intra-familial phenotypic differences in siblings, *Am. J. Med. Gen.* Part A, 170, 3033–3038.

So, E.Y. and Ouchi, T. (2014). BRAT1 deficiency causes increased glucose metabolism and mitochondrial malfunction, *BMC Cancer*, 14, 548.

Soldovieri, M.V., Cilio, M.R., Miceli, F., *et al.* (2007a). Atypical gating of M-type potassium channels conferred by mutations in uncharged residues in the S4 region of KCNQ2 causing benign familial neonatal convulsions, *J. Neurosci.*, 27, 4919–4928.

Soldovieri, M.V., Miceli, F., Bellini, G., *et al.* (2007b). Correlating the clinical and genetic features of Benign Familial Neonatal Seizures (BFNS) with the functional consequences of underlying mutations, *Channels (Austin)*, 1, 228–233.

Srivastava, S., Olson, H.E., Cohen, J.S., *et al.* (2016). BRAT1 mutations present with a spectrum of clinical severity, *Am. J. Med. Gen.* Part A, 170, 2265–2273.

Stamberger, H., Nikanorova, M., Willemsen, M.H., *et al.* (2016). STXBP1 encephalopathy, *Neurology*, 86, 954–962.

Stosser, M.B., Lindy, A.S., Butler, E., *et al.* (2017). High frequency of mosaic pathogenic variants in genes causing epilepsy-related neurodevelopmental disorders, *Genet. Med.*, 20, 403–410.

Straussberg, R., Ganelin-Cohen, E., Goldberg-Stern, H., *et al.* (2015). Lethal neonatal rigidity and multifocal seizure syndrome — Report of another family with a BRAT1 mutation, *Eur. J. Paediatr. Neurol.*, 19, 240–242.

Toonen, R.F.G., Wierda, K., Sons, M.S., *et al.* (2006). Munc18-1 expression levels control synapse recovery by regulating readily releasable pool size, *Proc. Natl. Acad. Sci. USA*, 103, 18332–18337.

Uddin, M., Woodbury-Smith, M., Chan, A., *et al.* (2017). Germline and somatic mutations in STXBP1 with diverse neurodevelopmental phenotypes, *Neurol. Gen.*, 3, e199.

Van De Pol, L.A., Wolf, N.I., Van Weissenbruch, M.M., *et al.* (2015). Early-onset severe encephalopathy with epilepsy: the BRAT1 gene should be added to the List of Causes, *Neuropediatrics*, 46, 392–400.

Vilan, A., Mendes Ribeiro, J., Striano, P., *et al.* (2017). A distinctive ictal amplitude-integrated electroencephalography pattern in newborns with neonatal epilepsy associated with KCNQ2 mutations, *Neonatology*, 112, 387–393.

Wang, I.-T.J., Allen, M., Goffin, D., *et al.* (2012). Loss of CDKL5 disrupts kinome profile and event-related potentials leading to autistic-like phenotypes in mice, *Proc. Natl. Acad. Sci. USA*, 109, 21516–21521.

Weckhuysen, S., Ivanovic, V., Hendrickx, R., *et al.* (2013). Extending the KCNQ2 encephalopathy spectrum: clinical and neuroimaging findings in 17 patients, *Neurology*, 81, 1697–1703.

Weckhuysen, S., Mandelstam, S., Suls, A., *et al.* (2012). KCNQ2 encephalopathy: emerging phenotype of a neonatal epileptic encephalopathy, *Ann. Neurol.*, 71, 15–25.

Wolff, M., Johannesen, K.M., Hedrich, U.B.S.S., *et al.* (2017). Genetic and phenotypic heterogeneity suggest therapeutic implications in SCN2A-related disorders, *Brain*, 140, 1316–1336.

Yue, C. and Yaari, Y. (2006). Axo-somatic and apical dendritic Kv7/M channels differentially regulate the intrinsic excitability of adult rat CA1 pyramidal cells, *J. Neurophysiol.*, 95, 3480–3495.

Zhou, P., Pang, Z.P., Yang, X., *et al.* (2013). Syntaxin-1 N-peptide and Habc-domain perform distinct essential functions in synaptic vesicle fusion, *EMBO J.*, 32, 159–171.

Chapter 4
Treatment Aspects of Developmental Epilepsies

Ryan Ghusayni, MD
Mohamad A. Mikati, MD

Division of Pediatric Neurology and Pediatric Epilepsy Program, Duke University Medical Center, Durham, NC, USA

4.1 Introduction

4.1.1 *General principles*

When first approaching a patient who has had a seizure, a decision must be made on whether to start an antiepileptic drug (AED) or not. The first step is to determine if the patient has had an epileptic seizure or a paroxysmal event that mimics seizures such as syncope. The second is to identify if there is any underlying etiology for symptomatic seizures, such as electrolyte disturbances, hypoglycemia, drug withdrawal, infection or acute head trauma. As a rule, only epileptic seizures are treated with long-term AED therapy, except if they are brief, infrequent and self-limiting, in which case one may choose to withhold or delay long-term AED therapy. The decision to treat or not to treat should be individualized taking into account factors such as seizure type, EEG, family history of seizures, possible etiology, driving status and type of work. The possible adverse effects of AEDs must be weighed against the benefits of preventing another seizure [Mikati and Tchapyjnikov, 2018; Pellock *et al.*, 2016]. Mechanisms of action of selected AEDs are illustrated in Figure 4.1.

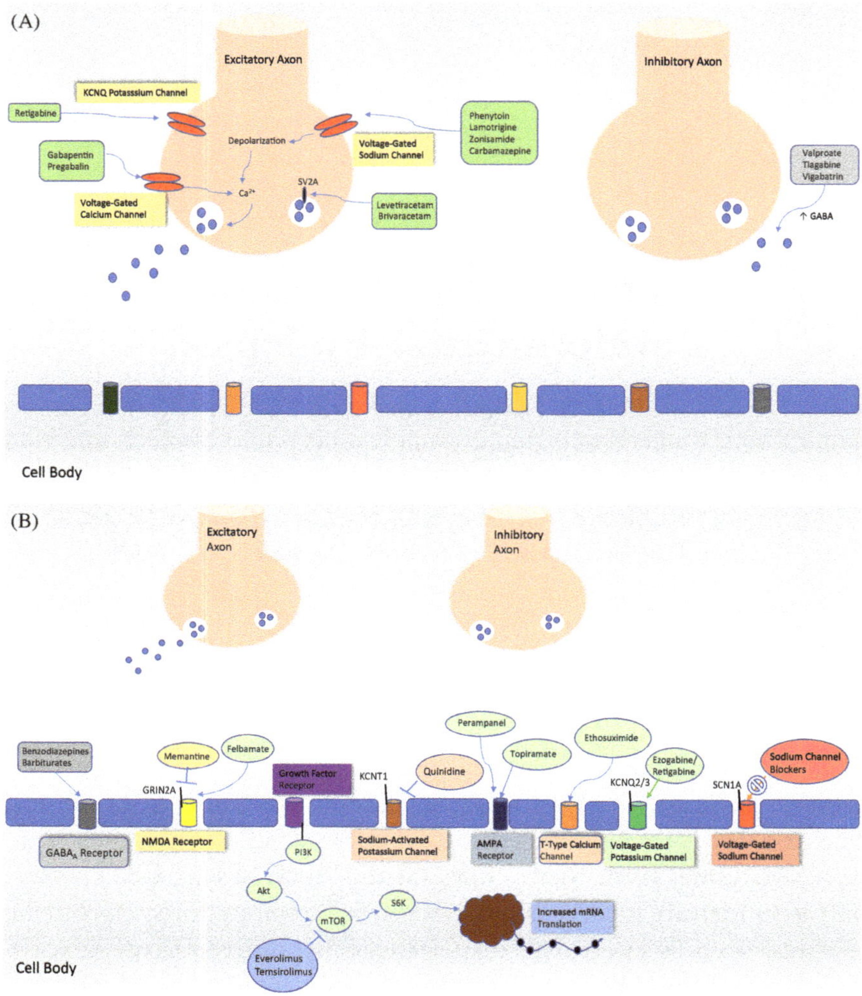

Figure 4.1. Mechanisms of action of selected antiepileptic drugs on presynaptic (A) and postsynaptic (A&B) receptors. Valproate inhibits GABA degradative enzymes, tiagabine blocks GABA transporter 1 and vigabatrin inhibits GABA transaminase, which catabolizes GABA, all contributing to increased GABA in the synaptic cleft.

It is at times preferable to start acute treatment with an AED that can later be given as maintenance therapy but this is not necessarily the best option all the time. In addition, it is the rule to start one medication and if it fails use another alternative again as monotherapy.

If two medications fail then the alternative is to start combining medications or to still try another monotherapy with an appropriate drug. For neonatal seizures, the most commonly used first-line drug for long term therapy is phenobarbital, followed by phenytoin or fosphenytoin but increasingly levetiracetam is being used as an earlier choice or even as an initial choice. In older children, focal seizures and epilepsies are usually initially treated with oxcarbazepine or levetiracetam, absence seizures with ethosuximide, juvenile myoclonic epilepsy with valproate or levetiracetam, with other choices being lamotrigine, zonisamide, topiramate and perampanel [Mikati and Tchapyjnikov, 2018]. Counseling families about the pros and cons of starting therapy including side effects of medications and risk of recurrence and complications of seizures including Sudden Unexpected Death in Epilepsy (SUDEP) are essential steps in the management of children with epilepsy.

Focal resective epilepsy surgery should be considered for patients with focal epilepsy not controlled despite the proper use of two AEDs. Patients with corresponding focal lesions on MRI usually have higher chances for seizure freedom than those with negative MRIs. Those not suited for focal resection surgery because their focus is not localizable or resectable, because they have multiple foci or because they have generalized epilepsy, may be candidates for one or more of several palliative procedures. These include vagus nerve stimulation, reactive neurostiumulation or corpus callosotomy [Wilmshurst *et al.*, 2015]. In children with epileptic encephalopathies or certain types of epilepsy, other options include dietary therapy such as with the classic ketogenic diet or its variants, or with immunotherapy such as steroids or adrenocorticotropic hormone (ACTH).

There are a number of factors to consider before withdrawal of AEDs. The decision should be tailored to the individual patient taking into account the etiology, EEG findings and clinical picture. The conventional wisdom has been to consider withdrawal two years after the last seizure. However, EEG is usually done at this time point to rule out continued predisposition for having seizures which may preclude withdrawal of therapy. Other predictors that increase the risk of recurrence after withdrawal are the presence of a structural underlying etiology and a history of a period of drug resistance before control was achieved.

A systematic review and meta-analysis has identified several independent predictors of seizure recurrence after drug withdrawal [Lamberink *et al.*, 2017]. These include the following: duration of the epileptic disease, seizure-free interval, number of antiepileptic drugs trialed, female sex, family history of epilepsy, number of seizures, focal seizures, and epileptiform abnormalities on EEG. All factors were positively correlated with seizure recurrence except seizure-free interval, which was negatively correlated with seizure recurrence. The review presented normograms and a scoring system that can assist clinicians in the difficult decision of withdrawing antiepileptic therapy.

4.1.2 *Epileptic and developmental encephalopathies*

In the International League Against Epilepsy's (ILAE) most recent position paper, a distinction was made among three types of encephalopathies: epileptic, developmental, and epileptic *and* developmental. Epileptic encephalopathy is a condition whereby epileptic activity leads to severe neurobehavioral consequences. Examples of an epileptic encephalopathy include West syndrome and Lennox-Gastaut syndrome. Developmental encephalopathy is defined as a condition with developmental impairment without the presence of epileptiform activity, as seen in patients with a number of gene mutations that may not be causing epilepsy. Developmental *and* epileptic encephalopathy consists of a combination of the previous two conditions whereby a genetic disorder leads to developmental delay which is complicated by frequent epileptiform activity contributing to developmental regression or plateau. An illustrative example of this type of encephalopathy is the developmental slowing or regression that occurs in Dravet syndrome one or two years before epileptiform activity is seen on EEG. This points to a separate developmental disorder secondary to SCN1A mutation, which also leads to epilepsy [Scheffer *et al.*, 2017].

The treatment of epileptic encephalopathies must be initiated quickly to avoid long term neurological sequelae and achieve improvement in cognition and behavior. Usually, the sooner therapy is commenced the better the long-term outcome. Immunotherapy with

ACTH or steroids is the treatment of first choice for many epileptic encephalopathies. The ketogenic diet is also often considered in cases of epileptic encephalopathy and is the treatment of first choice for glucose transporter I deficiency syndrome and pyruvate dehydrogenase deficiency [Wilmshurst *et al.*, 2015].

4.2 Neonatal-onset epilepsies

4.2.1 *Benign epilepsies*

Often the first therapy in neonatal seizures is to administer short-acting doses of benzodiazepines and monitor for seizure recurrence. Lorazepam is frequently used in this situation. Alternatives include diazepam and midazolam. If there is no recurrence, then there is often no need for long-term therapy. The most commonly used long acting first-line drug for neonatal seizures is phenobarbital, followed by phenytoin or fosphenytoin. Other AEDs usually given as alternatives or adjuvants include levetiracetam, topiramate, or lidocaine. IV lidocaine, as a rule, is not given with phenytoin or fosphenytoin due to the risk of precipitating arrhythmias and hypotension. Long-term therapy, if needed, usually does not include phenytoin which is poorly absorbed from the gastrointestinal tract in neonates. Phenobarbital, topiramate or levetiracetam are often used as monotherapy. With benign familial neonatal epilepsy (BFNE) there is complete seizure resolution with time in most cases, so long-term therapy is often not needed. Only one-third of patients have recurrence of seizures after a few months, but these are again easily controlled. There are reports of oral carbamazepine being effective in these cases [Mikati and Tchapyjnikov, 2018; Pellock *et al.*, 2016; Sands *et al.*, 2016].

4.2.2 *Ohtahara syndrome*

AEDs that have some efficacy include zonisamide, vigabatrin, high-dose phenobarbital, and levetiracetam. Some cases may respond to the ketogenic diet. Being an age-dependent epileptic encephalopathy, ACTH is advocated by some as a treatment in this disorder, albeit less effective than in West syndrome or Lennox-Gastaut syndrome. The danger in this syndrome is its potential progression to West syndrome. Interestingly, this progression alters the brain's response to AEDs, so it is worth retrying previous drugs especially if one or more has had favorable results. Fortunately, patients with the STXBP1 mutation have a better therapeutic response to the AEDs used and are less likely to progress to West syndrome. Functional hemispherectomy or focal resection surgeries may be of use in cases where focal dysplasia, rather than diffuse brain malformation or a gene mutation is the underlying etiology [Hani and Mikati, 2016; Pellock *et al.*, 2016].

4.2.3 *Early myoclonic encephalopathy*

This encephalopathy may be caused by various metabolic disorders and thus these must be investigated diagnosed and, accordingly, treated. Examples include using ketogenic diet to treat non-ketotic hyperglycinemia and pyridoxine or pyridoxal phosphate to treat pyridoxine dependency or pyridoxal 5′-phosphate dependency, respectively. The treatment strategy and course are similar to those employed in Ohtahara syndrome (see above). It is important to use drugs prudently, such as valproic acid or vigabatrin, while avoiding those that may interfere with some of the aforementioned metabolic disorders. For example, there is a report of two patients with nonketotic hyperglycinemia who developed acute encephalopathy on vigabatrin. In these two patients it was postulated that vigabatrin inhibited GABA transaminase in the brain, elevated GABA levels and thus enhanced that encephalopathy [Tekgul *et al.*, 2006].

4.3 Infantile-onset epilepsies

4.3.1 *Benign epilepsies*

Phenobarbital and levetiracetam are often used as first-line, but carbamazepine, zonisamide and other medications are also effective. It is difficult to assess the efficacy of these AEDs as seizures often remit spontaneously. Although benign in nature, these seizures may be treated early as they occur in clusters, making it difficult to assess their gravity.

4.3.2 *Benign myoclonic epilepsy of infancy*

The myoclonic jerks can easily be controlled with valproic acid (after underlying metabolic problems that may predispose to hepatotoxicity have been ruled out) or with clonazepam. If there is initial resistance to valproate or to clonazepam, higher doses may be attempted (30–40 mg/kg). If the patient is still not responding, phenobarbital, topiramate, zonisamide or clobazam may be tried. This syndrome is generally easy to control with medication. Even those not treated with medication may experience spontaneous remission; thus, the need for treatment may be discussed with the family.

4.3.3 *West syndrome*

ACTH (or corticosteroids) is the usual drug of first choice, except in tuberous sclerosis, where vigabatrin is preferred. These remain the only two FDA-approved treatments for West syndrome, although there are more than 30 reported treatments and many physicians use oral steroids as their drug of first choice due to cost and convenience issues and efficacy similar to that of ACTH. The usual dose of ACTH is 150 units/m^2 IM divided into a twice daily dose for 2 weeks, followed by 30 units/m^2 for 3 days, then 15 units/m^2 for 3 days, then 10 units/m^2 for 3 days, then 10 units/m^2 every other day for 6 days, and then the medication is stopped. Steroids are often effective in the short-term control of spasms, although the optimal dosage and duration of therapy remain controversial. One protocol consists of the following: prednisolone at a dose of 40 mg/day given as 13.3 mg three times daily for two weeks, then 15 mg twice daily for 5 days, then 10 mg twice daily for 5 days, then 5 mg every other day for 5 days, then stop the prednisolone. If there was found to be no response to the initial 13.3 mg three times daily dose, one may increase to 20 mg three times daily for 2 weeks then reduce back to 13.3 mg three times daily for 2 weeks, then continue the protocol as described above [Lux *et al.*, 2005]. ACTH may result in better long-term outcomes than oral steroids in cryptogenic cases of West syndrome but this is controversial. ACTH and steroids may result in better long-term outcomes than vigabatrin except in patients with tuberous sclerosis. Sulthiame is used in some European countries and may be efficacious. Carbamazepine and oxcarbazepine may worsen the spasms and are generally avoided. Other therapies that have shown promise include topiramate at a dose >6 mg/kg/day, zonisamide at a dose of 10–12 mg/kg/day, lamotrigine, felbamate, IVIG and the ketogenic diet. Moreover, it is possible to have an underlying metabolic condition, such as pyridoxine dependency or pyridoxal-5-phosphate dependency, which can be corrected. Glucose transporter deficiency also responds well to the ketogenic diet. Focal cortical resection and hemispherectomy may be considered in patients with focal cortical lesions who have not responded to medical therapy [Hancock *et al.*, 2002; Hani and Mikati, 2016; Pellock *et al.*, 2016; Wilmshurst *et al.*, 2015]. Figure 4.2 summarizes the proposed mechanism of action of ACTH.

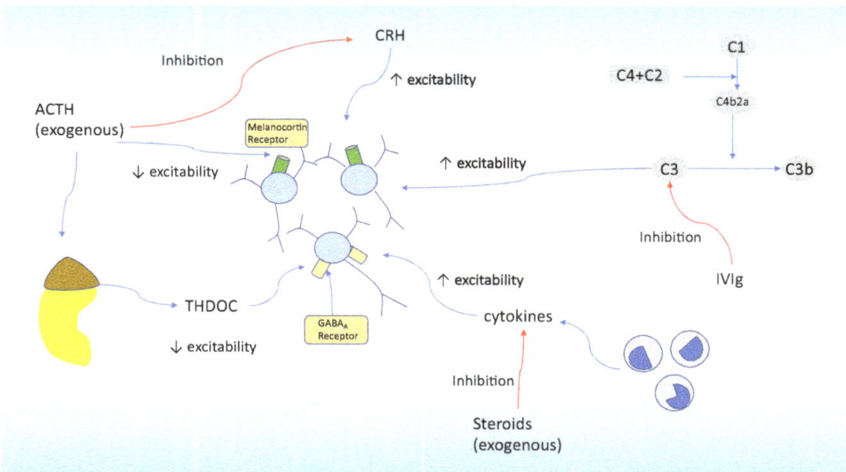

Figure 4.2. Proposed antiepileptic mechanisms of action of ACTH, corticosteroids & IVIG. C3 has been associated with epileptogenesis in a mouse model of temporal lobe epilepsy. Corticosteroids also decrease the synthesis of voltage-dependent calcium channels through transcription regulation. Immunomodulation is another mechanism of action not shown here (Verhelst *et al.*, 2005; Chen *et al.*, 2017). Abbreviations: THDOC: Tetrahydrodeoxy-corticosterone; IVIg: Intravenous Immunoglobulin.

It is important to re-emphasize that cessation of spasms and EEG improvement must be achieved as soon as possible to avoid or attenuate long-term sequelae of this illness and improve neurobehavioral outcomes. Thus, awake and asleep EEGs are often obtained 1, 2 and 4 weeks from the initiation of therapy to monitor drug response. If no response is seen, the drug must be tapered off and another one tried. If relapse occurs, it is preferable to restart the drug that showed the most favorable response, often with the option of a longer course of therapy.

4.3.4 *Dravet syndrome*

Valproate is usually prescribed for the first long-lasting seizure, and is considered to be first-line. GABAergic drugs are efficacious in this syndrome, including clonazepam, clobazam, valproate and stiripentol. Stiripentol and cannabidiol where available may be added onto the combination of valproate and benzodiazepines for refractory cases. Topiramate is used for convulsive or focal seizures. Levetiracetam, zonisamide, bromide, ethosuximide and the ketogenic diet may also be useful. Carbamazepine and lamotrigine should be avoided as they can aggravate convulsive or myoclonic seizures. Phenytoin and vigabatrin may also worsen myoclonic jerks. Fenfluramine is an orphan drug being assessed for its efficacy and safety. It is a serotonin agonist and serotonin reuptake inhibitor, thought to modulate NMDA receptor-mediated excitation. Vagus nerve stimulation reduces seizure frequency in this syndrome [Hani and Mikati, 2016; Pellock *et al.*, 2016; Wallace *et al.*, 2016].

The management of the comorbities associated with this syndrome is worth mentioning. Methylphenidate is at times prescribed for hyperactivity and impulsive behavior, and sleep disorders induced partially by nocturnal seizures may be treated with melatonin. However, one must be aware of the risk of cardiac arrhythmias and monitor that risk in Dravet syndrome particularly if such drugs are used. Orthopedic follow-up is necessary to screen for and treat associated kyphoscoliosis and foot deformities.

4.3.5 *Migrating focal seizures of infancy*

These seizures are difficult to control. If the seizures come under control within the first year, walking may be possible. Several treatments show variable efficacy, including clonazepam, stiripentol, bromide, levetiracetam, rufinamide, acetazolamide, vagus nerve stimulation and the ketogenic diet. Some patients with a mutation of the potassium channel gene *KCNT-1* have been reported to respond to quinidine. However, currently the data are not definitive for such efficacy [Abdelnour *et al.*, 2018].

4.4 Childhood-onset epilepsies

4.4.1 *Monogenic familial epilepsies*

Carbamazepine has been thought to be the most effective AED in autosomal dominant nocturnal frontal lobe epilepsy, with complete suppression of seizure activity in 70% of patients. The doses used are usually low (600 mg/day). Patients with CHRNA4 pathogenic variant p.Ser284Leu have been reported to respond to zonisamide. Those with a KCNT1 gain-of-function mutation have not benefited from quinidine therapy. There are case reports of acetazolamide and nicotine patches showing benefit when added to carbamazepine [Pellock *et al.*, 2016; Varadkar *et al.*, 2003; Willoughby *et al.*, 2003].

The optimal treatment of genetic epilepsy with febrile seizures plus is still vague. Rectal diazepam is prescribed as needed for those at risk for prolonged or recurrent febrile seizures. There are no guidelines for prophylactic therapy based on the pathophysiology of the disease, but most patients are treated with levetiracetam, valproate, topiramate or zonisamide.

Autosomal dominant epilepsy with auditory features (previously called familial lateral temporal lobe epilepsy) may be treated with any AED used for focal seizures. Drug resistance is rare. There is a case report from Japan about successful treatment of members of a family with focal resection and multiple subpial transection [Koizumi *et al.*, 2011; Pellock *et al.*, 2016].

4.4.2 *Multi-genic and other localized epilepsies*

Benign Rolandic Epilepsy (BRE) is often not treated as this is usually a benign, self-limited condition. The selection of AED for those who choose to treat varies widely among countries; sulthiame, carbamazepine and lamotrigine are preferred in Europe while levetiracetam is preferred in the United States. Oxcarbazepine is also often used. A survey done in the UK showed that carbamazepine was the drug of choice followed by valproic acid. For those found to develop electrical status during slow-wave sleep (ESES), the clinician must determine if a clinical deterioration occurred and should exclude exacerbation by ongoing therapy with sodium channel drugs. The treatment of ESES is not universally agreed upon, but the first step usually is to remove a medication that may be contributing to the generation of the ESES. Drugs like carbamazepine or oxcarbazepine are often the culprits. Nocturnal diazepam, continuous steroid therapy and intravenous gamma globulins (IVIG) are options, probably in that order. Ethosuximide, clobazam or valproate are other options. Often in BRE, medications are tapered after 2 years of seizure freedom even if the EEG has remained abnormal as the risk of recurrence is low in such cases irrespective of the EEG [Mellish *et al.*, 2015; Pellock *et al.*, 2016].

Occipital epilepsy of Gastaut is treated with valproic acid, carbamazepine, levetiracetam or oxcarbazepine. Panayiotopolous syndrome is a benign, self-limited disease; therefore, prophylactic antiepileptic therapy is often reserved for seizures that are impairing quality of life. Valproic acid and carbamazepine are likely equal in efficacy in treatment of Panayiotopolous syndrome. Lamotrigine may also be efficacious [Pellock *et al.*, 2016; Verrotti *et al.*, 2016].

4.4.3 *Multi-genic and other generalized epilepsies*

The primary drugs for the treatment of absence seizures are ethosuximide, valproic acid and lamotrigine. Ethosuximide is the preferred option as it is better tolerated than valproic acid and more effective than lamotrigine. Even though ethosuximide is equally effective to valproic acid in the control of the acute absence seizures, its use is associated with better chances for long term remissions. Valproic acid is the drug of choice for absence seizures combined with generalized tonic-clonic seizures since ethosuximide is not effective against such seizures. If the patient is refractory to monotherapy, a combination of ethosuximide and valproic acid is often tried. Other drugs that are usually not effective include gabapentin, carbamazepine, oxcarbazepine, phenobarbital, phenytoin, tiagabine and vigabatrin. Many of these medications can exacerbate absence seizures. The combination of valproic acid and clonazepam should also usually be avoided as it may precipitate absence status. Absence status is treated with IV benzodiazepines, IV valproic acid, or acetazolamide. Medication tapering should not be done before an EEG is obtained as even one-second generalized spike-wave (GSW) discharges may result in functional impairment by reducing reaction time during the discharges. Moreover, GSW discharges with hyperventilation indicate a high possibility of seizure recurrence and the clinician may often consider continuing medication. Finally, it is important to counsel the patient and family on injury prevention, including the use of bicycle helmets and refraining from unsupervised or inadequately supervised swimming.

As for the treatment of epilepsy with myoclonic absences, valproic acid alone or in combination with ethosuximide is preferred. Lamotrigine, levetiracetam, zonisamide or topiramate may be added to this combination. Alternatively, the combination of valproic acid and a benzodiazepine may be attempted. Rufinamide has been used as monotherapy. Phenytoin, vigabatrin and carbamazepine should be avoided as they may aggravate these seizures.

Valproic acid is the drug of choice for myoclonic-astatic epilepsy, as it is effective against the different seizure types in this syndrome. Although lamotrigine may be combined with valproic acid to give a synergistic effect, this combination has the potential to aggravate myoclonus and thus should be used with caution. It also increases the risk for potentially serious rashes due to lamotrigine. Ethosuximide may be beneficial in treating the myoclonic drop attacks in addition to absences. Steroids may be used if the patient experiences multiple astatic attacks and/or frequent non-convulsive status epilepticus. Other treatments that may be effective include ketogenic diet, zonisamide, IVIG, topiramate and levetiracetam. There is one report from Japan of a 7-year-old girl with myoclonic-astatic epilepsy refractory to treatment who improved with continuous infusion of IV lidocaine, which eventually was followed by remission and normalization of EEG abnormalities [Kanemura *et al.*, 1996]. The following drugs are known to potentially aggravate myoclonus: carbamazepine, vigabatrin, phenytoin, oxcarbazepine, tiagabine, gabapentin and pregabalin. There is a case report of a 3-year-old boy who developed myoclonic status epilepticus with levetiracetam given as monotherapy, although causality could not be proven [Kroll-Seger *et al.*, 2006]. However, there are also reports of levetiracetam aggravating other types of myoclonus, such as juvenile myoclonic epilepsy [Liu *et al.*, 2012]. Thus, levetiracetam may need to be used with caution.

4.4.4 *Lennox-Gastaut syndrome*

When the diagnosis of Lennox-Gastaut is made, the patient is usually already on multiple AEDs. Therefore, the strategy is to keep the AEDs that are benefitting the patient and remove those that are not or that have no evidence of efficacy. Seizures are rarely controlled with monotherapy.

This syndrome used to be treated with valproic acid as a first-line agent, topiramate as second-line and lamotrigine as third-line. However, clobazam is being used more often and earlier due to its potential better effectiveness than the other medications. Additionally, cannabidiol has recently been approved for therapy of seizures in Dravet syndrome and Lennox-Gastaut syndrome. Other drugs include rufinamide, felbamate and clonazepam. Existing randomized clinical trials (RCTs) have found that six drugs are efficacious in this syndrome: cannabidiol, clobazam, lamotrigine, topiramate, rufinamide and felbamate. These six drugs may be used as monotherapy or polytherapy. A good strategy is to start with a drug that has demonstrated efficacy in a given patient and has a favorable side effect profile for that patient, and then add other AEDs as necessary. Felbamate is not used regularly due to potentially dangerous idiosyncratic reactions such as aplastic anemia and hepatotoxicity. Also, carbamazepine may worsen drop attacks.

If medical management fails, vagus nerve stimulation and ketogenic diet are often helpful. Electrical stimulation of the centromedian thalamic nuclei is currently experimental. A retrospective review that looked at 71 children with Lennox-Gastaut syndrome started on ketogenic diet between 1994 and 2012 showed efficacy, with 51% of patients having at least 50% reduction in seizures and 23% having more than 90% reduction [Lemmon *et al.*, 2012]. Oral or intravenous steroids may be beneficial. Surgical options include corpus callosotomy, which has been shown to reduce drop attacks but not other seizures. Therefore, it is considered palliative rather than curative.

4.4.5 *Landau-Kleffner syndrome and epileptic encephalopathy with Continuous Spikes and Waves during Sleep (CSWS)*

The treatment of these two syndromes is quite similar. Initial therapy involves high-dose nocturnal diazepam or a course of oral steroids. These treatments are given over several months to avoid relapses. Another approach is to use standard AEDs; however, these do not improve language outcome as much as steroids. AEDs used include valproic acid, clobazam, ethosuximide, lamotrigine, levetiracetam, lacosamide and acetazolamide. Carbamazepine use is controversial as it may exacerbate the electrical seizure activity. IVIG and the ketogenic diet can also be beneficial [Fainberg *et al.*, 2016; Mikati *et al.*, 2002, 2010]. For patients found to have a *GRIN2A* gain-of-function mutation, memantine has been advocated. This is discussed further in section 4.8. There is a case report of a patient with this mutation experiencing improved speech upon treatment with prednisone and IVIG. For more information on *GRIN2A*-specific treatment, see Section 4.8.

The decision to pursue surgical treatment must be made based on localization and imaging findings. For lesional cases, focal cortical resection or hemispherectomy may be options depending on the extent of the pathology. There have been reports of left temporal masses, including subpial gliosis, astrocytomas and neocortical dysplasia, resulting in clinically intractable left-sided seizures that respond to resection [Blum *et al.*, 2007; Cole *et al.*, 1988; Nass *et al.*, 1993; Solomon *et al.*, 1993]. There is a unique case report of a 7-year-old girl who had a right temporal ganglioma resulting in falsely localizing left temporal status epilepticus and a picture of Landau-Kleffner syndrome and autism. Resection led to complete resolution of her seizures and improvement of her autistic features [Mikati *et al.*, 2009]. For non-lesional cases, multiple subpial transection may be beneficial. In one study, nine patients with electrical status epilepticus (ESES) during sleep underwent corpus callosotomy [Peltoloa *et al.*, 2011]. Two patients experienced seizure reduction, six patients had improved neurocognitive outcome and three patients had improved EEG recordings. This study suggested that corpus callosotomy may be beneficial for ESES patients who are not candidates for focal resection or multiple subpial transection [Peltola *et al.*, 2011]. Vagus nerve stimulation is also an option.

4.5 Juvenile-onset epilepsies

4.5.1 *Generalized epilepsies*

While ethosuximide and valproic acid are effective in childhood absence epilepsy, their effect in juvenile absence epilepsy is not well studied. If seizures prove to be intractable on these AEDs, zonisamide, topiramate or levetiracetam may be added. Zonisamide may be preferable because it acts by the same mechanism as ethosuximide, leading to inactivation of T-type calcium channels, and is therefore effective in this type of epilepsy. Carbamazepine, oxcarbazepine and phenytoin should be avoided as they may worsen the absence seizures.

According to the Standard and New Antiepileptic Drugs (SANAD) trial, valproic acid was shown to be superior to lamotrigine and topiramate in the treatment of juvenile myoclonic epilepsy and juvenile epilepsy with generalized tonic-clonic seizures only. However, lamotrigine is still efficacious and may be used in those who cannot take valproic acid and/or topiramate such as pregnant women or women with child bearing potential. Lamotrigine must be administered with caution as it may aggravate myoclonic jerks. Carbamazepine, oxcarbazepine and phenytoin have the same adverse potential. In refractory cases, levetiracetam can also be used [Marson *et al.*, 2007; Pellock *et al.*, 2016].

4.5.2 *Focal epilepsies*

Focal epilepsies in this age group are usually symptomatic and are usually treated with medications effective against focal seizures in general.

4.6 Variable-onset epilepsies

4.6.1 *Mesial temporal lobe epilepsy*

The treatment of mesial temporal sclerosis should begin with a trial of AEDs for focal epilepsies as detailed in Section 4.1.1. If medical management fails, which is often the case, then surgical resection is considered. Minimally invasive or alternative surgical techniques are currently options in addition to standard temporal lobectomy. These alternative procedures include selective amygdalohippocampectomy, gamma knife stereotactic radiosurgery and stereotactic laser thermoablation. Selective amygdalohippocampectomy involves a transsylvian or transcortical approach to temporal lobe structures thus avoiding an open approach. Stereotactic radiosurgery utilizes radioactive cobalt to deliver radiation to specific region of the brain. Stereotactic laser thermo-ablation uses thermal energy to induce cell death and is performed under MRI guidance. These procedures may offer less risk for neurocognitive side effects but also have generally less chance for seizure freedom than classical medial temporal lobectomy. For patients who are not surgical candidates, there are also minimally-invasive nonresective palliative procedures that can be employed, including vagus nerve stimulation, deep brain stimulation and responsive neurostimulation. The latter is a closed-loop stimulation system that analyzes regional electrocorticographic signals and delivers a current to terminate early seizure activity [Chang *et al.*, 2015; Waseem *et al.*, 2017].

4.6.2 *Progressive myoclonic epilepsies*

This is a group of difficult-to-manage epilepsies that have not been studied using RCTs due to the scarcity of patients. For myoclonus and seizures, valproic acid, benzodiazepines, zonisamide, levetiracetam, barbiturates, piracetam, are used. Ketognic diet and VNS may provide some benefit [Hajnsek *et al.*, 2013; Mikati and Tabbara, 2017; Smith *et al.*, 2000]. Metabolic disorders that may contraindicate the use of valproic acid should be ruled out before starting it. Adult patients may experience symptomatic relief with alcohol consumption and must be counseled to use alcohol moderately. Myoclonic epilepsy with ragged-red fibers (MERRF) patients benefit from coenzyme Q, L-tryptophan and N-acetylcysteine. In MERRF patients with stroke-like episodes, nitric oxide (NO)-precursors such as L-arginine and L-citrulline may be beneficial. Carbamazepine, vigabatrin, lamotrigine and gabapentin should be avoided in progressive myoclonic epilepsies as they have the potential to aggravate myoclonus. Moreover, precaution should be taken in treating specific diseases within this spectrum. AEDs that are mitochondrion-toxic include valproic acid, carbamazepine and phenytoin, and should not be given to MERRF patients. Phenytoin must be avoided in Unverricht-Lundborg disease. Gene therapy and augmentation of mitochondrial function are being studied. Intravenously administered enzyme therapy has been approved for the therapy of the CLN2 form of Batten disease [Finsterer and Zarrouk-Mahjoub, 2017; Pellock *et al.*, 2016; Shahwan *et al.*, 2005].

4.7 Autoimmune epilepsies

4.7.1 *Anti-NMDA encephalitis*

As discussed above, immunotherapy with IVIG and steroids may benefit some patients with epileptic encephalopathy. Immunotherapy is also used for the treatment of autoimmune epileptic encephalopathy or encephalitis.

The first step in a patient diagnosed with anti-NMDA receptor encephalitis is to search for an underlying teratoma, most commonly ovarian, as removal of such neoplasms may result in remission of the disease. First-line drug therapy is pulse intravenous methylprednisolone (30 mg/kg per day) for 3–5 days followed by IVIG (2 g/kg). If this does not work, rituximab or cyclophosphamide should be tried [Hallowell *et al.*, 2017; Pellock *et al.*, 2016].

4.7.2 *Other autoimmune encephalitidis*

Limbic encephalitis may be caused by anti-voltage gated potassium channel (VGKC) antibodies or other antibodies in children as well as in adults. Several types of immunotherapy have been used for this disease, including steroids with IVIG, IVIG alone, plasma exchange, 6-mercaptopurine, cyclophosphamide and mycophenolate mofetil [Dhamija *et al.*, 2011].

4.7.3 *Rasmussen encephalitis*

The only definitive treatment for Rasmussen's encephalitis thus far is either structural or functional hemispherectomy. 65–81% of patients remain seizure-free after this procedure. When the dominant hemisphere is involved, the decision on when to operate is difficult and warrants detailed discussion with the family. Homonymous hemianopsia and hemiplegia are inevitable consequences. Walking can be expected but fine motor control is usually impaired [Pellock *et al.*, 2016; Varadkar *et al.*, 2014].

Medical management is not very effective and a realistic goal should be to prevent severe seizures, namely bilateral convulsive seizures. Steroids, IVIG and plasmapheresis have demonstrated short-term but no long-term effect. Rituximab has shown promise as possible therapy. Tacrolimus has been shown to slow cerebral atrophy and neurological decline but does not change seizure frequency. Azathioprine has been reported to show positive results. Protein A immunoadsorption, a process by which protein A, a staphylococcal bacterial cell wall component, is used as an extracorporeal immunoadsorbent to remove IgG and immune complexes, has also shown favorable results. These therapies are often used to buy time before the diagnosis is confirmed clinically and or by brain biopsy particularly in children older than 5 years with a dominant hemisphere involvement [Pellock *et al.*, 2016; Varadkar *et al.*, 2014].

4.7.4 *Acute Disseminated Encephalomyelopathy (ADEM)*

ADEM is most often treated with steroids. The most widely used regimen is IV methylprednisolone 10–30 mg/kg/day for 5 days followed by an oral steroid taper over 4–6 weeks. IVIG can be used as second-line therapy for non-responders. For patients with fulminant, refractory disease, options include plasmapheresis, hypothermia and decompressive craniotomy [Pohl *et al.*, 2016].

4.8 Precision/personalized therapy

There has been an evolution in the use of the terms "precision medicine" and "personalized medicine"; indeed, these two terms are now used interchangeably with the preferred term being precision medicine. The use of the term "personalized medicine" started after the completion of the Human Genome Project, when scientists recognized the potential advantages of customizing medical treatment to an individual patient's genome. The trend is shifting towards the use of the term "precision medicine", which specifically means designing therapies based on the underlying molecular basis of disease, which may be shared by more than one person [Katsnelson, 2013].

mTOR inhibitors such as everolimus have been used to treat manifestations of tuberous sclerosis such as subependymal giant cell astrocytomas. Everolimus has recently been approved as a therapy of focal seizures in these patients as well. A phase III clinical trial named EXIST-3 (Examining Everolimus In a Study of Tuberous sclerosis) has recently been completed and found 29.3% reduction in seizures with 3–7 ng/ml of everolimus and 39.6% reduction with 9–15 ng/ml of everolimus. Moreover, this therapy may prove to be beneficial in cases of focal cortical dysplasia due to other genes related to the mTOR pathway, such as *DEPDC5*, *NPRL2*, and *NPRL3* [Delanty and Cavallleri, 2017; French *et al.*, 2016].

Patients with a *GRIN2A* mutation manifesting as Landau-Kleffner syndrome may benefit from treatment with the NMDA receptor antagonist, memantine. *GRIN2A* codes for one of the three subunits of the NMDA receptor (GluN1–3). In addition, a child with Ohtahara syndrome and a p.L812M mutation in the *GRIN2A* gene experienced reduced seizure frequency and improvement in interictal EEG upon treatment with memantine, while another patient with Ohtahara syndrome and a p.N615K mutation did not. Electrophysiological studies showed that the former mutation decreases the half-maximal effective concentration (EC_{50}) of glutamate and glycine but the latter mutation did not [Maljevic *et al.*, 2017; Pierson *et al.*, 2014].

Migrating focal seizures of infancy are often caused by a mutation in the *KCNT1* gene coding for a sodium-activated potassium channel and may be treated with quinidine, a potassium channel blocker. This therapy has also been tried in a patient with West syndrome and *KCNT1* mutation and was found to be beneficial. However, the beneficial effect of this therapy is not universal nor definitive given the open label nature of prior reports and the probability of bias to report positive results [Abdelnour *et al.*, 2018]. Quinidine can also prolong the QT interval and thus may predispose to cardiac arrhythmias. Therefore, any trial of such therapy must be given with caution and in coordination with a pediatric cardiologist [Chong *et al.*, 2016; Delanty and Cavallleri, 2017; Fukuoka *et al.*, 2017; Mikati *et al.*, 2015]. Bromides have also been reported to help control seizures in this syndrome.

Ezogabine (retigabine) is a medication that was used effectively for neonatal epileptic encephalopathies caused by *KCNQ2* mutations. *KCNQ2* and *KCNQ3* code for voltage-gated potassium channels and ezogabine was found to open these channels. However, this drug has been removed from the market due to adverse events, most importantly retinopathy [Brodie *et al.*, 2010; French *et al.*, 2011; Maljevic *et al.*, 2017; Tompson *et al.*, 2016].

GLUT1 deficiency syndrome is treated by placing the patient on a ketogenic diet. This diet focuses heavily on fats instead of carbohydrates, leading to the formation of ketone bodies as the primary source of energy for the brain, which is independent of the deficient GLUT1 glucose transporter in this syndrome [Maljevic *et al.*, 2017].

In some cases, knowledge of the causative mutation of a patient's epileptic syndrome leads to a more targeted use of classic AEDs. *PCDH19* gene mutations may be a cause of Dravet-like syndromes, epilepsy and mental retardation limited to females. A retrospective study found that in these patients, the most effective medications were clobazam and bromide. The presence of an *SCN1A* mutation in Dravet syndrome may make seizure control more sensitive to GABAergic drugs and fenfluramine. Animal studies on *SCN1A* mutations have found abnormalities in GABAergic cortical neurons. Sodium channel blocking agents such as lamotrigine should be avoided with this mutation, as it is a loss-of-function mutation of a sodium channel. A gain-of-function mutation in *SCN8A* causes the opposite phenomenon, as patients with these mutations are sensitive to treatment with phenytoin. Early Infantile Epileptic Encephalopathy due to an *SCN2A* mutation is another disorder responsive to sodium blocking agents such as phenytoin. If status develops in this disorder, lidocaine and acetazolamide are efficacious. Infantile epilepsy caused by Proline-rich transmembrane protein 2 (*PRRT2*) mutation responds to carbamazepine and oxcarbazepine. Malignant migrating partial seizures in infancy caused by 1-phosphatidylinositol-4,5-bisphosphate phosphodiesterase beta-1 (*PLCB1*) mutation responds to inositol. Finally, valproate must be avoided in polymerase gamma (*POLG*)-related disease because the risk of valproate-induced hepatotoxicity is increased in this disorder [Boerma *et al.*, 2016; Lotte *et al.*, 2016; Martin *et al.*, 2010; Menzler *et al.*, 2014; Oakley *et al.*, 2013; Poduri, 2017].

Pharmacogenomics falls under the umbrella term of precision/personalized therapy. Polymorphisms in the cytochrome P450 (CYP) enzymes of patients can potentially be used to guide the choice and dosing of AEDs. For example, defective CYP2C19 allelic variants lead to decreased phenobarbital clearance and higher serum concentration.

Other allelic variants that may affect the level of AEDs include CYP2D6, CYP2C9, and CYP3A4. The clinician must take a thorough medication history, as several medications act as stimulants or repressors of these enzymes. The P-glycoprotein pump can also be induced by medication, leading to an efflux of AEDs from cells. Calcium channel blockers are known to be P-glycoprotein pump inhibitors, and several studies have looked at the utility of verapamil and nimodipine as adjunct therapy for medically refractory epilepsy. In one open-label study with low-dose verapamil, 53% (10/19) of patients had a >50% reduction in seizure frequency. In another study, verapamil was given as adjunct therapy for refractory temporal lobe epilepsy and resulted in 36.84% of patients achieving >50% reduction in seizure frequency. Finally, a prospective randomized control trial of nimodipine as add-on therapy in focal refractory epilepsy resulted in 61.5% of patients achieving >50% reduction in seizure frequency [Asadi-Pooya *et al.*, 2013; Machado *et al.*, 2013; Narayanan *et al.*, 2016].

One important association is the HLA-B*15:02 allele found in Southeast Asian individuals with severe carbamazepine-induced adverse drug reactions, including the Steven Johnson Syndrome / Toxic Epidermal Necrolysis (SJS/TEN) spectrum. In fact, this allele is now being used as a biomarker by some authorities. A more globally found allele, HLA-A*31:01, was also found to be associated with carbamazepine-induced hypersensitivity reactions in Northern European subjects, albeit less severe than the reactions seen in HLA-B*15:02 individuals. Chinese studies have reported oxcarbazepine-induced SJS/TEN in HLA-B*15:02 patients, but no such reports exist for HLA-A*31:01 patients. These examples underscore the potential utility of using individual genomic differences as biomarkers when selecting AED therapy [de Leon, 2015; Kaniwa and Saito, 2013; Lopez-Garcia *et al.*, 2017; Striano *et al.*, 2016].

4.9 Future directions

The future of therapy for epilepsy is aiming towards controlling the level of expression of disease-causing mutations by delivering or stimulating the expression of an under-expressed gene or by silencing an over-expressed one. Antisense oligonucleotides (antagomirs) and small interfering RNA (siRNA) can be transfected into cells via a viral vector and bind to existing RNA in the cell to alter gene expression. For gain-of-function mutations, these antagomirs bind to mRNA and prevent its translation. For loss-of-function mutations, antisense RNA transcripts were found to occur naturally in cells and can be blocked to increase gene expression. This approach has been successful in treating Dravet syndrome caused by *SCN1A* loss-of-function mutation in animal models. The antagomir of miR-134 microRNA has the potential to be used in the treatment of intractable temporal lobe epilepsy as injection of this antagomir reduced kainic acid-induced seizure activity in mice. AAV-mediated gene therapy has been used in animal models of Rett syndrome, late-onset neuronal ceroid lipofuscinosis, Canavan disease and other neurogenetic disorders. Gene editing techniques may be used in the future treatment of epilepsy, among which the CRISPR/Cas9 system shows the most promise. This is a system composed of a nuclease, Cas9, able to cut double-stranded DNA and a guide RNA which targets a specific genomic segment. So far, this system has been used to introduce mutations in induced pluripotential stem cells (iPSCs) to better study and understand genetic diseases such as Dravet syndrome (introduction of the *SCN1A* mutation). There is hope that CRISPR/Cas9 may be used to correct genetic defects in both somatic and germline cells [Hsiao *et al.*, 2016; Jimenez-Mateos *et al.*, 2012; Wykes and Lignani, 2017].

References

Abdelnour, E., Gallentine, W., McDonald, M., Sachdev, M., Jiang, Y.H., and Mikati, M.A. (2018). Does age affect response to quinidine in patients with KCNT1 mutations? Report of three new cases and review of the literature, *Seizure*, 55, 1–3.

Asadi-Pooya, A.A., Razavizadegan, S.M., Abdi-Ardekani, A., and Sperling, M.R. (2013). Adjunctive use of verapamil in patients with refractory temporal lobe epilepsy: a pilot study, *Epilepsy Behav.*, 29, 150–154.

Bertram, J.H., Snyder, H.W., Jr., Gill, P.S., Shulman, I., Henry, D.H., Jenkins, D., and Kiprov, D.D. (1988). Protein A immunoadsorption therapy in HIV-related immune thrombocytopenia: a preliminary report, *Artif. Organs*, 12, 484–490.

Blum, A., Tremont, G., Donahue, J., Tung, G., Duncan, J., Buchbinder, B., and Gascon, G. (2007). Landau-Kleffner syndrome with lateral temporal focal cortical dysplasia and mesial temporal sclerosis: a 30-year follow-up, *Epilepsy Behav.*, 10, 495–503.

Boerma, R.S., Braun, K.P., van den Broek, M.P., van Berkestijn, F.M., Swinkels, M.E., Hagebeuk, E.O., Lindhout, D., van Kempen, M., Boon, M., Nicolai, J., *et al.* (2016). Erratum to: Remarkable Phenytoin Sensitivity in 4 Children with SCN8A-related Epilepsy: A Molecular Neuropharmacological Approach, *Neurotherapeutics*, 13, 238.

Brodie, M.J., Lerche, H., Gil-Nagel, A., Elger, C., Hall, S., Shin, P., Nohria, V., Mansbach, H., and Group, R.S. (2010). Efficacy and safety of adjunctive ezogabine (retigabine) in refractory partial epilepsy, *Neurology*, 75, 1817–1824.

Chang, E.F., Englot, D.J., and Vadera, S. (2015). Minimally invasive surgical approaches for temporal lobe epilepsy, *Epilepsy Behav.*, 47, 24–33.

Chen M, Arumugam TV, Leanage G, *et al.* (2017). Disease-modifying effect of intravenous immunoglobulin in an experimental model of epilepsy. *Sci Rep.*, 7, 40528.

Chong, P.F., Nakamura, R., Saitsu, H., Matsumoto, N., and Kira, R. (2016). Ineffective quinidine therapy in early onset epileptic encephalopathy with KCNT1 mutation, *Ann. Neurol.*, 79, 502–503.

Cole, A.J., Andermann, F., Taylor, L., Olivier, A., Rasmussen, T., Robitaille, Y., and Spire, J.P. (1988). The Landau-Kleffner syndrome of acquired epileptic aphasia: unusual clinical outcome, surgical experience, and absence of encephalitis, *Neurology*, 38, 31–38.

de Leon, J. (2015). The effects of antiepileptic inducers in neuropsychopharmacology, a neglected issue. Part II: Pharmacological issues and further understanding, *Rev. Psiquiatr. Salud. Ment.*, 8, 167–188.

Delanty, N. and Cavallleri, G. (2017). Genomics-guided precise anti-epileptic drug development, *Neurochem. Res.*, 42, 2084–2088.

Dhamija, R., Renaud, D.L., Pittock, S.J., McKeon, A., Lachance, D.H., Nickels, K.C., Wirrell, E.C., Kuntz, N.L., King, M.D., and Lennon, V.A. (2011). Neuronal voltage-gated potassium channel complex autoimmunity in children, *Pediatr. Neurol.*, 44, 275–281.

Fainberg, N., Harper, A., Tchapyjnikov, D., and Mikati, M.A. (2016). Response to immunotherapy in a patient with Landau-Kleffner syndrome and GRIN2A mutation, *Epileptic Disord.*, 18, 97–100.

Finsterer, J. and Zarrouk-Mahjoub, S. (2017). Management of epilepsy in MERRF syndrome, *Seizure*, 50, 166–170.

French, J.A., Abou-Khalil, B.W., Leroy, R.F., Yacubian, E.M., Shin, P., Hall, S., Mansbach, H., Nohria, V., and Investigators, R.S. (2011). Randomized, double-blind, placebo-controlled trial of ezogabine (retigabine) in partial epilepsy, *Neurology*, 76, 1555–1563.

French, J.A., Lawson, J.A., Yapici, Z., Ikeda, H., Polster, T., Nabbout, R., Curatolo, P., de Vries, P.J., Dlugos, D.J., Berkowitz, N., *et al.* (2016). Adjunctive everolimus therapy for treatment-resistant focal-onset seizures associated with tuberous sclerosis (EXIST-3): a phase 3, randomised, double-blind, placebo-controlled study, *Lancet*, 388, 2153–2163.

Fukuoka, M., Kuki, I., Kawawaki, H., Okazaki, S., Kim, K., Hattori, Y., Tsuji, H., Nukui, M., Inoue, T., Yoshida, Y., *et al.* (2017). Quinidine therapy for West syndrome with KCNTI mutation: A case report, *Brain Dev.*, 39, 80–83.

Hajnsek, S., Petelin Gadze, Z., Borovecki, F., Nankovic, S., Mrak, G., Gotovac, K., Sulentic, V., Kovacevic, I., and Bujan Kovac, A. (2013). Vagus nerve stimulation in Lafora body disease, *Epilepsy Behav. Case Rep.*, 1, 150–152.

Hallowell, S., Tebedge, E., Oates, M., and Hand, E. (2017). Rituximab for treatment of refractory anti-NMDA receptor encephalitis in a pediatric patient, *J. Pediatr. Pharmacol. Ther.*, 22, 118–123.

Hancock, E., Osborne, J.P., and Milner, P. (2002). Treatment of infantile spasms, *Cochrane Database Syst. Rev.*, CD001770.

Hani, A.J. and Mikati, M.A. (2016). Current and emerging therapies of severe epileptic encephalopathies, *Semin. Pediatr. Neurol.*, 23, 180–186.

Hsiao, J., Yuan, T.Y., Tsai, M.S., Lu, C.Y., Lin, Y.C., Lee, M.L., Lin, S.W., Chang, F.C., Liu Pimentel, H., Olive, C., *et al.* (2016). Upregulation of haploinsufficient gene expression in the brain by targeting a long noncoding RNA improves seizure phenotype in a model of Dravet syndrome, *EBioMedicine*, 9, 257–277.

Jimenez-Mateos, E.M., Engel, T., Merino-Serrais, P., McKiernan, R.C., Tanaka, K., Mouri, G., Sano, T., O'Tuathaigh, C., Waddington, J.L., Prenter, S., *et al.* (2012). Silencing microRNA-134 produces neuroprotective and prolonged seizure-suppressive effects, *Nat. Med.*, 18, 1087–1094.

Kanemura, H., Aihara, M., Sata, Y., Hatakeyama, K., Hinohara, Y., Kamiya, Y., Shimoda, C., and Nakazawa, S. (1996). [A successful treatment with a continuous intravenous lidocaine for a cluster of minor seizures in a patient with Doose syndrome], *No To Hattatsu*, 28, 325–331.

Kaniwa, N. and Saito, Y. (2013). The risk of cutaneous adverse reactions among patients with the HLA-A* 31:01 allele who are given carbamazepine, oxcarbazepine or eslicarbazepine: a perspective review, *Ther. Adv. Drug Saf.*, 4, 246–253.

Katsnelson, A. (2013). Momentum grows to make 'personalized' medicine more "precise", *Nat. Med.*, 19, 249.

Koizumi, S., Kawai, K., Asano, S., Ueki, K., Suzuki, I., and Saito, N. (2011). Familial lateral temporal lobe epilepsy confirmed with intracranial electroencephalography and successfully treated by surgery, *Neurol. Med. Chir.*, 51, 604–610.

Kroll-Seger, J., Mothersill, I.W., Novak, S., Salke-Kellermann, R.A., and Kramer, G. (2006). Levetiracetam-induced myoclonic status epilepticus in myoclonic-astatic epilepsy: a case report, *Epileptic Disord.*, 8, 213–218.

Lamberink, H.J., Otte, W.M., Geerts, A.T., Pavlovic, M., Ramos-Lizana, J., Marson, A.G., Overweg, J., Sauma, L., Specchio, L.M., Tennison, M., *et al.* (2017). Individualised prediction model of seizure recurrence and long-term outcomes after withdrawal of antiepileptic drugs in seizure-free patients: a systematic review and individual participant data meta-analysis, *Lancet Neurol.*, 16, 523–531.

Lemmon, M.E., Terao, N.N., Ng, Y.T., Reisig, W., Rubenstein, J.E., and Kossoff, E.H. (2012). Efficacy of the ketogenic diet in Lennox-Gastaut syndrome: a retrospective review of one institution's experience and summary of the literature, *Dev. Med. Child Neurol.*, 54, 464–468.

Liu, Y.H., Wang, X.L., Deng, Y.C., and Zhao, G. (2012). Levetiracetam-associated aggravation of myoclonic seizure in children, *Seizure*, 21, 807–809.

Lopez-Garcia, M.A., Feria-Romero, I.A., Serrano, H., Rayo-Mares, D., Fagiolino, P., Vazquez, M., Escamilla-Nunez, C., Grijalva, I., Escalante-Santiago, D., and Orozco-Suarez, S. (2017). Influence of genetic variants of CYP2D6, CYP2C9, CYP2C19 and CYP3A4 on antiepileptic drug metabolism in pediatric patients with refractory epilepsy, *Pharmacol. Rep.*, 69, 504–511.

Lotte, J., Bast, T., Borusiak, P., Coppola, A., Cross, J.H., Dimova, P., Fogarasi, A., Graness, I., Guerrini, R., Hjalgrim, H., *et al.* (2016). Effectiveness of antiepileptic therapy in patients with PCDH19 mutations, *Seizure*, 35, 106–110.

Lux, A.L., Edwards, S.W., Hancock, E., Johnson, A.L., Kennedy, C.R., Newton, R.W., O'Callaghan, F.J., Verity, C.M., Osborne, J.P., and United Kingdom Infantile Spasms, S. (2005). The United Kingdom Infantile Spasms Study (UKISS) comparing hormone treatment with vigabatrin on developmental and epilepsy outcomes to age 14 months: a multicentre randomised trial, *Lancet Neurol.*, 4, 712–717.

Machado RA, Romero EB, Astencio AMG, Santos AS, Cuartas VB, *et al.* (2013) Prospective randomized controlled trial of nimodipine as add-on therapy in the treatment of focal refractory epilepsy patients: a pilot study, *J. Neurol. Neurophysiol.*, 4:151.

Maljevic, S., Reid, C.A., and Petrou, S. (2017). Models for discovery of targeted therapy in genetic epileptic encephalopathies, *J. Neurochem.*, 143, 30–48.

Marson, A.G., Al-Kharusi, A.M., Alwaidh, M., Appleton, R., Baker, G.A., Chadwick, D.W., Cramp, C., Cockerell, O.C., Cooper, P.N., Doughty, J., *et al.* (2007). The SANAD study of effectiveness of valproate, lamotrigine, or topiramate for generalised and unclassifiable epilepsy: an unblinded randomised controlled trial, *Lancet*, 369, 1016–1026.

Martin, M.S., Dutt, K., Papale, L.A., Dube, C.M., Dutton, S.B., de Haan, G., Shankar, A., Tufik, S., Meisler, M.H., Baram, T.Z., *et al.* (2010). Altered function of the SCN1A voltage-gated sodium channel leads to gamma-aminobutyric acid-ergic (GABAergic) interneuron abnormalities, *J. Biol. Chem.*, 285, 9823–9834.

Mellish, L.C., Dunkley, C., Ferrie, C.D., and Pal, D.K. (2015). Antiepileptic drug treatment of rolandic epilepsy and Panayiotopoulos syndrome: clinical practice survey and clinical trial feasibility, *Arch. Dis. Child*, 100, 62–67.

Menzler, K., Hermsen, A., Balkenhol, K., Duddek, C., Bugiel, H., Bauer, S., Schorge, S., Reif, P.S., Klein, K.M., Haag, A., *et al.* (2014). A common SCN1A splice-site polymorphism modifies the effect of carbamazepine on cortical excitability — a pharmacogenetic transcranial magnetic stimulation study, *Epilepsia*, 55, 362–369.

Mikati, M. and Tchapyjnikov, D. (2018). Seizures in Childhood. In Nelson's Textbook of Pediatrics (Philadelphia, PA: Elsevier).

Mikati, M.A., El-Bitar, M.K., Najjar, M.W., Rbeiz, J.J., Barada, W.H., Najjar, V.F., Yaktin, U., and Tourjuman, O. (2009). A child with refractory complex partial seizures, right temporal ganglioglioma, contralateral continuous electrical status epilepticus, and a secondary Landau-Kleffner autistic syndrome, *Epilepsy Behav.*, 14, 411–417.

Mikati, M.A., Jiang, Y.H., Carboni, M., Shashi, V., Petrovski, S., Spillmann, R., Milligan, C.J., Li, M., Grefe, A., McConkie, A., *et al.* (2015). Quinidine in the treatment of KCNT1-positive epilepsies, *Ann. Neurol.*, 78, 995–999.

Mikati, M.A., Kurdi, R., El-Khoury, Z., Rahi, A., and Raad, W. (2010). Intravenous immunoglobulin therapy in intractable childhood epilepsy: open-label study and review of the literature, *Epilepsy Behav.*, 17, 90–94.

Mikati, M.A., Saab, R., Fayad, M.N., and Choueiri, R.N. (2002). Efficacy of intravenous immunoglobulin in Landau-Kleffner syndrome, *Pediatr Neurol.*, 26, 298–300.

Mikati, M.A. and Tabbara, F. (2017). Managing Lafora body disease with vagal nerve stimulation, *Epileptic Disord.*, 19, 82–86.

Narayanan, J., Frech, R., Walters, S., Patel, V., Frigerio, R., and Maraganore, D.M. (2016). Low dose verapamil as an adjunct therapy for medically refractory epilepsy — An open label pilot study, *Epilepsy Res.*, 126, 197–200.

Nass, R., Heier, L., and Walker, R. (1993). Landau-Kleffner syndrome: temporal lobe tumor resection results in good outcome, *Pediatr. Neurol.*, 9, 303–305.

Oakley, J.C., Cho, A.R., Cheah, C.S., Scheuer, T., and Catterall, W.A. (2013). Synergistic GABA-enhancing therapy against seizures in a mouse model of Dravet syndrome, *J. Pharmacol. Exp. Ther.*, 345, 215–224.

Pellock, J.M., Nordli, D.R., Sankar, R., and Wheless, J.W. (2016). Pellock's pediatric epilepsy: diagnosis and therapy, Fourth edition (New York, NY: Demos Medical Publishing).

Peltola, M.E., Liukkonen, E., Granstrom, M.L., Paetau, R., Kantola-Sorsa, E., Valanne, L., Falck, B., Blomstedt, G., and Gaily, E. (2011). The effect of surgery in encephalopathy with electrical status epilepticus during sleep, *Epilepsia*, 52, 602–609.

Pierson, T.M., Yuan, H., Marsh, E.D., Fuentes-Fajardo, K., Adams, D.R., Markello, T., Golas, G., Simeonov, D.R., Holloman, C., Tankovic, A., *et al.* (2014). GRIN2A mutation and early-onset epileptic encephalopathy: personalized therapy with memantine, Ann Clin Transl Neurol *1*, 190–198.

Poduri, A. (2017). When should genetic testing be performed in epilepsy patients?, *Epilepsy Curr.*, *17*, 16–22.

Pohl, D., Alper, G., Van Haren, K., Kornberg, A.J., Lucchinetti, C.F., Tenembaum, S., and Belman, A.L. (2016). Acute disseminated encephalomyelitis: Updates on an inflammatory CNS syndrome, *Neurology*, 87, S38–45.

Sands, T.T., Balestri, M., Bellini, G., Mulkey, S.B., Danhaive, O., Bakken, E.H., Taglialatela, M., Oldham, M.S., Vigevano, F., Holmes, G.L., *et al.*

(2016). Rapid and safe response to low-dose carbamazepine in neonatal epilepsy, *Epilepsia*, 57, 2019–2030.

Scheffer, I.E., Berkovic, S., Capovilla, G., Connolly, M.B., French, J., Guilhoto, L., Hirsch, E., Jain, S., Mathern, G.W., Moshe, S.L., *et al.* (2017). ILAE classification of the epilepsies: Position paper of the ILAE Commission for Classification and Terminology, *Epilepsia*, 58, 512–521.

Shahwan, A., Farrell, M., and Delanty, N. (2005). Progressive myoclonic epilepsies: a review of genetic and therapeutic aspects, *Lancet Neurol.*, 4, 239–248.

Smith, B., Shatz, R., Elisevich, K., Bespalova, I.N., and Burmeister, M. (2000). Effects of vagus nerve stimulation on progressive myoclonus epilepsy of Unverricht-Lundborg type, *Epilepsia*, 41, 1046–1048.

Solomon, G.E., Carson, D., Pavlakis, S., Fraser, R., and Labar, D. (1993). Intracranial EEG monitoring in Landau-Kleffner syndrome associated with left temporal lobe astrocytoma, *Epilepsia*, 34, 557–560.

Striano, P., Vari, M.S., Mazzocchetti, C., Verrotti, A., and Zara, F. (2016). Management of genetic epilepsies: From empirical treatment to precision medicine, *Pharmacol Res.*, 107, 426–429.

Tekgul, H., Serdaroglu, G., Karapinar, B., Polat, M., Yurtsever, S., Tosun, A., Coker, M., and Gokben, S. (2006). Vigabatrin caused rapidly progressive deterioration in two cases with early myoclonic encephalopathy associated with nonketotic hyperglycinemia, *J. Child. Neurol.*, 21, 82–84.

Tompson, D.J., Buraglio, M., Andrews, S.M., and Wheless, J.W. (2016). Adolescent Clinical Development of Ezogabine/Retigabine as Adjunctive Therapy for Partial-Onset Seizures: Pharmacokinetics and Tolerability, *J. Pediatr Pharmacol. Ther.*, 21, 404–412.

Varadkar, S., Bien, C.G., Kruse, C.A., Jensen, F.E., Bauer, J., Pardo, C.A., Vincent, A., Mathern, G.W., and Cross, J.H. (2014). Rasmussen's encephalitis: clinical features, pathobiology, and treatment advances, *Lancet Neurol.*, 13, 195–205.

Varadkar, S., Duncan, J.S., and Cross, J.H. (2003). Acetazolamide and autosomal dominant nocturnal frontal lobe epilepsy, *Epilepsia*, 44, 986–987.

Verhelst H, Boon P, Buyse G, *et al.* (2005). Steroids in intractable childhood epilepsy: clinical experience and review of the literature, *Seizure*, 14, 412–421.

Verrotti, A., Laino, D., Rinaldi, V.E., Suppiej, A., Giordano, L., Toldo, I., Margari, L., Parisi, P., Rizzo, R., Matricardi, S., *et al.* (2016). Clinical dissection of childhood occipital epilepsy of Gastaut and prognostic implication, *Eur. J. Neurol.*, 23, 241–246.

Wallace, A., Wirrell, E., and Kenney-Jung, D.L. (2016). Pharmacotherapy for Dravet syndrome, *Paediatr. Drugs*, 18, 197–208.

Waseem, H., Vivas, A.C., and Vale, F.L. (2017). MRI-guided laser interstitial thermal therapy for treatment of medically refractory non-lesional mesial temporal lobe epilepsy: outcomes, complications, and current limitations: A review, *J. Clin. Neurosci.*, 38, 1–7.

Willoughby, J., Pope, K., and Eaton, V. (2003). Nicotine as an antiepileptic agent in ADNFLE: an N-of-one study, *Epilepsia*, 44, 1238–1240.

Wilmshurst, J.M., Gaillard, W.D., Vinayan, K.P., Tsuchida, T.N., Plouin, P., Van Bogaert, P., Carrizosa, J., Elia, M., Craiu, D., Jovic, N.J., *et al.* (2015). Summary of recommendations for the management of infantile seizures: Task Force Report for the ILAE Commission of Pediatrics, *Epilepsia*, 56, 1185–1197.

Wykes, R.C. and Lignani, G. (2018). Gene therapy and editing: Novel potential treatments for neuronal channelopathies, *Neuropharmacology*, 132, 108–117.

Chapter 5

Febrile Seizures and Their Contribution to Temporal Lobe Epilepsy and Associated Cognitive Problems

Megan M. Curran,* PhD
Tallie Z. Baram,*,†,‡ MD, PhD

Departments of Anatomy/Neurobiology, Pediatrics† and Neurology‡, University of California, Irvine; Irvine, California, USA*

5.1 Introduction: Temporal lobe epilepsy and its antecedents

Spontaneous seizures are the most overt manifestation of epilepsy, a disorder that affects ~1% of the general population [Browne and Holmes, 2008; Hesdorffer *et al.*, 2011a; Zack and Kobau, 2017]. The seizures, and their unpredictability, lead to decreased quality of life in affected individuals, who are often unable to drive and may experience stigmatization from peers in the community. Temporal lobe epilepsy (TLE), a type of epilepsy involving the hippocampal-limbic circuit, is particularly difficult to treat, and one-third of patients with TLE experience seizures that are refractory to anticonvulsant medication [Schmidt and Löscher, 2005]. TLE often arises in adolescence, leading to decades of decreased quality of life and medical costs.

In addition to the overt burden of the seizures themselves, epileptic seizures are frequently accompanied by problems in memory and executive functions that contribute to poor quality of life [Loiselle *et al.*, 2016]. This is particularly a problem in TLE, because the temporal lobe is comprised of many brain circuits that are required for learning and memory function. These cognitive deficits, including memory and decision-making difficulties, often begin while patients are still in school, further hampering their education and future career potential [Helmstaedter *et al.*, 2003]. In fact, whereas the seizures in TLE have been considered the cause of memory problems, recent studies show that memory deficits often arise either before the onset, or independently of spontaneous seizures [Aikia *et al.*, 2001; Chowdhury *et al.*, 2014; Elger *et al.*, 2004; Hoppe *et al.*, 2007; Weiss *et al.*, 2017]. This suggests that cognitive deficits in chronic epilepsy cannot be exclusively interpreted as long-term effects of the seizures or anticonvulsant drugs. In addition to learning and memory related difficulties, children with epilepsy have significantly higher rates of depression (23%) and anxiety (36%) than their healthy peers, and these disorders can appear prior to or within months of the first epileptic seizure [Jones *et al.*, 2007].

TLE most commonly arises in individuals with a history of long childhood febrile seizures or febrile status epilepticus (FSE) [French *et al.*, 1993; Harvey *et al.*, 1995]. An ongoing study, the FEBSTAT study, has been following 199 children from the onset of FSE. This is the first large-scale prospective research on children that combines early brain imaging, cognitive and medical outcome measures. Results from this groundbreaking study, which started in 2002, have recently begun to emerge. It has confirmed previous findings in animal and human studies that FSE directly provokes hippocampal injury [Lewis *et al.*, 2014; McClelland *et al.*, 2016; Provenzale *et al.*, 2008; Shinnar *et al.*, 2012] and memory impairments [Martinos *et al.*, 2012; Weiss *et al.*, 2017]. Here we discuss the emerging evidence that FSE may contribute to both the seizures and the cognitive problems that are often an intrinsic component of TLE.

5.2 FSE contributes to the development of the seizures that define temporal lobe epilepsy: Support from human and experimental approaches

A subset of individuals with TLE, the most common epilepsy syndrome in adults, have a history of prolonged childhood febrile seizures [Hesdorffer *et al.*, 2011b]. Febrile seizures (FS) are defined as seizures that are associated with a fever without a central nervous system infection or acute electrolyte imbalance in a child without a previous afebrile seizure. Febrile seizures occur in children between six months and five years of age, with the peak incidence at 18 months (AAP Subcommittee on Febrile Seizures, 2008). Febrile seizures are common (affecting 2–5% of the population) and are normally brief and benign — there are no long-term consequences of a single short episode. A subset of FSs are long, lasting >30 minutes, and are categorized as FSE. This type of seizure comprises 25% of all pediatric status epilepticus and is estimated to affect between 25,000–30,000 children annually [Shinnar *et al.*, 1997]. For decades, we have known of a connection between early life FSE and the later development of TLE. In recent years, the FEBSTAT study and additional reports have begun to uncover that FSE may directly cause epilepsy, likely in concert with and in addition to genetic factors. There is an average of an 8–12 year period of network remodeling known as the latent period between FSE and the first epileptic seizure (Berg and Shinnar, 1996; Dubé *et al.*, 2007; Mathern *et al.*, 1995).

Prospective human studies enable us to identify a defining relationship between FSE and the risk of developing TLE or cognitive deficits. Human studies do not allow determination of whether FSE is a causal factor in TLE as clearly, genetic and other factors are contributors [Eckhaus *et al.*, 2013; Hildebrand *et al.*, 2016; Martin *et al.*, 2010a; Nur *et al.*, 2012]. As outlined in Figure 5.1, there are three plausible scenarios: A) FSE is the direct cause of TLE and/or cognitive deficits, and the brain would have developed normally without the febrile seizure; B) FSE develops in an already predisposed brain, but also contributes independently to the development of TLE and/or

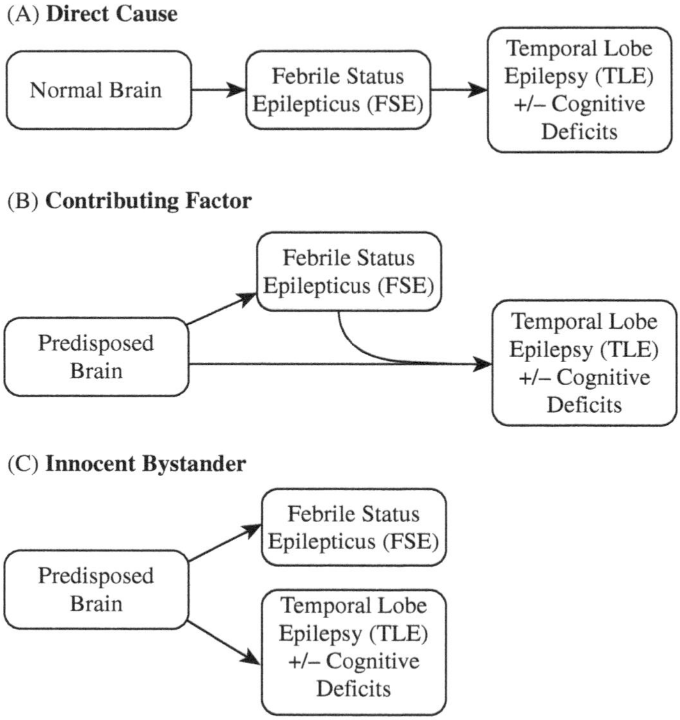

Figure 5.1. Development of febrile status epilepticus and later temporal lobe epilepsy and cognitive deficits.

cognitive deficits; or C) TLE and/or cognitive deficits develop via an independent process from the FSE, and FSE is just an "innocent bystander." We have generated a rodent model of experimental (e)FSE that provides a powerful tool to probe these alternatives.

Specifically, we have employed an age-appropriate model in rats, and found that eFSE directly causes limbic, temporal lobe-like epilepsy [Choy *et al.*, 2014; Dubé *et al.*, 2006, 2010]. The model is based on the hyperthermia that is the most obvious symptom of fever in children. Additionally, in children, the fever is normally caused by inflammation due to an infection, and the same inflammatory mediators are also both involved and required for the invocation of seizures in eFSE [Dubé *et al.*, 2005]. Hyperthermia is induced in rat pups via a regulated stream of warm air for 60 minutes. Heating time is adjusted to keep their core temperature within the range that invokes febrile seizures as recorded via electroencephalography (EEG), between 38.5–41.0°C [Baram *et al.*, 1997]. Both wild-type and genetically susceptible stains of mice have been used in these experiments, revealing that while genetics increases predisposition to FSE [van Gassen *et al.*, 2008; Martin *et al.*, 2010b], genetic susceptibility is not required for the generation of FSE or the permanent brain changes that FSE can cause [Dubé *et al.*, 2006, 2010; Lemmens *et al.*, 2009]. The age of immature rats (postnatal day 10–11, P10–11) that is used in eFSE reflects the developmental stage when the majority of human FSE occurs [Dubé *et al.*, 2007]. Behavioral seizures in immature rats include the arrest of hyperthermia-induced hyperkinesis followed by facial automatisms. Starting within months after FSE, 30–40% of the rats begin to develop spontaneous limbic seizures (temporal lobe epilepsy), a number similar to the human population [Annegers *et al.*, 1987; Choy *et al.*, 2014; Dubé *et al.*, 2006, 2010; Hesdorffer *et al.*, 2011a]. Therefore, the experimental approach provides strong support for a direct contribution of FSE to the development of TLE rather than TLE being caused by genetics, a supposition supported also by human twin studies [Jackson *et al.*, 1998].

5.3 FSE generates cognitive deficits in a subset of individuals: Support from human and experimental studies

The prevailing dogma in the child neurology literature has been that FSE does not lead to cognitive problems, but instead, memory problems are a result of the brain pathology that also underlies FSE [Chang *et al.*, 2000; Verity *et al.*, 1998]. Over the past decade, compelling information from both human studies [Martinos *et al.*, 2012; Nørgaard *et al.*, 2009; Shinnar *et al.*, 2012] and rodent models [Barry *et al.*, 2016; Dubé *et al.*, 2009; Patterson *et al.*, 2017] has challenged this prevailing dogma. Translational and clinical research has begun to uncover the relationship between TLE and cognitive

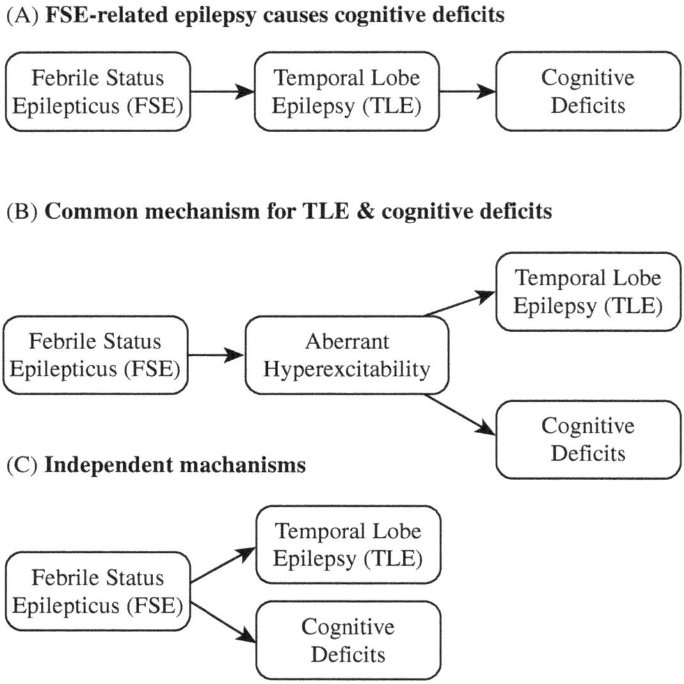

Figure 5.2. Relationship between the origins of temporal lobe epilepsy and cognitive deficits following febrile status epilepticus.

deficits (Figure 5.2) to examine if: A) FSE leads to TLE, which then causes the development of cognitive deficits; B) FSE causes changes within neuronal structure and connections, most likely aberrant hyperexcitability, which then separately (or via overlapping mechanisms) causes TLE and cognitive deficits; or C) TLE and cognitive deficits independently develop via two non-overlapping mechanisms following FSE.

Animal studies have allowed us to separate whether the effect of FSE directly causes cognitive difficulties or if the cognitive difficulties would have developed independent of the febrile seizure, as shown in Figure 5.1C. When rats experience FSE early in life and then are allowed to grow to adulthood, their performance on a variety of cognitive tests including Morris water maze [Dubé *et al.*, 2009], active avoidance task [Patterson *et al.*, 2017], and novel object location (Curran *et al.*, unpublished) is impaired compared to their littermate controls. By controlling for any genetic or environmental variance that could contribute to performance on cognitive tasks, we can clearly state that FSE directly causes the development of cognitive deficits that continue into adulthood.

Recent work in children has demonstrated that cognitive deficits in children can arise after an epilepsy-inducing insult, but before spontaneous seizures or independently from them [Bender *et al.*, 2013; Elger *et al.*, 2004; Hoppe *et al.*, 2007]. Human studies have revealed that when testing six weeks and one year after FSE, there are deficits in language, motor, and cognitive outcomes, even in children who had no known developmental delays prior to the FSE [Martinos *et al.*, 2013; Weiss *et al.*, 2016]. These findings suggest that FSE-induced memory problems do not depend on a resultant epilepsy that may follow these seizures. Of course, the same limbic/hippocampal networks contribute to memory processes and epilepsy, yet the networks might be affected by independent or partially overlapping processes. Indeed, data from the FEBSTAT study indicate that hippocampal injury following FSE and the memory problems co-exist in the same child [Weiss *et al.*, 2017], lending strong support for the notion that FSE injures the hippocampal circuit and thus induces memory problems. These findings provide major impetus for studying how FSE influences the hippocampal-cortical circuit and how cellular and molecular mechanisms provoke memory deficits.

5.4 Potential mechanisms for FSE-induced seizures and cognitive deficits

5.4.1 *Contribution of inflammation to the consequences of FSE*

Preventing or abrogating the contribution of an acquired insult such as FSE to hyperexcitability and memory problems should be a tractable goal, providing major impetus to study how FSE leads to these outcomes. Inflammatory processes are excellent candidates for mediating the effects of FSE on both epileptogenesis and memory problems. It has long been known that increased levels of inflammatory cytokines are seen in the brain of both epileptic animals as well as in brain tissue removed from patients with epilepsy [Aronica and Gorter, 2007; Balosso *et al.*, 2013] (also see Chapter 10). Inflammation is a good marker of the abnormal epileptic brain but analyzing differences in tissue after epilepsy has commenced does not allow distinguishing if inflammation is the cause of the spontaneous seizures or an effect of the seizing brain.

As a result of its role in the production of fever, inflammation is inherently linked to the initial febrile seizures [Eskilsson *et al.*, 2014; Heida and Pittman, 2005; Heida *et al.*, 2009; Luheshi *et al.*, 1997; Riazi *et al.*, 2010]. Inflammation not only produces the fever itself, but it also has a direct role in increasing the likelihood of spontaneous seizures from the limbic circuit [Dubé *et al.*, 2007; Patterson *et al.*, 2015; Vezzani *et al.*, 2011].

Not only is inflammation inherent in the febrile basis of FSE, there is an increase in inflammatory markers within the brain following FSE as well as febrile seizures in children. In the experimental model, the onset of the inflammation is fairly rapid, with a measurable increase in messenger RNA (mRNA) as early as one hour after the end of the febrile seizure and nearly completely disappearing by 96 hours post-seizure [Dubé *et al.*, 2010]. This increase is found in the same limbic regions and in the same animals in which an epilepsy-predictive magnetic resonance imaging (MRI) signal is observed [Choy *et al.*, 2014; Patterson *et al.*, 2015]. The inflammatory response consists of a variety of immune markers including cyclooxygenase 2 (COX2), GFAP (an astrocyte activation marker), TNF-α, Interleukin-1β (IL-1β), and Interleukin-1 Receptor 1 (IL-1R1) [Patterson *et al.*, 2015]. Without this increase in inflammation within the brain, particularly IL-1β, the brain is significantly more resistant to febrile seizure, as seen in mice deficient in IL-1β [Dubé *et al.*, 2005]. Thus, inflammation may be both a cause and a reflection of the permanent epileptogenic changes that occur in the brain following FSE.

Inflammation is a particularly enticing target for prevention of epileptogenesis because there are many drugs that are either available clinically or in development that directly interact with the inflammatory cascade. These range from broad anti-inflammatory agents such as dexamethasone (a glucocorticoid receptor agonist), to over-the-counter non-steroidal anti-inflammatory drugs (NSAIDs) including ibuprofen, to drugs that interact specifically with downstream components of the anti-inflammatory cascade, for example TG6-10-1, which blocks prostaglandin E_2 (PGE_2) from binding the EP2 receptor. Many studies in humans and animal models have investigated the use of anti-inflammatory drugs to prevent epileptogenesis with both encouraging [Akula *et al.*, 2008; Gobbo and O'Mara, 2004; Jiang *et al.*, 2015] and negative results [Claycomb *et al.*, 2011; Holtman *et al.*, 2010; Polascheck *et al.*, 2010]. This is likely a result of the fact that while inflammation can cause epileptogenic damage, portions of the inflammatory cascade may be neuroprotective and important for restoring normal neuronal function [Schwartz and Kipnis, 2005].

5.4.2 *Cellular and molecular level changes underlying epilepsy and cognitive problems*

The effects of insults, including long seizures such as FSE, on neurons and brain circuits are highly age dependent. Whereas adult seizures are known to promote neuronal death [Fujikawa, 1996], even prolonged seizures lead to minimal cell death during the early postnatal period [Dubé *et al.*, 2010; Sankar *et al.*, 1998; Toth *et al.*, 1998]. Indeed, the lack of cell death was perennially used as an argument that seizures had little consequence on the developing brain, and that any cognitive impairments observed following long developmental seizures were a result of pre-existing factors [Baram *et al.*, 2011].

Over the past decade, compelling data from both human studies and rodent models [Dubé *et al.*, 2004; Patterson *et al.*, 2015] suggest that functional consequences of early-life insult can arise without cell death. Indeed, whereas the developing brain is more resilient to seizure-induced excitotoxicity [Sullivan *et al.*, 2003], the immaturity of neuronal populations and networks engenders specific vulnerability of the developing brain [Haut *et al.*, 2004]. There is a widespread consensus, based on diverse approaches in rats and mice, that developing dentate gyrus granule cells (GCs) exhibit maturation-dependent vulnerability to SE: a subpopulation of GCs undergoes structural and functional reorganization following a pro-epileptic insult [Hosford *et al.*, 2016; Kron *et al.*, 2010]. Cells born roughly two weeks before to two weeks after the SE insult either develop hilar basal dendrites (HBD), migrate into the hilus or both, thus contributing to the aberrant circuitry [Goldberg and Coulter, 2013] underlying hyperexcitability and loss of precision in the DG. HBDs are apparent on newborn granule cells, but are normally lost with GC maturation and are targets of both autaptic excitatory synapses as well as excitatory synapses from neighboring GCs [Kron *et al.*, 2010]. This leads to an increase of excitation and increased susceptibility to seizures. We have evidence of retention of immature HBDs in GCs exposed to "SE" in vitro and of abnormal numbers of GCs with this immature feature in adult rats that experienced FSE as pups [Patterson *et al.*, 2017].

Additionally, we discovered that FSE leads to dendritic stunting in hippocampal pyramidal cells [Choy *et al.*, 2014; Patterson *et al.*, 2017] without evidence for cell loss [Dubé *et al.*, 2010; Patterson *et al.*, 2015; Toth *et al.*, 1998]. Other developmental insults such as chronic early-life stress were also found to promote impoverishment of apical dendritic trees and loss of synapses in hippocampal CA1 and CA3 that correlated directly with memory problems [Brunson *et al.*, 2005; Ivy *et al.*, 2010]. Accordingly, interventions that rescued dendrites and synapses ameliorated the memory problems [Ivy *et al.*, 2010]. Because of the close, apparently causal relationship of dendritic and synapse loss and memory problems [Chen *et al.*, 2004; Ivy *et al.*, 2010; Patterson *et al.*, 2017], this structural change provides a reproducible biomarker and target for intervention.

We have now begun to identify neuronal pathways that contribute directly to FSE-induced cognitive impairments, as their blockade rescues cognition. We performed transcriptomic analyses followed by bioinformatics and discovered coordinated transcriptionally-regulated changes in the expression of multiple genes that govern neuronal behavior. Importantly, this pro-epileptogenic transcriptional program involved Neuron-Restrictive Silencing Factor (NRSF), which is uniquely poised to mediate neuronal plasticity. Originally, NRSF expression was described in non-neuronal tissues where it suppresses neuron-specific genes [Chen *et al.*, 1998; Schoenherr and Anderson, 1995], indicating that neuronal genes carry NRSF-response elements (NRSEs) and are repressed by augmented NRSF levels to prevent expression in non-neuronal tissue [McClelland *et al.*, 2014]. Recently, NRSF expression in mature neurons has been described, where the factor may be crucial for normal function [Ballas and Mandel, 2005; Gao *et al.*, 2011; Singh-Taylor *et al.*, 2017]. NRSF's function is especially crucial in developing neurons, where expression of NRSF-regulated genes contributes to several aspects of maturation, including development of excitatory synapses [Chen *et al.*, 1998; Schoenherr and Anderson, 1995]. This is important, because during the developmental epoch when FSE takes place (infancy and early childhood in humans, P10-11 in the rat [Avishai-Eliner *et al.*, 2002]), many brain neurons are largely mature, but specific neuronal populations including granule cells (GCs) in the dentate gyrus (DG) are still differentiating and maturing [Schlessinger *et al.*, 1975; Thind *et al.*, 2008]. GCs should therefore be more affected by aberrantly increased levels of NRSF.

Seizures may increase NRSF levels and activity [Brennan *et al.*, 2016; Garriga-Canut *et al.*, 2006; McClelland *et al.*, 2011, 2014; Rodenas-Ruano *et al.*, 2012; Roopra *et al.*, 2001]. We found that this was also the case for FSE [Patterson *et al.*, 2017], and then measured the effects of NRSF blockade on cognition in adulthood. Rats that had NRSF binding blocked acutely for two days following FSE performed at the same levels as control rats on the active avoidance task, and significantly better than the rats that had FSE without NRSF blockade. These performance enhancements were already apparent on the second day of training and persisted for at least a month [Patterson *et al.*, 2017].

Acute NRSF blockade not only prevented memory problems, but also rescued the normal maturation of DG-GCs following FSE as measured by the number of abnormal hilar basal dendrites. Together, these facts suggest that gene-sets repressed by NRSF are a promising candidate mechanism for the FSE–induced abnormal structure and function of the hippocampal-cortical network. Importantly, the number of involved genes is likely to be relatively small; whereas ~600 hippocampal genes are potential targets of NRSF, increased NRSF levels after SE repressed only ~30 target genes in adult hippocampus, governed by the affinity of these genes to NRSF [McClelland *et al.*, 2014].

5.5 Predicting which child with FSE will develop epilepsy and/or cognitive problems

Currently, there is no practical way to predict the epilepsy or cognitive problems that follow FSE. Prediction would enable the development of a way to halt the epileptogenic and cognitive changes before they occur, and then to focus treatment on the children that are at risk. One of the most promising techniques available to track epileptogenic brain changes is MRI. MRI is non-invasive, clinically available, and is a direct measurement of underlying biological structure. It has long been known that there are MRI changes in the following FSE [Dubé *et al.*, 2004; Scott *et al.*, 2003; Shinnar *et al.*, 2012], but these changes have not been able to accurately predict future development of TLE. We described a non-invasive magnetic resonance imaging (MRI) signal that predicts which immature rats exposed to eFSE will develop epilepsy and which will remain unaffected [Choy *et al.*, 2014; Curran *et al.*, 2018]. These MRI scans were taken at a much earlier time point than previous studies, within four hours after eFSE, and reveal a reduced T_2 signal throughout the limbic circuit, and the reduction in the basolateral amygdala (BLA) was strongly predictive of development of epilepsy.

The signal change was initially found on an 11.7T high magnetic field T_2 MRI, but can also be found in a lower-strength 4.7T scanner using a T_2* signal, which can measure changes in deoxyhemoglobin [Chavhan *et al.*, 2009]. The signal reduction likely represents paramagnetic susceptibility effects derived from increasing unsaturated venous deoxyhemoglobin, supported by a strong inverse correlation of deoxyhemoglobin in venous blood with brain T_2 values in a strong magnetic field (11.7T) [Choy *et al.*, 2014]. Investigation of the mechanisms that underlie the predictive signal changes and continue enhancing their predictive value will hopefully be able to help us inform parents if their child is at increased risk of epilepsy or cognitive deficits and ideally be able to intervene and prevent these.

In the past decade, our knowledge and understanding of how a single long febrile seizure, and specifically febrile status epilepticus, can lead to permanent brain changes has advanced considerably. We have begun to understand the molecular and cellular level changes that begin within minutes of febrile status epilepticus and are changed into adulthood. These changes lead to increased risk of epilepsy and permanent learning and memory deficits, but recent advances move us closer to being able to prevent them.

Acknowledgments

This work was supported by NIH grants NS35439; NS78279 T32 NS45540; and T32 GM008620.

References

Aikia, M., Salmenpera, T., Partanen, K., and Kalviainen, R. (2001). Verbal memory in newly diagnosed patients and patients with chronic left temporal lobe epilepsy, *Epilepsy Behav.*, 2, 20–27.

Akula, K.K., Dhir, A., and Kulkarni, S.K. (2008). Rofecoxib, a selective cyclooxygenase-2 (COX-2) inhibitor increases pentylenetetrazol seizure threshold in mice: Possible involvement of adenosinergic mechanism, *Epilepsy Res.*, 78, 60–70.

Annegers, J.F., Hauser, W.A., Shirts, S.B., and Kurland, L.T. (1987). Factors prognostic of unprovoked seizures after febrile convulsions, *N. Engl. J. Med.*, 316, 493–498.

Aronica, E. and Gorter, J.A (2007). Gene expression profile in temporal lobe epilepsy, *Neuroscientist*, 13, 100–108.

Avishai-Eliner, S., Brunson, K.L., Sandman, C. A., and Baram, T.Z. (2002). Stressed-out, or in (utero)?, *Trends Neurosci.*, 25, 518–524.

Ballas, N. and Mandel, G. (2005). The many faces of REST oversee epigenetic programming of neuronal genes, *Curr. Opin. Neurobiol.*, 15, 500–506.

Balosso, S., Ravizza, T., Aronica, E., and Vezzani, A. (2013). The dual role of TNF-α and its receptors in seizures, *Exp. Neurol.* 247, 267–271.

Baram, T.Z., Gerth, A., and Schultz, L. (1997). Febrile seizures: an appropriate-aged model suitable for long-term studies, *Brain Res. Dev. Brain Res.*, 98, 265–270.

Baram, T.Z., Jensen, F.E., and Brooks-Kayal, A. (2011). Does acquired epileptogenesis in the immature brain require neuronal death, *Epilepsy Curr.*, 11, 21–26.

Barry, J.M., Sakkaki, S., Barriere, S.J., Patterson, K.P., Lenck-Santini, P.P., Scott, R.C., Baram, T.Z., and Holmes, G.L. (2016). Temporal coordination of hippocampal neurons reflects cognitive outcome post-febrile status epilepticus, *EBioMedicine*, 7, 175–190.

Bender, A.C., Natola, H., Ndong, C., Holmes, G.L., Scott, R.C., and Lenck-Santini, P.P. (2013). Focal Scn1a knockdown induces cognitive impairment without seizures, *Neurobiol. Dis.*, 54, 297–307.

Berg, A.T. and Shinnar, S. (1996). Complex febrile seizures, *Epilepsia*, 37, 126–133.

Brennan, G.P., Dey, D., Chen, Y., Patterson, K.P., Magnetta, E.J., Hall, A.M., Dube, C.M., Mei, Y.T., and Baram, T.Z. (2016). Dual and opposing roles of microRNA-124 in epilepsy are mediated through inflammatory and NRSF-dependent gene networks, *Cell Rep.*, 14, 2402–2412.

Browne, T.R. and Holmes, G.L. (2008). Handbook of Epilepsy (Jones & Bartlett Learning).

Brunson, K.L., Baram, T.Z., and Bender, R.A. (2005). Hippocampal neurogenesis is not enhanced by lifelong reduction of glucocorticoid levels, *Hippocampus,* 15, 491–501.

Chang, Y.C., Guo, N.W., Huang, C.C., Wang, S.T., and Tsai, J.J. (2000). Neurocognitive attention and behavior outcome of school-age children with a history of febrile convulsions: a population study, *Epilepsia*, 41, 412–420.

Chavhan, G.B., Babyn, P.S., Thomas, B., Shroff, M.M., and Haacke, E.M. (2009). Principles, techniques, and applications of T2*-based MR imaging and its special applications, *Radiographics*, 29, 1433–1449.

Chen, Y., Bender, R.A., Brunson, K.L., Pomper, J.K., Grigoriadis, D.E., Wurst, W., and Baram, T.Z. (2004). Modulation of dendritic differentiation by corticotropin-releasing factor in the developing hippocampus, *Proc. Natl. Acad. Sci. U. S. A.*, 101, 15782–15787.

Chen, Z.-F., Paquette, A.J., and Anderson, D.J. (1998). NRSF/REST is required in vivo for repression of multiple neuronaltarget genes during embryogenesis, *Nat. Genet.*, 20, 136–142.

Chowdhury, F.A., Elwes, R.D.C., Koutroumanidis, M., Morris, R.G., Nashef, L., and Richardson, M.P. (2014). Impaired cognitive function in idiopathic generalized epilepsy and unaffected family members: An epilepsy endophenotype, *Epilepsia*, 55, 835–840.

Choy, M., Dubé, C.M., Patterson, K., Barnes, S.R., Maras, P., Blood, A.B., Hasso, A.N., Obenaus, A., and Baram, T.Z. (2014). A novel, noninvasive, predictive epilepsy biomarker with clinical potential, *J. Neurosci.*, 34, 8672–8684.

Claycomb, R.J., Hewett, S.J., and Hewett, J.A. (2011). Prophylactic, prandial rofecoxib treatment lacks efficacy against acute PTZ-induced seizure generation and kindling acquisition, *Epilepsia*, 52, 273–283.

Curran, M.M., Haddad, E., Patterson, K.P., Choy, M., Dubé, C.M., Baram, T.Z., and Obenaus, A. (2018). Epilepsy-predictive magnetic resonance imaging changes following experimental febrile status epilepticus: Are they translatable to the clinic?, *Epilepsia*, 59, 2005–2018.

Dubé, C., Yu, H., Nalcioglu, O., and Baram, T.Z. (2004). Serial MRI after experimental febrile seizures: altered T2 signal without neuronal death, *Ann. Neurol.*, 56, 709–714.

Dubé, C., Vezzani, A., Behrens, M., Bartfai, T., and Baram, T.Z. (2005). Interleukin-1beta contributes to the generation of experimental febrile seizures, *Ann. Neurol.*, 57, 152–155.

Dubé, C., Richichi, C., Bender, R.A., Chung, G., Litt, B., and Baram, T.Z. (2006). Temporal lobe epilepsy after experimental prolonged febrile seizures: prospective analysis, *Brain*, 129, 911–922.

Dubé, C.M., Brewster, A.L., Richichi, C., Zha, Q., and Baram, T.Z. (2007). Fever, febrile seizures and epilepsy, *Trends Neurosci.*, 30, 490–496.

Dubé, C.M., Zhou, J., Hamamura, M., Zhao, Q., Ring, A., Abrahams, J., McIntyre, K., Nalcioglu, O., Shatskih, T., Baram, T.Z., *et al.* (2009). Cognitive dysfunction after experimental febrile seizures, *Exp. Neurol.*, 215, 167–177.

Dubé, C.M., Ravizza, T., Hamamura, M., Zha, Q., Keebaugh, A., Fok, K., Andres, A.L., Nalcioglu, O., Obenaus, A., Vezzani, A., *et al.* (2010). Epileptogenesis provoked by prolonged experimental febrile seizures: mechanisms and biomarkers, J. *Neurosci.*, 30, 7484–7494.

Eckhaus, J., Lawrence, K.M., Helbig, I., Bui, M., Vadlamudi, L., Hopper, J.L., Scheffer, I.E., and Berkovic, S.F. (2013). Genetics of febrile seizure subtypes and syndromes: A twin study, *Epilepsy Res.*, 105, 103–109.

Elger, C.E., Helmstaedter, C., and Kurthen, M. (2004). Chronic epilepsy and cognition, *Lancet Neurol.*, 3, 663–672.

Eskilsson, A., Mirrasekhian, E., Dufour, S., Schwaninger, M., Engblom, D., and Blomqvist, A. (2014). Immune-induced fever is mediated by IL-6 receptors on brain endothelial cells coupled to STAT3-dependent induction of brain endothelial prostaglandin synthesis, *J. Neurosci.*, 34, 15957–15961.

French, J.A., Williamson, P.D., Thadani, V.M., Darcey, T.M., Mattson, R.H., Spencer, S.S., and Spencer, D.D. (1993). Characteristics of medial temporal lobe epilepsy: I. Results of history and physical examination, *Ann. Neurol.*, 34, 774–780.

Fujikawa, D.G. (1996). The temporal evolution of neuronal damage from pilocarpine-induced status epilepticus, *Brain Res.*, 725, 11–22.

Gao, Z., Ure, K., Ding, P., Nashaat, M., Yuan, L., Ma, J., Hammer, R.E., and Hsieh, J. (2011). The master negative regulator REST/NRSF controls adult neurogenesis by restraining the neurogenic program in quiescent stem cells, *J. Neurosci.*, 31, 9772–9786.

Garriga-Canut, M., Schoenike, B., Qazi, R., Bergendahl, K., Daley, T.J., Pfender, R.M., Morrison, J.F., Ockuly, J., Stafstrom, C., Sutula, T., *et al.* (2006). 2-Deoxy-D-glucose reduces epilepsy progression by NRSF-CtBP–dependent metabolic regulation of chromatin structure, *Nat. Neurosci.*, 9, 1382–1387.

van Gassen, K.L.I., Hessel, E.V.S., Ramakers, G.M.J., Notenboom, R.G.E., Wolterink-Donselaar, I.G., Brakkee, J.H., Godschalk, T.C., Qiao, X., Spruijt, B.M., van Nieuwenhuizen, O., *et al.* (2008). Characterization of febrile seizures and febrile seizure susceptibility in mouse inbred strains, *Genes, Brain Behav.*, 7, 578–586.

Gobbo, O.L. and O'Mara, S.M. (2004). Post-treatment, but not pre-treatment, with the selective cyclooxygenase-2 inhibitor celecoxib markedly enhances functional recovery from kainic acid-induced neurodegeneration, *Neuroscience*, 125, 317–327.

Goldberg, E.M. and Coulter, D.A. (2013). Mechanisms of epileptogenesis: a convergence on neural circuit dysfunction, *Nat. Rev. Neurosci.*, 14, 337–349.

Harvey, A.S., Grattan-Smith, J.D., Desmond, P.M., Chow, C.W., and Berkovic, S.F. (1995). Febrile seizures and hippocampal sclerosis:

Frequent and related findings in intractable temporal lobe epilepsy of childhood, *Pediatr. Neurol.*, 12, 201–206.

Haut, S.R., Velíšsková, J., and Moshé, S.L. (2004). Susceptibility of immature and adult brains to seizure effects, *Lancet Neurol.*, 3, 608–617.

Heida, J.G. and Pittman, Q.J. (2005). Causal links between brain cytokines and experimental febrile convulsions in the rat, *Epilepsia*, 46, 1906–1913.

Heida, J.G., Moshé, S.L., and Pittman, Q.J. (2009). The role of interleukin-1beta in febrile seizures, *Brain Dev.*, 31, 388–393.

Helmstaedter, C., Kurthen, M., Lux, S., Reuber, M., and Elger, C.E. (2003). Chronic epilepsy and cognition: a longitudinal study in temporal lobe epilepsy, *Ann. Neurol.*, 54, 425–432.

Hesdorffer, D.C., Logroscino, G., Benn, E.K.T., Katri, N., Cascino, G., and Hauser, W.A. (2011a). Estimating risk for developing epilepsy: A population-based study in Rochester, Minnesota, *Neurology*, 76, 23–27.

Hesdorffer, D.C., Benn, E.K.T., Bagiella, E., Nordli, D., Pellock, J., Hinton, V., and Shinnar, S. (2011b). Distribution of febrile seizure duration and associations with development, *Ann. Neurol.*, 70, 93–100.

Hildebrand, M.S., Phillips, A.M., Mullen, S.A., Adlard, P.A., Hardies, K., Damiano, J.A., Wimmer, V., Bellows, S.T., McMahon, J.M., Burgess, R., *et al.* (2016). Loss of synaptic Zn2+ transporter function increases risk of febrile seizures, *Sci. Rep.*, 5, 17816.

Holtman, L., Van Vliet, E.A., Edelbroek, P.M., Aronica, E., and Gorter, J.A. (2010). Cox-2 inhibition can lead to adverse effects in a rat model for temporal lobe epilepsy, *Epilepsy Res.*, 91, 49–56.

Hoppe, C., Elger, C.E., and Helmstaedter, C. (2007). Long-term memory impairment in patients with focal epilepsy, *Epilepsia*, 48 Suppl. 9, 26–29.

Hosford, B.E., Liska, J.P., and Danzer, S.C. (2016). Ablation of newly generated hippocampal granule cells has disease-modifying effects in epilepsy, *J. Neurosci.*, 36, 11013–11023.

Ivy, A.S., Rex, C.S., Chen, Y., Dubé, C., Maras, P.M., Grigoriadis, D.E., Gall, C.M., Lynch, G., and Baram, T.Z. (2010). Hippocampal dysfunction and cognitive impairments provoked by chronic early-life stress involve excessive activation of CRH receptors, *J. Neurosci.*, 30, 13005–13015.

Jackson, G.D., McIntosh, A.M., Briellmann, R.S., and Berkovic, S.F. (1998). Hippocampal sclerosis studied in identical twins, *Neurology*, 51, 78–84.

Jiang, J., Yang, M., Quan, Y., Gueorguieva, P., Ganesh, T., and Dingledine, R. (2015). Therapeutic window for cyclooxygenase-2 related anti-inflammatory therapy after status epilepticus, *Neurobiol. Dis.*, 76, 126–136.

Jones, J.E., Watson, R., Sheth, R., Caplan, R., Koehn, M., Seidenberg, M., and Hermann, B. (2007). Psychiatric comorbidity in children with new onset epilepsy, *Dev. Med. Child Neurol.*, 49, 493–497.

Kron, M.M., Zhang, H., and Parent, J.M. (2010). The developmental stage of dentate granule cells dictates their contribution to seizure-induced plasticity, *J. Neurosci.*, 30, 2051–2059.

Lemmens, E.M.P., Aendekerk, B., Schijns, O.E.M.G., Blokland, A., Beuls, E.A.M., and Hoogland, G. (2009). Long-term behavioral outcome after early-life hyperthermia-induced seizures, *Epilepsy Behav.*, 14, 309–315.

Lewis, D. V, Shinnar, S., Hesdorffer, D.C., Bagiella, E., Bello, J.A., Chan, S., Xu, Y., MacFall, J., Gomes, W. a, Moshé, S.L., *et al.* (2014). Hippocampal sclerosis after febrile status epilepticus: the FEBSTAT study, *Ann. Neurol.*, 75, 178–185.

Loiselle, K.A., Ramsey, R.R., Rausch, J.R., and Modi, A.C. (2016). Trajectories of health-related quality of life among children with newly diagnosed epilepsy, *J. Pediatr. Psychol.*, 41, 1011–1021.

Luheshi, G.N., Stefferl, A., Turnbull, A. V, Dascombe, M.J., Brouwer, S., Hopkins, S.J., and Rothwell, N.J. (1997). Febrile response to tissue inflammation involves both peripheral and brain IL-1 and TNF-alpha in the rat, *Am. J. Physiol.*, 272, R862–8.

Martin, M.S., Dutt, K., Papale, L.A., Dubé, C.M., Dutton, S.B., de Haan, G., Shankar, A., Tufik, S., Meisler, M.H., Baram, T.Z., *et al.* (2010a). Altered function of the SCN1A voltage-gated sodium channel leads to γ-aminobutyric acid-ergic (GABAergic) interneuron abnormalities, *J. Biol. Chem.*, 285, 9823–9834.

Martin, M.S., Dutt, K., Papale, L.A., Dubé, C.M., Dutton, S.B., de Haan, G., Shankar, A., Tufik, S., Meisler, M.H., Baram, T.Z., *et al.* (2010b). Altered Function of the SCN1A Voltage-gated Sodium Channel Leads to γ-Aminobutyric Acid-ergic (GABAergic) Interneuron Abnormalities, *J. Biol. Chem.*, 285, 9823–9834.

Martinos, M.M., Yoong, M., Patil, S., Chin, R.F.M., Neville, B.G., Scott, R.C., and De Haan, M. (2012). Recognition memory is impaired in children after prolonged febrile seizures, *Brain*, 135, 3153–3164.

Martinos, M.M., Yoong, M., Patil, S., Chong, W.K., Mardari, R., Chin, R.F.M., Neville, B.G.R., De Haan, M., and Scott, R.C. (2013). Early developmental outcomes in children following convulsive status epilepticus: A longitudinal study, *Epilepsia*, 54, 1012–1019.

Mathern, G.W., Babb, T.L., Vickrey, B.G., Melendez, M., and Pretorius, J.K. (1995). The clinical-pathogenic mechanisms of hippocampal neuron loss and surgical outcomes in temporal lobe epilepsy, *Brain*, 118, 105–118.

McClelland, A.C., Gomes, W.A., Shinnar, S., Hesdorffer, D.C., Bagiella, E., Lewis, D.V, Bello, J.A., Chan, S., MacFall, J., Chen, M., *et al.* (2016). Quantitative evaluation of medial temporal lobe morphology in children with febrile status epilepticus: Results of the FEBSTAT study, *Am. J. Neuroradiol.*, 37, 2356–2362.

McClelland, S., Flynn, C., Dubé, C., Richichi, C., Zha, Q., Ghestem, A., Esclapez, M., Bernard, C., and Baram, T.Z. (2011). Neuron-restrictive silencer factor-mediated hyperpolarization-activated cyclic nucleotide gated channelopathy in experimental temporal lobe epilepsy, *Ann. Neurol.*, 70, 454–464.

McClelland, S., Brennan, G.P., Dubé, C., Rajpara, S., Iyer, S., Richichi, C., Bernard, C., and Baram, T.Z. (2014). The transcription factor NRSF contributes to epileptogenesis by selective repression of a subset of target genes, *Elife*, 3, e01267.

Nørgaard, M., Ehrenstein, V., Mahon, B.E., Nielsen, G.L., Rothman, K.J., and Sørensen, H.T. (2009). Febrile seizures and cognitive function in young adult life: a prevalence study in Danish conscripts, *J. Pediatr.*, 155, 404–409.

Nur, B.G., Kahramaner, Z., Duman, O., Dundar, N.O., Sallakcı, N., Yavuzer, U., and Haspolat, S. (2012). Interleukin-6 gene polymorphism in febrile seizures, *Pediatr. Neurol.*, 46, 36–38.

Patterson, K.P., Brennan, G.P., Curran, M., Kinney-lang, E., Dubé, C., Ly, C., Obenaus, A., and Baram, T.Z. (2015). Rapid, coordinate inflammatory responses after experimental febrile status epilepticus: Implications for epileptogenesis, *ENeuro*, 2, 1–12.

Patterson, K.P., Barry, J.M., Curran, M.M., Singh-Taylor, A., Brennan, G., Rismanchi, N., Page, M., Noam, Y., Holmes, G.L., and Baram, T.Z. (2017). Enduring memory impairments provoked by developmental febrile seizures are mediated by functional and structural effects of neuronal restrictive silencing factor, *J. Neurosci.*, 37, 3748–16.

Polascheck, N., Bankstahl, M., and Löscher, W. (2010). The COX-2 inhibitor parecoxib is neuroprotective but not antiepileptogenic in the pilocarpine model of temporal lobe epilepsy, *Exp. Neurol.*, 224, 219–233.

Provenzale, J.M., Barboriak, D.P., VanLandingham, K., MacFall, J., Delong, D., and Lewis, D. V. (2008). Hippocampal MRI signal hyperintensity after febrile status epilepticus is predictive of subsequent mesial temporal sclerosis, *Am. J. Roentgenol.*, 190, 976–983.

Riazi, K., Galic, M.A., and Pittman, Q.J. (2010). Contributions of peripheral inflammation to seizure susceptibility: Cytokines and brain excitability, *Epilepsy Res.*, 89, 34–42.

Rodenas-Ruano, A., Chávez, A.E., Cossio, M.J., Castillo, P.E., and Zukin, R.S. (2012). REST-dependent epigenetic remodeling promotes the developmental switch in synaptic NMDA receptors, *Nat. Neurosci.*, 15, 1382–1390.

Roopra, A., Huang, Y., and Dingledine, R. (2001). Neurological disease: listening to gene silencers, *Mol. Interv.*, 1, 219–228.

Sankar, R., Shin, D.H., Liu, H., Mazarati, A., Pereira de Vasconcelos, A., and Wasterlain, C.G. (1998). Patterns of status epilepticus-induced neuronal injury during development and long-term consequences, *J. Neurosci.*, 18, 8382–8393.

Schlessinger, A.R., Cowan, W.M., and Gottlieb, D.I. (1975). An autoradiographic study of the time of origin and the pattern of granule cell migration in the dentate gyrus of the rat, *J. Comp. Neurol.*, 159, 149–175.

Schmidt, D. and Löscher, W. (2005). Drug resistance in epilepsy: putative neurobiologic and clinical mechanisms, *Epilepsia*, 46, 858–877.

Schoenherr, C.J., and Anderson, D.J. (1995). The neuron-restrictive silencer factor (NRSF): a coordinate repressor of multiple neuron-specific genes, *Science*, 267, 1360–1363.

Schwartz, M. and Kipnis, J. (2005). Protective autoimmunity and neuroprotection in inflammatory and noninflammatory neurodegenerative diseases, *J. Neurol. Sci.*, 233, 163–166.

Scott, R.C., King, M.D., Gadian, D.G., Neville, B.G.R., and Connelly, A. (2003). Hippocampal abnormalities after prolonged febrile convulsion: A longitudinal MRI study, *Brain*, 126, 2551–2557.

Shinnar, S., Pellock, J.M., Moshé, S.L., Maytal, J., O'Dell, C., Driscoll, S.M., Alemany, M., Newstein, D., and DeLorenzo, R.J. (1997). In whom does status epilepticus occur: Age-related differences in children, *Epilepsia*, 38, 907–914.

Shinnar, S., Bello, J.A., Chan, S., Hesdorffer, D.C., Lewis, D. V, Macfall, J., Pellock, J.M., Nordli, D.R., Frank, L.M., Moshe, S.L., *et al.* (2012). MRI abnormalities following febrile status epilepticus in children: the FEBSTAT study, *Neurology*, 79, 871–877.

Singh-Taylor, A., Molet, J., Jiang, S., Korosi, A., Bolton, J.L., Noam, Y., Simeone, K., Cope, J., Chen, Y., Mortazavi, A., *et al.* (2017).

NRSF-dependent epigenetic mechanisms contribute to programming of stress-sensitive neurons by neonatal experience, promoting resilience, *Mol. Psychiatry*, 23, 648–657.

Steering Committee on Quality Improvement and Management, and Subcommittee on Febrile Seizures (2008). Febrile seizures: clinical practice guideline for the long-term management of the child with simple febrile seizures, *Pediatrics*, 121, 1281–1286.

Sullivan, P.G., Dubé, C., Dorenbos, K., Steward, O., and Baram, T.Z. (2003). Mitochondrial uncoupling protein-2 protects the immature brain from excitotoxic neuronal death, *Ann. Neurol.*, 53, 711–717.

Thind, K.K., Ribak, C.E., and Buckmaster, P.S. (2008). Synaptic input to dentate granule cell basal dendrites in a rat model of temporal lobe epilepsy, *J. Comp. Neurol.*, 509, 190–202.

Toth, Z., Yan, X.X., Haftoglou, S., Ribak, C.E., and Baram, T.Z. (1998). Seizure-induced neuronal injury: vulnerability to febrile seizures in an immature rat model, *J. Neurosci.*, 18, 4285–4294.

Verity, C.M., Greenwood, R., and Golding, J. (1998). Long-term intellectual and behavioral outcomes of children with febrile convulsions, *N. Engl. J. Med.*, 338, 1723–1728.

Vezzani, A., French, J., Bartfai, T., and Baram, T.Z. (2011). The role of inflammation in epilepsy, *Nat. Rev. Neurol.*, 7, 31–40.

Weiss, E., DM, M., Shinnar, S., Hesdorffer, D., Lewis, D., Shinnar, R., Bello, J., Chan, S., Seinfeld, S., Gallentine, W., *et al.* (2017). Memory function following febrile status epilepticus: Results of the FEBSTAT Study. In American Epilepsy Society Annual Meeting (Washington DC), Abst. 2.368.

Weiss, E.F., Masur, D., Shinnar, S., Hesdorffer, D.C., Hinton, V.J., Bonner, M., Rinaldi, J., Van de Water, V., Culbert, J., Shinnar, R.C., *et al.* (2016). Cognitive functioning one month and one year following febrile status epilepticus, *Epilepsy Behav.*, 64, 283–288.

Zack, M.M. and Kobau, R. (2017). National and state estimates of the numbers of adults and children with active epilepsy — United States, 2015, *Morb. Mortal. Wkly. Rep.*, 66, 821–825.

Chapter 6

BRD2: The First Locus Discovered for a Common Epilepsy (Juvenile Myoclonic Epilepsy): What Was Right, What Was Wrong, and How Studies of IGE Make Progress

David A. Greenberg, PhD
Shilpa Pathak, PhD

Department of Pediatrics, Ohio State University and Nationwide Children's Hospital, Columbus, Ohio 43215, USA

6.1 The discovery of the genetic locus

This chapter discusses 30 years of work on the discovery, replication, population genetics, and basic mechanisms attributable to *BRD2* that influence the expression of Juvenile Myoclonic Epilepsy (JME). We divide the chapter into the following topics:

(1) The discovery of the first genetic locus for any form of epilepsy.
(2) Replication of the finding.

(3) The relationship of the locus for JME to other IGE[1] syndromes.
(4) Identification of *BRD2*, more replications of *BRD2's* effect, and expansion to endophenotypes.
(5) The difficulties in collecting family data.
(6) The effect of the "channelopathy hypothesis" on IGE research.
(7) The JME mouse model: Proving *BRD2* is the gene.
(8) What changes to *BRD2's* DNA cause JME susceptibility? The epigenetic hypothesis.
(9) Implications of the *BRD2* finding for studies of IGE.

Juvenile Myoclonic Epilepsy (OMIM 608816) is among the most common of the adolescent onset generalized epilepsy syndromes and has a prevalence of ~1 in 1000 people worldwide ([Camfield *et al.*, 2013], NIH). JME is characterized clinically by uncontrollable myoclonic jerks (mostly on awakening). The interictal electroencephalogram (EEG) in untreated patients shows generalized spikes-and-waves (4–6 Hz) and polyspike-and-wave discharges [Janz, 1997; Kasteleijn-Nolst Trenite *et al.*, 2013]. Although most patients respond to pharmacological treatment, the frequency of symptom recurrence is high when antiepileptic medication is discontinued [Pavlovic *et al.*, 2011].

JME is highly familial. Also, the most common interictal EEG finding in JME patients is a 4–6 Hz spike-and-wave complex that is also seen in family members of JME patients, members without frank epilepsy [Tsuboi and Christian, 1973].

---

[1] In this chapter, we deliberately use the term Idiopathic Generalized Epilepsy (IGE) rather than the more current Genetic Generalized Epilepsy (GGE). This is partly to emphasize that the term "genetic" being used in the designation GGE obscures the fact that there is a lack of identified, proven genes. While IGE(s), collectively, have been shown to be *familial*, the actual *genetic* contribution has remained elusive. For example, despite an apparently herculean effort and the many reports of genes supposedly causing IGEs such as JME, almost none have been proven. The recent report of Santos *et al.* [2017] in which the evidence for 229 proposed genes for JME was examined, highlights our view that the designation of "genetic" in the GGE acronym is premature. IGE is a collection of different syndromes, some of which will be genetic but some perhaps not. We must distinguish them, one from the other, first.

In 1988, we published evidence for a genetic locus for an idiopathic generalized epilepsy (IGE), which was the first locus, not only for an IGE but for any form of epilepsy. The epilepsy we had chosen to study was Juvenile Myoclonic Epilepsy (JME), or the Syndrome of Janz (named after Dr. Dieter Janz who first described it in 1957 [Janz and Christian, 1957]); Prof. Janz had called it Impulsive Petit Mal.

There were specific reasons for studying the genetics of JME. These include: 1) it is a common form of adolescent-onset seizures that does not show simple Mendelian inheritance, and our interest was in common, complex forms of epilepsy; 2) it had been shown to be highly familial [Tsuboi and Christian, 1973]; 3) Dr. A.V. Delgado-Escueta, who was the director of the Epilepsy Center at the Wadsworth Veterans' Administration Hospital, had, without knowledge of Janz's work, independently identified the syndrome and named it JME (some years after Janz had published his description of the syndrome). Because of his interest in the syndrome, Dr. Delgado-Escueta had identified a number of JME families, which made a linkage analysis feasible.

We typed 24 families for 30(!) protein markers then available throughout the genome. (This was well before the human genome had been sequenced and even before microsatellite markers became available, so our ability to search the genome was limited.) All families were identified through a JME patient, carefully diagnosed according to strict criteria. We also interviewed, collected DNA, and administered EEGs to every cooperating family member and counted as "affected" any family member with a spike-and-wave EEG trait, whether that EEG-positive family member was affected with seizures or had no seizure history. On occasion, a family member admitted to having had jerks. ("Oh, I've had those for years! It's no big deal.") Our analysis yielded a statistically significant indication of linkage of JME to the HLA region of chromosome 6 (6p21) [Greenberg *et al.*, 1988b].

6.2 Replication of the finding

About three years later, Professor Janz in Berlin analyzed his larger number of families and confirmed the linkage to the 6p21 region [Weissbecker *et al.*, 1991]. In that analysis, as in the original analysis, abnormal EEGs found in any family member, affected or not, was also counted as "affected" for the analysis. Because the Berlin data set was larger than our original data set, a subsequent publication was able to further analyze the data, testing the effect of classifying the abnormal EEGs in unaffected family members as "affected" or "unaffected". By performing analyses that changed the classification of family members with an abnormal EEG, but who had no seizures, we tested the hypothesis that the abnormal EEGs in unaffected family members represented a subclinical marker or "endophenotype" of the epilepsy [Durner *et al.*, 1991], i.e., that the abnormal EEG trait was influenced by the same gene(s) as was JME. The analysis found that classifying the EEG-positive family members without frank seizures as "affected" increased the evidence for linkage, and classifying them as "unaffected" reduced the linkage evidence. Because linkage analysis is highly sensitive to correct phenotypic classification (unlike association analysis[2]), the observation that the lod score increased when EEG-positive individuals were classified as "affected" indicated that classification was the one most consistent with the inheritance of the epilepsy in the family, i.e. the same gene influenced both the epilepsy and the EEG trait.

6.3 The relationship of the locus for JME to other IGE syndromes

After these findings were published, some epileptologists speculated that this locus for JME was also responsible for susceptibility to

---

[2]Linkage analysis is sensitive to incorrect phenotype classification because linkage traces genes as they move from one generation to the next. Incorrect phenotype classification (classifying a subject without the phenotype as having the phenotype) has a high probability of inducing a "no coinheritance of marker and phenotype" in the family, thus reducing the evidence in favor of linkage or even turning it to evidence against linkage. An incorrect phenotype classification in an association analysis has much less impact on the final result because the analysis is a tally of "cases" and "controls", not the family. The current belief, that collecting large samples overwhelms the misclassification, can be questioned. Thus, the impact of a single misclassification on findings is much less in an association analysis. On the other hand, linkage has a methodology to detect and compensate for heterogeneity, called the "heterogeneity lod score" (hetlod or Hlod). Association analysis has no such methodology.

other forms of IGE. To answer this question, we collected data on families identified through patients with an adolescent-onset IGE that was not JME (and who had no JME in their families) and performed the same analysis we did with the JME data. (We confined our efforts to the already-identified chromosome 6 region.) In families identified through a patient with adolescent-onset tonic-clonic seizures (but, again, without awakening myoclonic jerks) or through a patient with adolescent-onset absence seizures, we found strong evidence *against* linkage to the chr. 6 locus [Greenberg *et al.*, 1995]. This is important because almost all JME cases we examined came to medical attention not because of the symptom of myoclonic jerks but because these JME patients presented with tonic-clonic seizures or juvenile absence epilepsy. (In those days, JME was not well recognized as a separate epilepsy syndrome. The initial diagnosis of most patients who proved to be JME was usually "grand mal" or "epilepsy with generalized tonic-clonic seizures" (EGTCS) and occasionally "focal epilepsy".) The importance of the evidence showing there is a genetic difference between JME and non-JME IGEs cannot be overstated: What we call IGE (or now genetic generalized epilepsy (GGE)) is a collection of separate conditions with clinical presentations that may differ only slightly from one another (e.g., with/without awakening myoclonus) and with differing, yet likely overlapping, etiologies, some of which will be genetic [Durner *et al.*, 2001a]. The implication of this finding of genetic heterogeneity within IGE (i.e., multiple diseases with similar presentation but different etiologies) is that, without careful diagnosis and symptom classification, finding the genetic contributions to epilepsy syndromes will be difficult because genetic heterogeneity will mask indications of a gene's contribution to the etiology no matter what the method employed to find genetic influences. Recent studies in epilepsy genetics has borne this out (see below).

A later analysis of new Berlin data also showed interesting results [Sander *et al.*, 1997]. The new Berlin data continued to confirm the linkage to chr. 6 but also suggested that there is an ethnic component; families from non-European countries did not show linkage to the region.

6.4 Identification of *BRD2*, more replications, and expansion to endophenotypes

In 2000, after a decade of collecting new IGE data in the New York area, Greenberg *et al.* [2000a] were able to confirm several aspects of previous observations and add new information. 1) The New York data set again confirmed the linkage of JME to chr. 6p21 that had originally been published 12 years previously and had been replicated in the Berlin data analysis. 2) The data confirmed the observation that linkage to 6p21 could be detected only in European-origin families; excluding African-American and Hispanic families from the data increased the evidence for linkage and analysis of those non-European-origin families alone produced evidence against linkage. 3) The new data also showed evidence for *association* of JME with markers in the region of 6p21. What is particularly interesting about that last finding is that, in the case-control association study, we used *non-JME probands* as controls. Thus, this finding was not only the first demonstration of an association of JME in the same region as the linkage, it underscored that JME and the non-JME IGE epilepsy diatheses are different. In order to achieve a statistically significant result using a phenotype in which "controls" differed from cases only in that "controls" had no myoclonic jerks, the genetic bases of the diseases had to be different at that locus. However, while the discovery of association underscored the genetic evidence for the location of the gene, it did not pinpoint the exact location.

To discover the identity of *EJM1*, as the gene was now called, we undertook a detailed SNP analysis. With extensive SNP typing in the HLA region, and the good fortune to have identified two recombinant events (one in our data and one in the published Berlin data), we were able to narrow the candidate region to less than ½ a megabase just distal to the HLA-DP gene. In [Pal *et al.*, 2003], we reported that the evidence pointed to a gene called, at that time, RING3 (for "really interesting new gene") that was later shown to be *BRD2*. At the time, the function of this gene was mostly unknown, but the protein produced by this gene was known to bind histones and was involved with the transcription of DNA to RNA. Eventually, we found that the microsatellite marker for which we first found the association turned out to be in intron2a, in the middle of *BRD2* (see Figure 6.1).

Shortly thereafter, more findings from other laboratories supported *BRD2*'s involvement in epilepsy and epilepsy-related phenomena. Tauer *et al.* [2005] analyzed linkage data from families with photoparoxysmal response (PPR, or photosensitivity), i.e., abnormal EEG responses to light flashes. Their genome-wide linkage scan showed that this trait, like JME, mapped to the chr. 6p21 region. In follow-up work published a year later, the *BRD2* locus was found to be associated with this trait [Lorenz *et al.*, 2006]. Shortly after the Tauer *et al.* and Lorenz *et al.* findings, Cavalleri *et al.* [2007] published a study that illustrated both the heterogeneity within JME and the issue of ethnicity-based confounding. These authors examined association of *BRD2* with JME in five separate populations: English, Irish, German, Australian, and Indian. Both the English and Irish populations not only confirmed association of JME with *BRD2*, but identified a SNP as associated with JME that the Pal *et al.* work had also found, a SNP located in the promoter region of *BRD2* (more details below). The Indian population did not support association with JME, which is not surprising given the evidence that the effect of *BRD2* on JME susceptibility was confined to those of European origin. The Australian population did not find association evidence but, like the United States, Australia is ethnically diverse and without a careful delineation of the backgrounds of the subjects, it is difficult to draw conclusions. The puzzling finding was the German data, which had not only replicated the linkage — twice — but also found both linkage and association of *BRD2* with PPR. It is impossible, in hindsight, to answer the question as to why the German data did not find association when the data set used in the original German study easily found linkage and another subset found both linkage and association (the PPR finding). However, the data had substantially enlarged by collecting families from multiple locations following Dr. Janz's retirement. (Dr. Janz was greatly assisted in his data collection by Dr. Gertrude Beck-Managetta, both were superb epileptologists who have since passed away.) Given the effect of heterogeneity on genetic studies, especially when multiple sites and possible diagnostic variance are taken into account, the difficulty of replication cannot be minimized.

6.5 The difficulties in diagnosis for genetic studies and collecting family data

Our experience in data collection for the IGE project underscores the importance — and difficulty — of careful, consistent, clinical evaluation before including a case/family in the data. While ascertaining families used in the Greenberg *et al.* study, which came mostly from large, U.S., east coast cities, we rejected, based on the medical records alone, about 50% of cases as not meeting criteria even before interviews and EEGs. It must be emphasized that these diagnoses were not necessarily incorrect for treatment purposes but, as shown by subsequent data analysis, JME, as a nosological unit, is a heterogeneous disorder. Just from the linkage data (discussed above), we know that there is heterogeneity based on ethnicity, and subsequent analysis (discussed below) shows further evidence of heterogeneity. (It is important to underscore that diagnosis for treatment is different from diagnosis for genetic studies. In diagnosing for treatment, one determines if the symptoms fit the standard criteria and chooses a treatment appropriate to the diagnosis. If the treatment is successful, the diagnosis is considered "correct." If the treatment is unsuccessful, one reconsiders the diagnosis or changes treatments. To assure reliable results, hypothesis testing in genetic studies has much less leeway.) In our experience, not all physicians diagnose JME the same way, which adds to the data collection problem. For example, we have seen so-called JME patients referred to our study who were given their diagnoses of JME for some of the following reasons: the patient responded to valproic acid; the patient had no jerks but had 4–6 Hz spike and wave on EEG; the patient reported "twitches"; jerks occurred only in response to flashing lights; jerks occurred any time of day (not only or mostly on awakening); and jerks occurred at night in sleep. The first three symptoms on this list are insufficient for a diagnosis of JME. The others *might* indicate JME but would not be correct for a genetic study. If they are *not* JME but are included, then one is introducing heterogeneity and potentially destroying the genetic signal in the data. Also, inclusion of non-Caucasian cases (for our studies) would degrade any genetic signal at *BRD2*. By using a data set with sufficient heterogeneity, one can disprove every gene identification.

6.6 The effect of the "channelopathy hypothesis" on IGE research

Over time, it has proven difficult to identify genes for any common disease. The genes that have been accepted as causing some form of epilepsy have almost all been for epilepsies that are rare and genetically simple (e.g., Dravet's Syndrome, GLUT1-related epilepsy); these have enjoyed the level of replication seen for *BRD2*'s relationship to JME. Of the genetically complex epilepsies, besides JME, only studies of Rolandic epilepsy [Strug *et al.*, 2009] have found as strong linkage and association signals, but even the Rolandic epilepsy data has yet to be replicated independently. The EFHC1 locus on chr. 6p12 [Suzuki *et al.*, 2004] has been independently linkage-replicated [Pinto *et al.*, 2006], but the purportedly seizure-related mutations in *EFHC1* turned out to be common in other populations [Subaran *et al.*, 2014] and genetic association has not been observed [Bai *et al.*, 2009], but it is clear there is *some* gene in the region linked to seizures in Hispanic patients. That gene may or may not be *EFHC1*.

Yet despite the multiple replications of the 6p21 linkage, the multiple replications of the *BRD2* association, the expansion of the phenotype to include photosensitivity and abnormal EEGs, and (as discussed below) the evidence from the mouse model, until recently, *BRD2* has not been included on lists of genes related to epilepsy, for complex, largely unknown reasons.

In the time between the initial discovery of *BRD2*'s relationship to JME (1988, first replication in 1991) and the later replications in linkage and association that occurred after 2000, the channelopathy hypothesis came to dominate thinking about the cause of most epilepsy. The channelopathy hypothesis, which posited that all epilepsy results from mutations in ion channel genes, was promulgated in the late 1990's and was accepted to such an extent that, when an epilepsy-related genetic study found evidence of a seizure-related locus, if a channel gene was not nearby, the region was ignored. (Elsewhere, we have discussed the setbacks to the field from the uncritical acceptance of this hypothesis [Greenberg, 2011; Subaran *et al.*, 2014].) *BRD2* is not a channel gene and so did not fit the then-prevalent paradigm, thus limiting its acceptance as an influence on JME expression.

To add to the problem, since the *BRD2* findings were published, the entire field of human genetics, as well as IGE studies, has gone down a path that we view as limiting approaches to genetic problem-solving, just as the channelopathy hypothesis was limiting for IGE research. Previous emphasis on the importance of phenotype has been discarded and more recent studies have treated IGE as though it were a single disease. This approach is based on the idea that, if enough genomes are SNP-typed or sequenced and used in association studies (Genome-Wide Association Studies, or GWAS), the genes will be found, irrespective of confounders. This belief resembles a cult of "big data" based on GWAS studies of very large samples of cases and controls. In studies of common epilepsies, the yield of this approach has been negligible [Heinzen *et al.*, 2012; Leu *et al.*, 2012; Steffens *et al.*, 2012]. In today's studies of common disease, if an association with a marker is found to be statistically significant, the odds ratio is seldom greater than 1.5, and usually lower [Wray *et al.*, 2008]. These low odds ratios (a measure of the overall "effect" of the gene on the disease) has been interpreted it two ways: 1) Either there are so many genes interacting (the so-called polygenic model) that any given locus identified contributes only a small fraction of the disease risk, which, it is said, explains the low odds ratio (usually thousands of cases and controls are needed to have enough data to detect such a small effect); or, 2) there are a small number of cases in which the gene discovered is *causative* for, or a major contributor to, the disease but leads to a phenotype not distinguishable clinically from the mass of common diseases. Thus, this gene stands out because of its strong effect on a small fraction of the total sample. However, the size of that effect is diluted by the heterogeneity in the entire sample. Thus, without the detailed individual *clinical* information to discover how the disease "caused" by the associated marker may differ clinically from the other disease forms, the subtype of disease leading to the association cannot be separated out. The former (polygenic) explanation holds sway at the moment, despite analyses showing that even the polygenic model cannot explain the low odds ratios seen in GWAS studies [Hodge and Greenberg, 2016]. Thus, genetic heterogeneity, together with ignoring the critical importance of the phenotype, continues to undermine usefulness of the technical strides that have been made in genome sequencing, among other advances in generating genome-related data.

Another recent finding regarding gene searches warrants mention. Santos *et al.* [2017] reviewed reports of genes involved in JME. Fifty studies, almost all of which used a candidate gene approach, provided data on 229 polymorphisms in or near 55 different genes. Of those 55 genes, the authors report that only three held up to scrutiny, rs2029461 SNP in GRM4, rs3743123 in CX36, and the above-mentioned rs3918149 in *BRD2*. This report also raises themes we discuss here and notes that, despite the enormous effort that has gone into finding JME-related loci, few solid results have emerged. However, as we discuss in this report, our extensive results on *BRD2* have proven replicable and led to testable biological hypotheses.

6.7 The JME mouse model: Proving *BRD2* is the gene influencing JME

The accumulated data convinced us that *BRD2* was influencing JME expression. We then asked: How is *BRD2* producing epilepsy susceptibility? The answer could provide a key to understanding the mechanism underlying other forms of IGE as well as JME. Recall, JME presentation is usually not only myoclonic jerks; in fact it is the tonic-clonic seizures that usually cause patients to seek medical attention, even if the jerks begin before these major seizures. In addition, about 30% of JME patients also have absence seizures, so it is likely that knowledge of whatever *BRD2* is doing or not doing in the brain will generate information about the underlying neurological basis of other forms of IGE. Since one of our goals was to determine how *BRD2* influences the brain, we decided to create a mouse model in which one or both *BRD2* alleles were turned off. The mouse model provided some surprising results:

(I) Homozygous null (*Brd2–/–*) (that is, lacking any *Brd2*) mice succumb in utero about day 8–10 of gestation, demonstrating that *Brd2* is an essential gene for viability. *Brd2* null embryos have a nervous system that is highly underdeveloped, with an open neural tube and involuted and disorganized growth, while the other observable organ systems have a more-or-less normal appearance [Gyuris *et al.*, 2009; Shang *et al.*, 2009]. Equally surprising is that, in normal (*Brd2+/+*) embryos at about gestational day 8, the majority of the *Brd2 that* is expressed in the embryo is found in the developing nervous system [Shang *et al.*, 2009]. Whatever *Brd2*'s involvement in promoting epilepsy expression, its function is critical for proper brain maturation.

(II) Heterozygous mice (*Brd2+/–*, lacking one of the two *Brd2* alleles) are normal in appearance and superficially normal in development, behavior, fecundity, cognition, and other measures of health. However, on testing, they have both spontaneous seizures and abnormal EEGs, and are also more susceptible to flurothyl-induced seizures [Velisek *et al.*, 2011] than are wild-type mice. This sensitivity to chemical-induced seizures does not begin until after the onset of puberty, analogous to JME, which shows adolescent onset. There are also marked male-female differences in timing of tonic-clonic seizures, with female mice showing more sensitivity to major seizures than male mice, again similar to JME, in which there is female preponderance [Asadi-Pooya *et al.*, 2015; Camfield *et al.*, 2013; Genton P, 2000; Janz D, 1989; Kleveland and Engelsen, 1998; Pal *et al.*, 2006; Pedersen and Petersen, 1998; Tsuboi and Christian, 1973].

(III) *Brd2+/–* mice also show behaviors that can be viewed as similar to JME patients, who have been reported to have certain behavioral characteristics notable enough to define a "JME personality" [Chachua, 2014; Moschetta *et al.*, 2011]. The mice have normal cognition but show impulsive/aggressive behavior.

(IV) Perhaps most compelling, *Brd2+/–* mice show deficits of GABAergic neurons in specific brain areas that, in normal mice, are related to seizure suppression [Velisek *et al.*, 2011]. Such deficits are also seen in selected other brain regions (e.g., amygdala [Chachua, 2014] but not others (e.g., hippocampus).

From these observations, we infer, first, that lack of *Brd2* produces a mouse with seizure characteristics remarkably similar to JME. Second, the GABAergic system is primarily affected by that lack, with a clear deficit of GABAergic neurons in certain brain regions but not in others. Third, the fast-spiking parvalbumin GABAergic neuron population is affected primarily. The observation that onset of seizure sensitivity only begins after puberty emphasizes the neurodevelopmental aspects of JME and, likely, other IGEs.

While this work is far from complete (e.g, how *does* a deficit of *Brd2* lead to reduced numbers of parvalbumin neurons?) it gives us a starting place for understanding how IGE susceptibility comes about. We infer that, with reduced amounts of BRD2, an entire chain of the developmental process does not go to completion. Recall that a complete absence of *Brd2* leads to brain developmental chaos during embryogenesis. One can easily imagine developmental processes, for which *Brd2* is essential, also applying to other molecules that can subtly disrupt brain development, producing similar deficits and outcomes but different phenotypes. As we have stated elsewhere [Greenberg *et al.*, 1992], all indications are that IGE in general and JME in particular, require *multiple* genetic inputs, that is, are oligogenic conditions. Our first work on JME [Greenberg *et al.*, 1988a] supported the hypothesis that at least two genes need to interact to produce the phenotype. We have evidence that other gene encodes malic enzyme 2 [Durner *et al.*, 2001b; Greenberg *et al.*, 2005; Wang *et al.*, 2019].

6.8 What DNA changes to *BRD2* cause JME susceptibility? The epigenetic hypothesis

When *BRD2* was first identified as a culprit in JME, we believed that mutations would be found in *BRD2*'s exons. Not only did we not find any such mutations. Until recently, there were very few reported mutations anywhere in *BRD2*, no epilepsy-related mutations [Genetic Testing Registry, accessed in December, 2018]. Recently, Maniyar *et al.* [2017] reported that, in the Southern Indian population, three novel missense mutations were found in 2.2% of JME patients after sequencing all 12 exons. No mutations were found in controls. It is noteworthy that, in previous work, *BRD2*'s influence on JME expression appears predominantly in Caucasian patients and, as we discuss below, epigenetic phenomena, rather than exonic mutations, appear to be involved in Caucasian JME patients.

Careful examination of the DNA sequence revealed an alternatively spliced exon between exons two and three, which we designated exon2a [Shang *et al.*, 2011] (Figure 6.1). Exon2a, if present in the mRNA, would induce a stop codon, likely causing no protein to be produced. Remarkably, this alternatively-spliced exon was evolutionarily highly conserved, having the same sequence going back to marsupials, suggesting this piece of DNA was important for the gene to carry out its function. Thus, we considered the presence of this alternatively spliced exon as a possible mechanism for a decrease in *BRD2* expression in human JME patients analogous to the decrease in the mouse model.

We also discovered that, in human DNA, the *intron* between exon2a and exon 3 had a surprising number of variants: there were at least five locations in this intron that were polymorphic. (Among

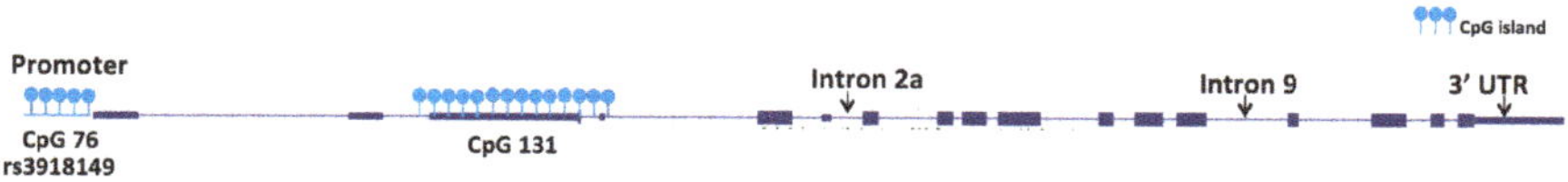

Figure 6.1. Schematic of *BRD2* locus showing positions of CpG islands, SNP and other landmark features.

these variants was the microsatellite marker that was used for the original association study [Greenberg *et al.*, 2000a].) There were 240 possible variant combinations, although only about 20 different combinations were actually identified in approximately 100 JME study subjects in our cohort. This observation suggested that different combinations of variants might influence splicing of exon2a and thus could lead to BRD2 protein reduction. Initial work on this question suggested that different variant combinations did influence the regular-splice:alternative-splice ratio [Shang *et al.*, 2011], but the original findings could not be confirmed. We were not able to detect any differences in mRNA abundance in the different intron2a configurations, although the testing might not have had sufficient sensitivity. Thus, while the possibility that the intronic variants contribute to a reduction of *BRD2* expression cannot be excluded, the evidence we had was not convincing enough.

Eventually, we investigated another possible explanation for *BRD2*'s connection to JME besides exon2a splicing. When we re-examined the evidence for *BRD2* differences in cases and controls we noticed that in both our association study [Pal *et al.*, 2003] and in the Cavalleri *et al.* study [Cavalleri *et al.*, 2007], there was a SNP associated with JME, *rs3918149*. This SNP is located in (one of) *BRD2*'s promoter regions. Furthermore, it is in a CpG island, CpG76, a region that can be epigenetically modified by methylation. (Methylation can cause gene silencing.) We therefore investigated methylation of the region using lymphoblasts collected from JME patients and family members. Figure 6.1 shows the structure of the *BRD2* DNA and the positions of the gene structure elements noted above.

We compared methylation of the CpG76 island in the promoter region of *BRD2* in three groups: 1) JME patients vs unaffected family members; 2) JME vs non-JME forms of IGE (the adolescent onset non-JME IGEs included epilepsy with tonic-clonic seizures and adolescent-onset absence); 3) Caucasian JME patients vs non-Caucasian JME patients (non-Caucasians included African-American, Hispanic, or mixed ancestry). In addition, we compared methylation levels in JME patients vs. unaffected family members in families showing

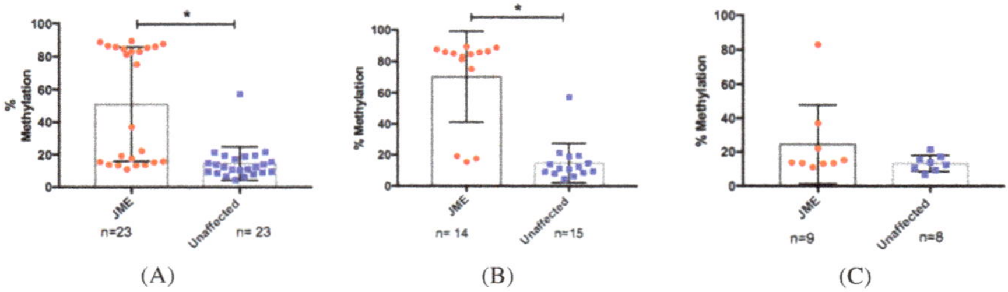

Figure 6.2. Status of DNA methylation of the *BRD2* promoter in human families identified through a JME patient.

2A-C: Box plots showing CpG76 methylation levels in Caucasian JME patients and unaffected family members (A), Caucasian JME patients with positive evidence of linkage to *BRD2* and unaffected family members (B) and Caucasian JME patients without positive linkage evidence to *BRD2* and unaffected family members (C). Data represented as means ± SEM. * indicates significant comparison.

evidence of linkage vs. families that showed evidence against linkage [Greenberg *et al.*, 2000b].

The results [Pathak *et al.*, 2018] were striking. The methylation of the CpG76 island in the promoter region correlated with the expression of JME in about half of Caucasian JME patients compared to methylation levels in unaffected family members as controls (Figure 6.2A). Furthermore, the correlation was even stronger when only probands from families that also showed positive evidence of linkage (i.e., cosegregation of JME with markers in the region) were compared with those families showing no such correlation (Figures 6.2B & 6.2C).

Among Caucasian JME patients, there is a clear bimodal distribution in methylation levels, with slightly more than half of the patients showing high levels of methylation and the remainder showing methylation levels similar to unaffected family members (Figure 6.2A). Furthermore, those showing methylation come overwhelmingly from families showing linkage of *BRD2*-region markers to JME (Figure 6.2B); those with no methylation come from families with evidence against linkage of JME to *BRD2*-region markers (Figure 6.2C).

At least as striking are the results for non-JME forms of adolescent-onset IGEs (Figure 6.3A) and for JME families of non-Caucasian

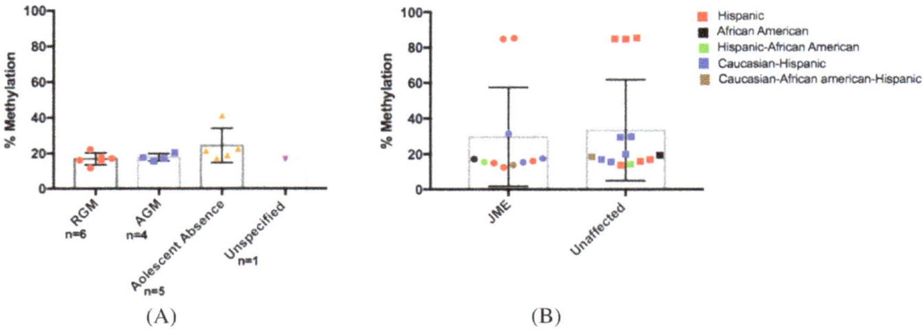

Figure 6.3. DNA methylation analysis of CpG76 by pyrosequencing on DNA from lymphoblastoid cells in Caucasian non-JME Idiopathic Generalized Epilepsy patients (A) and non-Caucasian JME families (B).

origin (Figure 6.3B). None of the non-JME IGE patients have methylation levels comparable to what we see in the linked JME patients. In the ethnicity difference graph, non-Caucausian JME patients are compared with unaffected family members, showing little difference between the two groups. It is still noteworthy that there are five subjects, two classified as JME and three unaffected family members (all Hispanic) who have high methylation levels, further emphasizing why the issue of heterogeneity is so critical in studies of IGE. (The EEG status of the unaffected family members with high methylation levels is unknown.)

6.9 Implications of *BRD2* findings for studies of IGE

These striking results strengthen all the previous findings about the ethnic specificity of *BRD2*-related JME [Cavalleri *et al.*, 2007; Greenberg *et al.*, 2000b; Sander, 1996], and confirm that JME among Caucasians is a genetically distinct form of IGE, despite the similarity of its clinical presentation to other forms of adolescent-onset IGEs [Greenberg *et al.*, 1995]. The results also emphasize that reducing heterogeneity and obtaining meticulous demographic data (especially family data) are critical to solving the origins of IGE.

What are the implications of these issues for studies of IGE?

First and perhaps foremost, these results show that just looking for mutations in exons, as has been the current approach, will not reveal the subtle changes in gene expression that may be responsible for IGE susceptibility. As argued elsewhere [Greenberg, 2011], subtle changes in gene control regions (e.g., introns, promoters, siRNA, etc.) in multiple genes are likely to be involved in common disease expression in general and IGE in particular. The failure of simple exon sequencing and association studies to yield useful information about IGE should be sufficient to show that deeper thought about, and understanding of, the genome is essential, understanding that goes beyond mere sequence.

Second, these results came from *family* studies and studies of *inheritance*. The current general approach to common disease is to look for *association* of disease and markers on hundreds, thousands, or tens of thousands of cases and controls but without having collected detailed clinical information. Without such information, it is nearly impossible to determine which phenotype, or combination of phenotypic traits, is the one influenced by the proposed marker/gene. One is left with a statistically significant p value pointing to a locus with a relative risk of, say, 1.1; that is, an indication of *something* in the genomic region that, with a large enough sample, has a detectable influence on disease expression but an influence that is miniscule and tells little about what is causing the disease. Even more difficult, such results provide little clue about how to use that information. What kind of changes can one look for in laboratory studies on a gene that has such a small influence on the phenotype? Furthermore, recent practice in IGE genetic studies has been to simply lump all IGEs together, treating them as one disease. Such an approach, which ignores the problem of heterogeneity and its effect on genetic studies, makes finding genetic loci for IGE difficult and, at least as critical, almost impossible to use as a starting point to understand the underlying neuronal/chemical/structural changes leading to seizure susceptibility.

One advantage of linkage analysis is that it is relatively insensitive to genes of minor effect ("genes of minor influence" refers to those that raise the relative risk only to approximately 2.0 or less [Greenberg,

1993]). Thus, when a solid linkage result is identified, it is fairly certain that, whichever gene in the linkage region is influencing the trait, it represents a strong influence on the phenotype and is therefore worth pursuing to find out how it contributes to disease. Association analysis is much more sensitive than linkage to minor effects and yields multiple gene indications but, as noted above, the phenotypic information required to separate important from unimportant effects is usually not available (note the 259 proposed JME genes examined by Santos *et al.* [2017]) because of the sample sizes involved. The larger the data set, the easier it is to detect smaller and smaller effects, i.e. obtain highly significant p values, but statistical significance is not the same as biological significance. This is especially true for common diseases such as IGE, in which heterogeneity, difficult phenotyping, and multiple genes are involved. Even genes with proven mendelian inheritance can require decades of work to determine both *how* they cause disease *and* understanding of the disease mechanism, knowledge required to design effective interventions. Association analyses that yield odds ratios barely above 1.0 suggest that it will be difficult to find out what the gene does but, even worse, that the follow-up work is likely of uncertain relevance to the common disease. When working with human data, as opposed to mouse data, there is also the question of which subjects to include in a follow-up, since, in an association analysis yielding low odds ratios, only a fraction of the affected carriers of the associated marker will have the relevant disease genotype and a large number, although affected, will be carriers of the associated marker only by chance. Transgenic mouse models can be created using candidate genes in the region, but these are expensive and there is no guarantee that the mouse will reflect the human disease process.

As this summary of the work on *BRD2* and epilepsy shows, even having a convincing, replicated linkage, population, association, and even mouse model evidence pointing to a gene, provides no certainty that there will be exonic mutations. Our work on exon2a (an exon that, when taken together with the large number of variants in the neighboring intron 2a, appears to lead to nonsense mediated decay) led us to devote resources to investigating the effects of those intronic variant configurations on *BRD2* expression. Only when those results proved inconclusive in our hands did we turn to examining the promoter region, which harbored a JME associated SNP. This led us to note the CpG island and the methylation differences quoted in this report. But, had we not been able to separate the different strata (linked vs. unlinked; JME vs. non-JME IGE; Caucasian JME vs. non-Caucasian) and examine them separately, we would not have had any clue about the possible involvement of epigenetic effects on JME expression.

References

Asadi-Pooya, A.A., Hashemzehi, Z., and Emami, M. (2015). Epidemiology and clinical manifestations of juvenile myoclonic epilepsy (JME) in Iran, *Neurol. Sci.*, 36, 713–716.

Bai, D., Bailey, J.N., Duron, R.M., Alonso, M.E., Medina, M.T., Martinez-Juarez, I.E., Suzuki, T., Machado-Salas, J., Ramos-Ramirez, R., Tanaka, M., Ortega, R.H., Lopez-Ruiz, M., Rasmussen, A., Ochoa, A., Jara-Prado, A., Yamakawa, K., and Delgado-Escueta, A.V. (2009). DNA variants in coding region of EFHC1: SNPs do not associate with juvenile myoclonic epilepsy, *Epilepsia*, 50, 1184–1190.

Camfield, C.S., Striano, P., and Camfield, P.R. (2013). Epidemiology of juvenile myoclonic epilepsy. *Epilepsy Behav.*, 28 Suppl 1, S15–17.

Cavalleri, G.L., Walley, N.M., Soranzo, N., Mulley, J., Doherty, C.P., Kapoor, A., Depondt, C., Lynch, J.M., Scheffer, I.E., Heils, A., Gehrmann, A., Kinirons, P., Gandhi, S., Satishchandra, P., Wood, N.W., Anand, A., Sander, T., Berkovic, S.F., Delanty, N., Goldstein, D.B., and Sisodiya, S.M. (2007). A Multicenter Study of BRD2 as a Risk Factor for Juvenile Myoclonic Epilepsy, *Epilepsia*, 48, 706–712.

Chachua, T., Goletiani, C., Maglakelidze, G., Sidyelyeva, G., Daniel, M., Morris, M., Miller, J., Shang, E., Wolgemuth, D., Greenberg, D.A., Velíšková, J., Velíšek, L. (2014). Sex-specific behavioral traits in the Brd2 mouse model of Juvenile Myoclonic Epilepsy, *Genes Brain Behav.*, 13, 702–712.

Durner, M., Keddache, M.A., Tomasini, L., Shinnar, S., Resor, S.R., Cohen, J., Harden, C., Moshe, S.L., Rosenbaum, D., Kang, H., Ballaban-Gil, K., Hertz, S., Labar, D.R., Luciano, D., Wallace, S., Yohai, D., Klotz, I., Dicker, E., and Greenberg, D.A. (2001a). Genome scan of idiopathic generalized epilepsy: evidence for major susceptibility gene and modifying genes influencing the seizure type, *Ann. Neurol.*, 49, 328–335.

Durner, M., Keddache, M.A., Tomasini, L., Shinnar, S., Resor, S.R., Cohen, J., Harden, C., Moshe, S.L., Rosenbaum, D., Kang, H., Ballaban-Gill, K., Hertz, S., Labar, D.R., Luciano, D., Wallace, S., Yohai, D., Klotz, I., Dicker, D., and Greenberg, D.A. (2001b). Genome scan of idiopathic generalised epilepsy: evidence for major susceptibility gene and modifying genes influencing the seizure type, *Ann. Neurol.*, 49, 328–335.

Durner, M., Sander, T., Greenberg, D.A., Johnson, K., Beck-Mannagetta, G., and Janz, D. (1991). Localization of idiopathic generalized epilepsy on chromosome 6p in families of juvenile myoclonic epilepsy patients, *Neurology*, 41, 1651–1655.

Genton, P., Thomas P. (2000). Juvenile myoclonic epilepsy today: current definition and limits. In *Juvenile Myoclonic Epilepsy: The Janz Syndrome*, Schmitz B., Sander T., eds. (Petersfield, UK: Wright Biomedical Publishing Ltd), pp. 12–32.

Greenberg, D.A. (1993). Linkage analysis of "necessary" disease loci versus "susceptibility" loci, *Am. J. Hum. Genet.*, 52, 135–143.

Greenberg, D.A., Cayanis, E., Strug, L., Marathe, S., Durner, M., Pal, D.K., Alvin, G.B., Klotz, I., Dicker, E., Shinnar, S., Bromfield, E.B., Resor, S., Cohen, J., Moshe, S.L., Harden, C., and Kang, H. (2005). Malic enzyme 2 may underlie susceptibility to adolescent-onset idiopathic generalized epilepsy, *Am. J. Hum. Genet.*, 76, 139–146.

Greenberg, D.A., Delgado-Escueta, A.V., Maldonado, H.M., and Widelitz, H. (1988a). Segregation analysis of juvenile myoclonic epilepsy, *Genet. Epidemiol.*, 5, 81–94.

Greenberg, D.A., Delgado-Escueta, A.V., Widelitz, H., Sparkes, R.S., Treiman, L., Maldonado, H.M., Park, M.S., and Terasaki, P.I. (1988b). Juvenile myoclonic epilepsy (JME) may be linked to the BF and HLA loci on human chromosome 6, *Am. J. Med. Genet.*, 31, 185–192.

Greenberg, D.A., Durner, M., and Delgado-Escueta, A.V. (1992). Evidence for multiple gene loci in the expression of the common generalized epilepsies, *Neurology*, 42, 56–62.

Greenberg, D.A., Durner, M., Keddache, M., Shinnar, S., Resor, S.R., Moshe, S.L., Rosenbaum, D., Cohen, J., Harden, C., Kang, H., Wallace, S., Luciano, D., Ballaban-Gil, K., Tomasini, L., Zhou, G., Klotz, I., and Dicker, E. (2000a). Reproducibility and complications in gene searches: linkage on chromosome 6, heterogeneity, association and maternal inheritance in juvenile myoclonic epilepsy, *Am. J. Hum. Genet.*, 66, 508–516.

Greenberg, D.A., Durner, M., Keddache, M., Shinnar, S., Resor, S.R., Moshe, S.L., Rosenbaum, D., Cohen, J., Harden, C., Kang, H., Wallace, S., Luciano, D., Ballaban-Gil, K., Tomasini, L., Zhou, G., Klotz, I., and Dicker, E. (2000b). Reproducibility and complications in gene searches: linkage on chromosome 6, heterogeneity, association, and maternal inheritance in juvenile myoclonic epilepsy, *Am. J. Hum. Genet.*, 66, 508–516.

Greenberg, D.A., Durner, M., Resor, S., Rosenbaum, D., and Shinnar, S. (1995). The genetics of idiopathic generalized epilepsies of adolescent onset: differences between juvenile myoclonic epilepsy and epilepsy with random grand mal and with awakening grand mal, *Neurology*, 45, 942–946.

Greenberg, D.A. and Subaran, R. (2011). Blinders, phenotype, and fashionable genetic analysis: a critical examination of the current state of epilepsy genetic studies, *Epilepsia*, 52, 1–9.

Gyuris, A., Donovan, D.J., Seymour, K.A., Lovasco, L.A., Smilowitz, N.R., Halperin, A.L., Klysik, J.E., and Freiman, R.N. (2009). The chromatin-targeting protein Brd2 is required for neural tube closure and embryogenesis, *Biochim. Biophys. Acta*, 1789, 413–421.

Heinzen, E.L., Depondt, C., Cavalleri, G.L., Ruzzo, E.K., Walley, N.M., Need, A.C., Ge, D., He, M., Cirulli, E.T., Zhao, Q., Cronin, K.D., Gumbs, C.E., Campbell, C.R., Hong, L.K., Maia, J.M., Shianna, K.V., McCormack, M., Radtke, R.A., O'Conner, G.D., Mikati, M.A., Gallentine, W.B., Husain, A.M., Sinha, S.R., Chinthapalli, K., Puranam, R.S., McNamara, J.O., Ottman, R., Sisodiya, S.M., Delanty, N., and Goldstein, D.B. (2012). Exome sequencing followed by large-scale genotyping fails to identify single rare variants of large effect in idiopathic generalized epilepsy, *Am. J. Hum. Genet.*, 91, 293–302.

Hodge, S.E., and Greenberg, D.A. (2016). How Can We Explain Very Low Odds Ratios in GWAS? I. Polygenic Models, *Hum. Hered.*, 81, 173–180.

Janz, D. (1997). The idiopathic generalised epilepsies of adolescence with childhood and juvenile age of onset, *Epilepsia*, 38, 4–11.

Janz D, B.-M.G., Pantazis, G. (1989). Family studies on the genetics of juvenile myoclonic epilepsy (epilepsy with impulsive petit-mal). In Genetics of the Epilepsies., A.V. Beck-Mannagetta G, Janz D, ed. (Berlin: Springer), pp. 43–66.

Janz, D. and Christian, W. (1957). Impulsiv-petit mal, *Dtsch. Z. Nervenheilk.*, 176, 348–386.

Kasteleijn-Nolst Trenite, D.G., Schmitz, B., Janz, D., Delgado-Escueta, A.V., Thomas, P., Hirsch, E., Lerche, H., Camfield, C., Baykan, B., Feucht, M., Martinez-Juarez, I.E., Duron, R.M., Medina, M.T., Rubboli, G., Jerney, J., Hermann, B., Yacubian, E., Koutroumanidis, M., Stephani, U., Salas-Puig, J., Reed, R.C., Woermann, F., Wandschneider, B., Bureau, M., Gambardella, A., Koepp, M.J., Gelisse, P., Gurses, C., Crespel, A., Nguyen-Michel, V.H., Ferlazzo, E., Grisar, T., Helbig, I., Koeleman, B.P., Striano, P., Trimble, M., Buono, R., Cossette, P., Represa, A., Dravet, C., Serafini, A., Berglund, I.S., Sisodiya, S.M., Yamakawa, K., and Genton, P. (2013). Consensus on diagnosis and management of JME: From founder's observations to current trends, *Epilepsy Behav.*, 28 Suppl 1, S87–90.

Kleveland, G. and Engelsen, B.A. (1998). Juvenile myoclonic epilepsy: clinical characteristics, treatment and prognosis in a Norwegian population of patients, *Seizure*, 7, 31–38.

Leu, C., de Kovel, C.G., Zara, F., Striano, P., Pezzella, M., Robbiano, A., Bianchi, A., Bisulli, F., Coppola, A., Giallonardo, A.T., Beccaria, F., Trenite, D.K., Lindhout, D., Gaus, V., Schmitz, B., Janz, D., Weber, Y.G., Becker, F., Lerche, H., Kleefuss-Lie, A.A., Hallman, K., Kunz, W.S., Elger, C.E., Muhle, H., Stephani, U., Moller, R.S., Hjalgrim, H., Mullen, S., Scheffer, I.E., Berkovic, S.F., Everett, K.V., Gardiner, M.R., Marini, C., Guerrini, R., Lehesjoki, A.E., Siren, A., Nabbout, R., Baulac, S., Leguern, E., Serratosa, J.M., Rosenow, F., Feucht, M., Unterberger, I., Covanis, A., Suls, A., Weckhuysen, S., Kaneva, R., Caglayan, H., Turkdogan, D., Baykan, B., Bebek, N., Ozbek, U., Hempelmann, A., Schulz, H., Ruschendorf, F., Trucks, H., Nurnberg, P., Avanzini, G., Koeleman, B.P., and Sander, T. (2012). Genome-wide linkage meta-analysis identifies susceptibility loci at 2q34 and 13q31.3 for genetic generalized epilepsies, *Epilepsia*, 53, 308–318.

Lorenz, S., Taylor, K.P., Gehrmann, A., Becker, T., Muhle, H., Gresch, M., Tauer, U., Sander, T., and Stephani, U. (2006). Association of BRD2 polymorphisms with photoparoxysmal response, *Neurosci. Lett.*, 400, 135–139.

Maniyar, R.Z., Dosi, M.A., Parveen Jahan, B.N. Umarji, Shivannaryan, Parthansaradhi G., Syed Muneer. (2017). Novel missense mutations in BRD2 gene of JME patients: A study from South India. *Int. J. Med. Health Res.*, 3(5), 5.

Moschetta, S., Fiore, L.A., Fuentes, D., Gois, J., and Valente, K.D. (2011). Personality traits in patients with juvenile myoclonic epilepsy, *Epilepsy Behav.*, 21, 473–477.

Pal, D.K., Durner, M., Klotz, I., Dicker, E., Shinnar, S., Resor, S., Cohen, J., Harden, C., Moshe, S.L., Ballaban-Gill, K., Bromfield, E.B., and Greenberg, D.A. (2006). Complex inheritance and parent-of-origin effect in juvenile myoclonic epilepsy, *Brain Dev.*, 28, 92–98.

Pal, D.K., Evgrafov, O.V., Tabares, P., Zhang, F., Durner, M., and Greenberg, D.A. (2003). BRD2 (RING3) is a probable major susceptibility gene for common juvenile myoclonic epilepsy, *Am. J. Hum. Genet.*, 73, 261–270.

Pathak, S., Miller, J., Morris, E.C., Stewart, W.C.L., Greenberg, D.A. (2018) DNA methylation of the BRD2 promoter is associated with juvenile myoclonic epilepsy in Caucasians. *Epilepsia*, 59, 1011–1019.

Pavlovic, M., Jovic, N., and Pekmezovic, T. (2011). Antiepileptic drugs withdrawal in patients with idiopathic generalized epilepsy, *Seizure*, 20, 520–525.

Pedersen, S.B. and Petersen, K.A. (1998). Juvenile myoclonic epilepsy: clinical and EEG features, *Acta Neurol. Scand.*, 97, 160–163.

Pinto, D., Louwaars, S., Westland, B., Volkers, L., de Haan, G.J., Trenite, D.G., Lindhout, D., and Koeleman, B.P. (2006). Heterogeneity at the JME 6p11-12 locus: absence of mutations in the EFHC1 gene in linked Dutch families, *Epilepsia*, 47, 1743–1746.

Sander, T. (1996). The genetics of idiopathic generalized epilepsy: implications for the understanding of its aetiology, *Mol. Med. Today*, 2, 173–180.

Sander, T., Bockenkamp, B., Hildmann, T., Blasczyk, R., Kretz, R., Wienker, T.F., Volz, A., Schmitz, B., Beck-Mannagetta, G., Riess, O., Epplen, J.T., Janz, D., and Ziegler, A. (1997). Refined mapping of the epilepsy susceptibility locus EJM1 on chromosome 6, *Neurology*, 49, 842–847.

Santos, B.P.D., Marinho, C.R.M., Marques, T., Angelo, L.K.G., Malta, M., Duzzioni, M., Castro, O.W., Leite, J.P., Barbosa, F.T., and Gitai, D.L.G. (2017). Genetic susceptibility in Juvenile Myoclonic Epilepsy: Systematic review of genetic association studies, *PLoS One*, 12, e0179629.

Shang, E., Cui, Q., Wang, X., Beseler, C., Greenberg, D.A., and Wolgemuth, D.J. (2011). The bromodomain-containing gene BRD2 is regulated at transcription, splicing, and translation levels, *J. Cell Biochem.*, 112, 2784–2793.

Shang, E., Wang, X., Wen, D., Greenberg, D.A., and Wolgemuth, D.J. (2009). Double bromodomain-containing gene Brd2 is essential for embryonic development in mouse, *Dev. Dyn.*, 238, 908–917.

Steffens, M., Leu, C., Ruppert, A.K., Zara, F., Striano, P., Robbiano, A., Capovilla, G., Tinuper, P., Gambardella, A., Bianchi, A., La Neve, A., Crichiutti, G., de Kovel, C.G., Kasteleijn-Nolst Trenite, D., de Haan, G.J., Lindhout, D., Gaus, V., Schmitz, B., Janz, D., Weber, Y.G., Becker, F., Lerche, H., Steinhoff, B.J., Kleefuss-Lie, A.A., Kunz, W.S., Surges, R., Elger, C.E., Muhle, H., von Spiczak, S., Ostertag, P., Helbig, I., Stephani, U., Moller, R.S., Hjalgrim, H., Dibbens, L.M., Bellows, S., Oliver, K., Mullen, S., Scheffer, I.E., Berkovic, S.F., Everett, K.V., Gardiner, M.R., Marini, C., Guerrini, R., Lehesjoki, A.E., Siren, A., Guipponi, M., Malafosse, A., Thomas, P., Nabbout, R., Baulac, S., Leguern, E., Guerrero, R., Serratosa, J.M., Reif, P.S., Rosenow, F., Morzinger, M., Feucht, M., Zimprich, F., Kapser, C., Schankin, C.J., Suls, A., Smets, K., De Jonghe, P., Jordanova, A., Caglayan, H., Yapici, Z., Yalcin, D.A., Baykan, B., Bebek, N., Ozbek, U., Gieger, C., Wichmann, H.E., Balschun, T., Ellinghaus, D., Franke, A., Meesters, C., Becker, T., Wienker, T.F., Hempelmann, A., Schulz, H., Ruschendorf, F., Leber, M., Pauck, S.M., Trucks, H., Toliat, M.R., Nurnberg, P., Avanzini, G., Koeleman, B.P., and Sander, T. (2012). Genome-wide association analysis of genetic generalized epilepsies implicates susceptibility loci at 1q43, 2p16.1, 2q22.3 and 17q21.32, *Hum. Mol. Genet.*, 21, 5359–5372.

Strug, L.J., Clarke, T., Chiang, T., Chien, M., Baskurt, Z., Li, W., Dorfman, R., Bali, B., Wirrell, E., Kugler, S.L., Mandelbaum, D.E., Wolf, S.M., McGoldrick, P., Hardison, H., Novotny, E.J., Ju, J., Greenberg, D.A., Russo, J.J., and Pal, D.K. (2009). Centrotemporal sharp wave EEG trait in rolandic epilepsy maps to Elongator Protein Complex 4 (ELP4), *Eur. J. Hum. Genet.*, 17, 1171–1181.

Subaran, R.L., Conte, J.M., Stewart, W.C., and Greenberg, D.A. (2014). Pathogenic EFHC1 mutations are tolerated in healthy individuals dependent on reported ancestry, *Epilepsia*, 56, 188–194.

Suzuki, T., Delgado-Escueta, A.V., Aguan, K., Alonso, M.E., Shi, J., Hara, Y., Nishida, M., Numata, T., Medina, M.T., Takeuchi, T., Morita, R., Bai, D., Ganesh, S., Sugimoto, Y., Inazawa, J., Bailey, J.N., Ochoa, A., Jara-Prado, A., Rasmussen, A., Ramos-Peek, J., Cordova, S., Rubio-Donnadieu, F., Inoue, Y., Osawa, M., Kaneko, S., Oguni, H., Mori, Y., and Yamakawa,

K. (2004). Mutations in EFHC1 cause juvenile myoclonic epilepsy, *Nat. Genet.*, 36, 842–849.

Tauer, U., Lorenz, S., Lenzen, K.P., Heils, A., Muhle, H., Gresch, M., Neubauer, B.A., Waltz, S., Rudolf, G., Mattheisen, M., Strauch, K., Nurnberg, P., Schmitz, B., Stephani, U., and Sander, T. (2005). Genetic dissection of photosensitivity and its relation to idiopathic generalized epilepsy, *Ann. Neurol.*, 57, 866–873.

Tsuboi, T. and Christian, W. (1973). On the genetics of primary generalized epilepsy with sporadic myoclonias of impulsive petit mal. A clinical and electroencephalographic study of 399 probands, *Humangenetik*, 19, 155–182.

Velíšek, L., Shang, E., Velíšková, J., Chachua, T., Macchiarulo, S., Maglakelidze, G., Wolgemuth, D.J., and Greenberg, D.A. (2011). GABAergic neuron deficit as an idiopathic generalized epilepsy mechanism: the role of BRD2 haploinsufficiency in juvenile myoclonic epilepsy, *PloS One*, 6, e23656.

Wang, M., Greenberg, D.A., Stewart, C.L.S. (2019). Replication, reanalysis, and gene expression: *ME2* and genetic generalized epilepsy, *Epilepsia* (in press).

Weissbecker, K.A., Durner, M., Janz, D., Scaramelli, A., Sparkes, R.S., and Spence, M.A. (1991). Confirmation of linkage between juvenile myoclonic epilepsy locus and the HLA region of chromosome 6, *Am. J. Med. Genet.*, 38, 32–36.

Wray, N.R., Goddard, M.E., and Visscher, P.M. (2008). Prediction of individual genetic risk of complex disease, *Curr. Opin. Genet. Dev.*, 18, 257–263.

Chapter 7

Epigenetics and Epilepsy in the Developing Brain

Detlev Boison, PhD

Legacy Research Institute, Portland, OR 97232, USA
Department of Neurology, Oregon Health and Science University, Portland, OR 97239, USA
Department of Neuroscience, Washington State University, Vancouver, WA 98686, USA

7.1 Introduction

Because genetics play an important role in developmental epilepsies (see preceding chapter) it is an implicit conclusion that epigenetic changes, which may affect the expression of the same 'epilepsy genes', likewise contribute to or modify the development of epilepsy. Unlike genetic mutations, which are most frequently inherited, epigenetic changes are acquired and potentially reversible through therapeutic intervention, even if carried on to offspring. The role of epigenetics in the epilepsies is a relatively new research area that contributes to our understanding of epileptogenic processes during brain development and in adulthood and offers hope for novel disease-modifying therapeutic interventions.

7.2 Epigenetics

Epigenetic gene regulation is mediated by chemical modifications of histones and DNA, such as histone methylation, histone acetylation, and DNA methylation. In addition, gene expression is under the control of non-coding RNAs. Those epigenetic modifications depend on enzyme reactions that catalyze the exchange of methyl groups or acetyl groups. The underlying biochemistry of epigenetic gene regulation is relatively simple and directly couples epigenetic changes to metabolism and the availability of methyl- or acetyl- group transferring metabolites, which in turn are influenced by environmental and dietary factors. Through those mechanisms, the genome can adapt rapidly to environmental changes. From an evolutionary perspective it is highly likely that epigenetic mechanisms evolved first as a rapid and efficient strategy to regulate gene expression globally [Boison, 2016]. This is because chemical modifications of DNA or histones are simple, reversible, and adaptable to environmental and energetic needs. Transcription factors that require a sophisticated network of G-protein coupled receptors and protein kinase pathways likely evolved much later in order to fine tune a preexisting primordial epigenetic system for gene regulation. Therefore, it is not surprising that this evolutionarily ancient epigenetic control system uniquely links metabolism with disease [Kaelin and McKnight, 2013] and thereby is of crucial importance for our understanding of normal physiological processes such as development and aging. On the other hand, maladaptive epigenetic changes contribute to a wide range of pathologies including cancer, epilepsy, and developmental disorders [Kinnaird *et al.*, 2016; Qureshi and Mehler, 2010b, 2014a, c].

7.3 Developmental and environmental factors that influence epigenetic signatures

As outlined above, the epigenetic regulatory system is designed to act as a rheostat to adjust physiological responses to changes in energy homeostasis or environmental factors. The following paragraphs describe the role of epigenetic mechanisms in brain development and known factors that influence epigenetic signatures.

7.3.1 *The epigenetics of brain development and function*

DNA methylation introduces a fundamental epigenetic barrier that guides and restricts developmental differentiation; thereby, epigenetic control of gene expression is essential for the generation of a multitude of cell and tissue types derived from a single fertilized egg. Reprogramming of epigenetic marks is of critical importance for many developmental processes. To reset the epigenome for totipotency, primordial germ cells undergo sequential epigenetic changes and genome wide demethylation [Hajkova *et al.*, 2010; Surani *et al.*, 2007]. However, certain genes, e.g. those that are required for neocortical development, have a late phase of reprogramming that occurs in the postnatal period [Tuesta and Zhang, 2014]. Therefore it is essential that cortical neurons maintain the ability to reprogram by demethylation/methylation cycles throughout adult life. Demethylation mediated through the enzyme Tet1 is associated with hippocampal learning and memory and adult neurogenesis [Colquitt *et al.*, 2013; Levenson *et al.*, 2006]. In line with those findings, the blockade of DNA methyltransferases (DNMT) impairs hippocampal long-term potentiation associated with altered DNA methylation in the promoter regions of Reelin and brain-derived neurotrophic factor (BDNF) [Levenson *et al.*, 2006]. Tet-mediated demethylation is prominently active in the brain and promotes DNA demethylation in the adult brain at activity-dependent hippocampal synapses [Kaas *et al.*, 2013]. Tight control of epigenetic processes is therefore crucial for normal brain development and function. Disruption of those mechanisms causes neurodevelopmental defects such as those found in Rett syndrome [Amir *et al.*, 1999], which is a prime example of an epigenetic disease. Dysfunction of MeCP2, a methylated DNA binding protein and transcriptional repressor, triggers Rett syndrome and some other forms of autism spectrum disorder [Cheng and Qiu, 2014]. Because various forms of prenatal stress are considered to be potent causative factors for the development of autism [Gardener *et al.*, 2011; Kolevzon *et al.*, 2007; Patterson, 2009], epigenetic alterations are obvious candidate mechanisms for the spectrum of autism-like and related developmental disorders. Because of the tight association between epigenetic changes and neurodevelopmental aberration, it is essential to explore mechanisms that impact on epigenetic changes and guide normal brain development.

7.3.2 *Environmental factors*

There is a strong association between environmental factors that influence both neurodevelopmental disorders and epigenetic changes, though causative mechanisms have not yet been delineated. Maternal immune activation (MIA), as caused by viral or bacterial infection during pregnancy, is widely considered a risk factor for the development of schizophrenia, autism, or developmental epilepsy in offspring [Estes and McAllister, 2016]. The timing appears to be instrumental for determining the nature and severity of the outcomes [Meyer, 2014] with mid-gestational time-points favoring the development of schizophrenia and later time points the development of autism spectrum disorder or developmental epilepsies [Mazarati *et al.*, 2017; Meyer, 2014; Pineda *et al.*, 2013; Washington *et al.*, 2015].

Sleep affects epigenetic functions, which in turn affect sleep and chronobiology [Qureshi and Mehler, 2014b]. Because many forms of epilepsy have distinct circadian patterns, particularly in children [Gurkas *et al.*, 2016; Ramgopal *et al.*, 2014; Ramgopal *et al.*, 2012], it is tempting to speculate that epigenetic mechanisms contribute to circadian patterns of seizure activity in children.

7.3.3 *Diet*

The interplay between diet and epigenetic outcome is well established and based largely on studies on diet-epigenome interactions in cancer [Mayne *et al.*, 2016]. Therefore, the phrase "you are what you eat" gets new meaning in the sense that diet regulates the expression of genes through epigenetic mechanisms. Of particular interest are high-fat, low-carbohydrate ketogenic diets (KDs) that are highly effective in the treatment of refractory seizures in the pediatric population [Freeman *et al.*, 2009; Kossoff and Rho, 2009; Kossoff *et al.*, 2009; Stafstrom, 2004; Stafstrom and Rho, 2012]. KD therapy enhances the production of two epigenetic modulators: beta-hydroxybutyrate, a potent histone deacetylase (HDAC) inhibitor [Shimazu *et al.*, 2013] and adenosine [Lusardi *et al.*, 2015; Masino *et al.*, 2011]. In line with this mechanism of action, and as will be discussed in more detail later, KD therapy not only suppresses seizures, but also exerts disease modifying effects in epilepsy, supporting the conclusion that epigenetic mechanisms might be involved.

7.3.4 *Adenosine*

The purine ribonucleoside adenosine is an evolutionary ancient metabolite with multiple functions [Boison, 2015, 2016; Park and Gupta, 2013]. As structural component of both ATP and RNA (including poly-A tails of messenger RNAs), it assumed an early evolutionary role acting as a rheostat to control energy homeostasis. Therefore, under conditions during which energy needs exceed energy supply, adenosine levels rise and dampen activities that consume energy. Being a 'retaliatory metabolite' [Newby, 1984], adenosine also assumed an early evolutionary role as regulator of gene expression through epigenetic mechanisms [Boison, 2016]. Adenosine receptors arose much later to further fine-tune a pre-existing metabolism-based regulatory control network [Park and Gupta, 2013]. DNA and histone methylation require the transfer of a methyl group from S-adenosylmethionine (SAM) resulting in the formation of S-adenosylhomocysteine, which is then cleaved into adenosine and homocysteine. We recently discovered that adenosine kinase (ADK), by removing adenosine, drives the flux of methyl groups through the transmethylation pathway thereby increasing the methylation status of the epigenome, whereas experimental or therapeutic adenosine augmentation prevents methylation reactions through mass action [Fedele *et al.*, 2004; Williams-Karnesky *et al.*, 2013]. This is an important mechanism that directly links environmental factors — via adenosine — to epigenetic alterations. For example, factors such as sleep [Huang *et al.*, 2011; Porkka-Heiskanen and Kalinchuk, 2011], injury [Clark *et al.*, 1997; Lusardi *et al.*, 2012], or diet [Lusardi *et al.*, 2015; Masino *et al.*, 2011], all affect adenosine, suggesting that adenosine might be a biochemical mediator that links epigenetic alterations to environmental cues.

7.4 The epigenetics of epilepsy

The epigenetics of epilepsy is a relatively new research area and has been covered in several review articles [Boison, 2016; Chen *et al.*, 2017a; Grote *et al.*, 2015; Henshall and Kobow, 2015; Hwang *et al.*, 2013; Kobow and Blumcke, 2014; Qureshi and Mehler, 2014d; Younus and Reddy, 2017]. Most studies to date have focused on adult epilepsies, in particular temporal lobe epilepsy, whereas developmental factors in developmental epilepsies remain under studied (see Chapter 1). Here I discuss the contribution of changes in DNA methylation, histone methylation and acetylation, as well as noncoding RNAs within the context of adult and developmental epilepsies.

7.4.1 *DNA methylation*

DNA methylation is catalyzed by a group of DNA methyltransferases (DNMT1, DNMT3a, and DNMT3b), which transfer methyl groups from SAM on cytosine residues in DNA — mostly within so called CpG islands — and result in the formation 5-methylcytosine (5mC). The 'methylation hypothesis of epileptogenesis' [Kobow and Blumcke, 2011] proposes that increased activity of DNMTs and resulting global DNA hypermethylation is implicated in the progression and maintenance of epilepsy. This hypothesis is based on initial findings that hypermethylation of the *reelin* gene is directly implicated in the pathophysiology of TLE [Kobow *et al.*, 2009]. Because Reelin plays a role in the maintenance of the laminar structure in the dentate gyrus, increased DNA methylation and resulting reduced expression of the *reelin* gene leads to characteristic histopathological alterations of granule cells in the dentate gyrus [Heinrich *et al.*, 2006].

In line with a critical role of DNA methylation changes as a contributing factor in epileptogenesis, upregulated DNMT activity and associated changes in DNA methylation have been reported in patients with TLE [Kobow and Blumcke, 2011, 2012; Kobow *et al.*, 2009, 2013a; Miller-Delaney *et al.*, 2015; Zhu *et al.*, 2012]. Genome-wide changes in global DNA methylation were also found in rodent models of status epilepticus-induced chronic epilepsy

[Kobow *et al.*, 2013b; Lusardi *et al.*, 2015; Williams-Karnesky *et al.*, 2013], supporting the clinical findings. Because adenosine provides negative feedback control of DNMT activity through mass action [Boison, 2016; Williams-Karnesky *et al.*, 2013], the overexpression of ADK, a characteristic pathological hallmark of TLE [Aronica *et al.*, 2011, 2013; Boison and Aronica, 2015; Gouder *et al.*, 2004; Li *et al.*, 2008] is expected to drive epileptogenesis by increasing the flux of methyl groups through the transmethylation pathway, resulting in increased global DNA methylation status. The notion that this mechanism plays a key role in epileptogenesis is supported by findings that a transient dose of adenosine, delivered to the hippocampal formation via engineered silk-based adenosine releasing polymers, prevents epilepsy progression long-term in the systemic kainic acid model of TLE [Williams-Karnesky *et al.*, 2013]. The amino acid and neurotransmitter glycine, which is likewise dysregulated in TLE [Shen *et al.*, 2015], plays also an important role in carbon metabolism and can act as acceptor of methyl groups, thereby shunting methyl groups away from the DNA methylation pathway [Boison, 2016]. Through this interaction, the glycine and adenosine systems are linked and the dysregulation of both systems in TLE is expected to have a significant impact on DNA methylation [Boison, 2016].

7.4.2 *Histone modifications*

Histone modifications associated with epilepsy and its development include histone phosphorylation, acetylation, and methylation. Thus, increased phosphorylation of histone H3 has been reported after pilocarpine- and kainic acid (KA)-induced seizures [Crosio *et al.*, 2003; Sng *et al.*, 2006]. Phosphorylation of H3 in turn is involved in complex crosstalk with other histone modifications [Banerjee and Chakravarti, 2011]. The same triggers, as well as electroconvulsive seizures, also induce the acetylation of H4, a process that is linked to upregulation of BDNF, c-fos, and c-jun [Huang *et al.*, 2002; Sng *et al.*, 2006; Tsankova *et al.*, 2004]. However, reduced H4 acetylation was also found after seizures at a different set of gene loci such as GluR2, a subunit of the α-amino-3-hydroxy-5-methyl-4-isoxazoleproprionic acid (AMPA) receptor [Huang *et al.*, 2002; Tsankova *et al.*, 2004], whose repression has been associated with the initiation of epileptogenesis and increased neuronal hyperexcitability [Tanaka *et al.*, 2000]. Thus, HDAC inhibitors that block deacetylation of the gene locus for GluR2 might exert their neuroprotective effects through this mechanism [Huang *et al.*, 2002]. Traumatic brain injury (TBI), a well-recognized trigger for subsequent epileptogenesis [Pitkanen and Lukasiuk, 2011], induces significant changes in histone acetylation patterns. For example, controlled cortical impact triggered a reduction in H3 acetylation, which could be reversed by HDAC inhibition [Dash *et al.*, 2009a,b, 2010; Rao *et al.*, 2006; Shein *et al.*, 2009; Zhang *et al.*, 2008].

As outlined above, environmental factors and adverse events in early life can have lasting effects on epigenetic marks. In particular, neurodevelopmental disorders such as schizophrenia or autism spectrum disorder have been linked to epigenetic changes that maintain long-lasting effects of prenatal stress [Cattane *et al.*, 2018]. Early life events can trigger changes in histone acetylation with lasting consequences for behavioral phenotypes including stress, anxiety, and increased activity levels [Weaver *et al.*, 2004]. Importantly, some of those phenotypes can be reversed by the administration of an HDAC inhibitor [Weaver *et al.*, 2006]. Those findings support the rationale for investigating a potential role of HDAC inhibitors such as valproic acid, sodium butyrate, or trichostatin A, for the prevention of epileptogenesis through interference with epigenetically determined gene expression profiles [Qureshi and Mehler, 2010a, b, 2014d].

7.4.3 *Non-coding RNAs*

Among non-coding RNAs implicated as epigenetic regulators in the epilepsies, microRNAs (miRNAs) have received most attention. MiRNAs target messenger RNAs (mRNAs) for degradation or translational repression and thereby modify gene expression. In a system of 'epigenetic-miRNA regulatory circuits', miRNA expression is regulated via DNA methylation and histone modification and thereby provides regulatory feedback by integrating several epigenetic mechanisms [Sato *et al.*, 2011]. A critical role of miRNAs in the process of neuroinflammation and neuroprotection has been identified in several studies [Bake *et al.*, 2014; Lopez-Ramirez *et al.*, 2014; Selvamani *et al.*, 2012; Yin *et al.*, 2014]. In line with a role in neuroinflammation and neuroprotection, both pro-epileptogenic [Hu *et al.*, 2011a, 2012; Jimenez-Mateos *et al.*, 2011, 2012; Sano *et al.*, 2012; Song *et al.*, 2011], and anti-epileptogenic [McKiernan *et al.*, 2012; Tan *et al.*, 2013] profiles have been described for certain miRNAs. In independent studies, status epilepticus induced the upregulation of miR-134 [Jimenez-Mateos *et al.*, 2012, 2015; Peng *et al.*, 2013], a miRNA responsible for the promotion of apoptosis [Zhang *et al.*, 2014]. In line with a pro-epileptogenic role of miR-134, the use of a miR-134 selective antagomir reduced the incidence of seizure development in a mouse model of status epilepticus [Jimenez-Mateos *et al.*, 2012, 2015. A link to neuroinflammatory processes implicated in epileptogenesis was provided by identifying consistent upregulation of miR-132, an anti-inflammation marker, in several epilepsy models [Shaked *et al.*, 2009; Vezzani *et al.*, 2011]. MiRNAs therefore emerge both as biomarkers as well as therapeutic targets for epileptogenesis.

7.4.4 *REST/NRSF*

In addition to non-selective biochemical mechanisms that determine the rate of chemical modifications on DNA or histones, more selective epigenetic changes are thought to be under the control of master regulators. One of those 'meta-regulators' is the repressor element 1-silencing transcription factor (REST) also known as neuron-restrictive silencer factor (NRSF). REST/NRSF controls over 1800 genes related to synaptic function and structure, neural plasticity and excitability [Ballas *et al.*, 2005; Ballas and Mandel, 2005; D'Alessandro *et al.*, 2009; Qureshi *et al.*, 2010; Qureshi and Mehler, 2009; Tahiliani *et al.*, 2007]. In line with a prominent role in epilepsy, several studies have documented robust upregulation of REST/NRSF after induced seizures [Gillies *et al.*, 2009; Palm *et al.*, 1998]. A seminal study demonstrated that REST/NRSF is also responsive to metabolic intervention. Garriga-Canut and colleagues demonstrated that the glycolytic inhibitor 2-deoxy-D-glucose (2DG) suppressed kindling epileptogenesis and the progression of seizure-induced upregulation of brain derived neurotrophic factor (BDNF). 2DG affected BDNF expression by reducing the expression of REST/NRSF, which created a repressive environment at the BDNF promoter [Garriga-Canut *et al.*, 2006]. However, further studies on the role of REST/NRSF in epilepsy using knockout models yielded conflicting results: The genetic disruption of REST/NRSF in glutamatergic forebrain neurons accelerated kindling epileptogenesis [Hu *et al.*, 2011b], whereas the genetic deletion of REST/NRSF in all neurons attenuated susceptibility to pentylenetetrazole (PTZ)-induced seizures and excitotoxicity. It is currently unclear whether differences are due to cell-type selectivity of effects, the animal models used, or strains and other biological and technical variables.

7.5 Epigenetic factors in developmental epilepsies

Because many developmental epilepsies are based on gene mutations [Howard and Baraban, 2017], epigenetic factors implicated in developmental epilepsies received less attention. However, because epigenetic modifications can affect the expression of genes known to be implicated in developmental epilepsies, it is tempting to conclude that a wide range of epigenetically active triggers during gestation, such as those discussed above, might contribute to the development of so called non-genetic developmental epilepsies. The interaction with the epigenome and gene mutations also implicates epigenetic modifications as potentially reversible and that genetic mutations can be 'silenced' by epigenetic alterations.

One example for possible epigenome–genome interactions is the methyl-CpG-binding protein 2 (MeCP2), which is a 'reader' of DNA methylation status [Fasolino and Zhou, 2017; Kriaucionis and Bird, 2003]. Mutations in the *Mecp2* gene have been identified as causative factors for the development of some forms of autism spectrum disorder (ASD), including Rett syndrome [Amir *et al.*, 1999; Wan *et al.*, 1999], a neurodevelopmental disorder comprised of regression of acquired motor skills, loss of purposeful activity, hand stereotypies, loss of acquired spoken language, and seizures [Ben Zeev Ghidoni, 2007; Chahrour and Zoghbi, 2007; Krajnc, 2015]. In line with a critical role of MeCP2 in the regulation of key neurodevelopmental processes, changes in DNA methylation status are now considered a potential contributing factor for the development of ASD and related neurodevelopmental disorders [Vogel Ciernia and LaSalle, 2016]. Similarly, epigenetic changes (transient histone hyperacetylation) induced by valproic acid have been associated with the development of ASD in rodent models [Mabunga *et al.*, 2015]. It is tempting to speculate that epigenetic alterations during fetal brain development may replicate effects caused by gene mutations (such as MeCP2). This concept has therapeutic implications, because epigenetic changes, in contrast to genetic mutations, are potentially reversible. It might even be possible to neutralize the effects of genetic mutations by targeted epigenetic therapies.

7.6 Epigenetic therapies

Epigenetic drugs such as HDAC inhibitors or DNMT inhibitors are already clinically used for the therapy of a variety of cancers, mostly lymphomas and myelomas [Singh *et al.*, 2013; Virani *et al.*, 2012]. In contrast, epigenetic therapies for the treatment of epilepsies are still in development.

7.6.1 *DNA methylation blockers*

Only a few studies have explored a role of DNA methylation blockers in models of epileptogenesis. As a proof of principle, DNMT inhibition via zebularine altered status epilepticus-induced hippocampal methylation and synaptic plasticity and restored decreases of binding of the transcription factor AP2alpha to the Nr2b gene promoter [Ryley Parrish *et al.*, 2013]. Similarly, the DNMT inhibitor RG108 blocked hypermethylation of the RASgrf1 promoter and suppressed acute epileptic activity in a mouse model of kainic acid-induced epilepsy [Chen *et al.*, 2017b]. A potential therapeutic use as an antiepileptogenic agent, the DNMT inhibitor 5-Aza-2dC was shown to increase PTZ seizure thresholds, attenuate seizures in fully kindled rats, and suppress kindling epileptogenesis [Williams-Karnesky *et al.*, 2013]. Together, those studies suggest that DNMT inhibitors might have a disease-modifying effect in epilepsy. One hurdle for the use of those agents for the prevention of epilepsy is that most known DNMT inhibitors induce DNA alterations, which lead to secondary inhibition of DNMTs. Therefore, the therapeutic action of those agents, although useful for the therapy of cancer, might be too nonspecific to afford significant therapeutic efficacy in epilepsy.

7.6.2 *HDAC inhibitors*

The well-known antiepileptic drug valproic acid (VPA) suppresses seizures by increasing the levels of GABA in the brain. In addition, VPA is also a potent HDAC inhibitor [Gottlicher, 2004]. Chronic treatment with VPA promotes increased H3 acetylation in the brain [Eleuteri *et al.*, 2009]. Thus, VPA combines antiepileptic with epigenetic properties. By inhibiting HDACs and normalizing HDAC-dependent gene expression within the epileptic dentate gyrus, VPA potently blocked seizure-induced neurogenesis. Importantly, the inhibition of aberrant neurogenesis protected the animals from seizure-induced cognitive impairment in a hippocampus-dependent learning task [Jessberger *et al.*, 2007]. Although epigenetic effects and direct effects on GABAergic neurotransmission could not be distinguished in this study, those findings support a possible disease-modifying effect of HDAC inhibition. Similarly, the HDAC inhibitor sodium butyrate has shown disease-modifying activity in stress responses [Deutsch *et al.*, 2008, 2009]. Twice daily treatment with sodium butyrate significantly delayed kindling epileptogenesis in mice as shown by a significant delay in the development of stage 4/5 seizures and reduced severity of behavioral seizures [Younus and Reddy, 2017]. Those findings suggest a potential antiepileptogenic efficacy of sodium butyrate.

7.6.3 *Adenosine*

Through interference with the transmethylation pathway, adenosine is uniquely suited to block both DNA methylation and histone methylation [Boison, 2016]. Epilepsy and its progression can be prevented by the transient augmentation of adenosine. Our past research has demonstrated that both focal adenosine augmentation through local adenosine-releasing silk- or cell- based brain implants [Li *et al.*, 2007, 2008; Szybala *et al.*, 2009; Williams-Karnesky *et al.*, 2013], as well as systemic adenosine augmentation through a small molecule ADK inhibitor, can prevent epilepsy or its progression in etiologically different rodent systems that model epileptogenesis in TLE, our clinical target. We have shown that therapeutic adenosine augmentation prevents kindling epileptogenesis in the rat [Li *et al.*, 2007; Szybala *et al.*, 2009], prevents epilepsy development in the mouse intraamygdaloid [Li *et al.*, 2008] and intrahippocampal KA models, and prevents epilepsy progression in the rat systemic KA model [Williams-Karnesky *et al.*, 2013]. We demonstrated that the robust antiepileptogenic effects of adenosine are based on an epigenetic mechanism, whereby increased levels adenosine reduce global DNA methylation levels through mass action [Williams-Karnesky *et al.*, 2013]. A key driving force for pathological increases in DNA methylation status are maladaptive changes in adenosine metabolism triggered by pathological overexpression of the key adenosine metabolizing enzyme ADK [Aronica *et al.*, 2013; Boison, 2008, 2013; Li *et al.*, 2008; Williams-Karnesky *et al.*, 2013]. Whereas drug development efforts previously targeted the cytoplasmic isoform ADK-S to enhance adenosine receptor activation, we recently showed that a specific isoform of ADK (ADK-L), located in the nucleus of the cell, plays a key role in the regulation of adenosine receptor-independent epigenetic functions of adenosine [Williams-Karnesky *et al.*, 2013]. In line with those findings, a transient dose of a small molecule ADK inhibitor prevents epileptogenesis in the mouse intrahippocampal KA model of TLE. Since ADK is overexpressed in the epileptic brain and is associated with epileptogenesis [Aronica *et al.*, 2011, 2013; Boison, 2012, 2013; de Groot *et al.*, 2012; Fedele *et al.*, 2005; Gouder *et al.*, 2004; Li *et al.*, 2008; Williams-Karnesky *et al.*, 2013], there is a strong rationale for the clinical development of ADK inhibitors that restore normal adenosine function. The development and validation of new ADK inhibitors that mobilize long-lasting antiepileptogenic epigenetic effects through transient ADK-L inhibition will enhance the contribution of desirable epigenetically-based antiepileptogenic effects of adenosine. Importantly, the transient therapeutic use of ADK inhibitors will allow us to mitigate risks associated with chronic ADK inhibition.

7.6.4 *Ketogenic diet*

KDs have successfully been used for almost one hundred years for the treatment of epilepsy. KDs are also of interest for antiepileptogenic therapy, because KDs lead to the generation of beta-hydroxybutyrate, a potent HDAC inhibitor [Shimazu *et al.*, 2013] and the production of adenosine [Lusardi *et al.*, 2015; Masino *et al.*, 2011]. Consistent with those mechanisms, KD therapy exerts disease-modifying effects both in genetic models of metabolic epilepsy as well as in rodent models of TLE through epigenetic mechanisms. KD therapy postponed disease progression, delayed the onset of severe seizures and increased the lifespan of *Kcna1* null mice, a model of progressive epilepsy [Simeone *et al.*, 2016]. A disease-modifying epigenetic mechanism of KD therapy is further supported by findings that KD therapy attenuated seizure progression and ameliorated DNA methylation-mediated changes in gene expression [Kobow *et al.*, 2013]. Subsequently, it was shown that transient KD therapy restored normal adenosine levels and global DNA methylation levels in the rat pilocarpine model of TLE, whereas epileptic control animals were adenosine deficient and hypermethylated; importantly, transient KD therapy reduced seizure activity long-term, even after reversal to a control diet [Lusardi *et al.*, 2015]. Because KD therapy increases adenosine [Lusardi *et al.*, 2015; Masino *et al.*, 2011] and because adenosine blocks DNA methylation [Williams-Karnesky *et al.*, 2013] KD therapy likely exerts its disease-modifying effects through an adenosine-dependent epigenetic mechanism.

7.7 Conclusions and future perspectives

There is compelling data that a variety of factors during fetal development can affect the brain long-term through epigenetic alterations. Because gene mutations are known to cause developmental epilepsies, it is tempting to speculate that environmentally-induced epigenetic changes, which affect the expression of genes critical for brain development, likewise are a plausible cause of neurodevelopmental epilepsies. More research is needed to investigate which developmental stressors and which epigenetic mechanisms might be implicated. If epigenetic changes can cause epilepsy, those changes — in contrast to gene mutations — are potentially reversible. Thus, there is a realistic potential for the development of novel disease-modifying therapeutics that target the epigenome to exert long-lasting changes in gene expression. The role of epigenetics in epilepsy is a nascent research area and more research is needed to answer compelling questions such as: Can epilepsy be prevented? Or: Is epilepsy reversible?

Acknowledgments

The author is funded through grants from the NINDS (NS084920, NS103740, NS065957) and the Good Samaritan Hospital Foundations.

References

Amir, R.E., Van den Veyver, I.B., Wan, M., Tran, C.Q., Francke, U., and Zoghbi, H.Y. (1999). Rett syndrome is caused by mutations in X-linked MECP2, encoding methyl-CpG-binding protein 2, *Nat. Genet.*, 23, 185–188.

Aronica, E., Sandau, U.S., Iyer, A., and Boison, D. (2013). Glial adenosine kinase — A neuropathological marker of the epileptic brain, *Neurochem. Int.*, 63, 688–695.

Aronica, E., Zurolo, E., Iyer, A., de Groot, M., Anink, J., Carbonell, C., van Vliet, E.A., Baayen, J.C., Boison, D., and Gorter, J.A. (2011). Upregulation of adenosine kinase in astrocytes in experimental and human temporal lobe epilepsy, *Epilepsia*, 52, 1645–1655.

Bake, S., Selvamani, A., Cherry, J., and Sohrabji, F. (2014). Blood brain barrier and neuroinflammation are critical targets of IGF-1-mediated neuroprotection in stroke for middle-aged female rats, *PloS One*, 9, e91427.

Ballas, N., Grunseich, C., Lu, D.D., Speh, J.C., and Mandel, G. (2005). REST and its corepressors mediate plasticity of neuronal gene chromatin throughout neurogenesis, *Cell*, 121, 645–657.

Ballas, N. and Mandel, G. (2005). The many faces of REST oversee epigenetic programming of neuronal genes, *Curr. Opin. Neurobiol.*, 15, 500–506.

Banerjee, T. and Chakravarti, D. (2011). A peek into the complex realm of histone phosphorylation, *Mol. Cell. Biol.*, 31, 4858–4873.

Ben Zeev Ghidoni, B. (2007). Rett syndrome, *Child Adolesc. Psychiatr. Clin. N. Am.*, 16, 723–743.

Boison, D. (2008). The adenosine kinase hypothesis of epileptogenesis, *Progr. Neurobiol.*, 84, 249–262.

Boison, D. (2012). Adenosine dysfunction in epilepsy, *Glia*, 60, 1234–1243.

Boison, D. (2013). Adenosine kinase: exploitation for therapeutic gain, *Pharmacol. Rev.*, 65, 906–943.

Boison, D. (2016). Adenosinergic signaling in epilepsy, *Neuropharmacology*, 104, 131–139.

Boison, D. (2016). The biochemistry and epigenetics of epilepsy: focus on adenosine and glycine, *Front. Mol. Neurosci.*, 9, 26.

Boison, D., and Aronica, E. (2015). Comorbidities in neurology: is adenosine the common link?, *Neuropharmacology*, 97, 18–34.

Cattane, N., Richetto, J., and Cattaneo, A. (2018). Prenatal exposure to environmental insults and enhanced risk of developing schizophrenia and autism spectrum disorder: focus on biological pathways and epigenetic mechanisms, *Neurosci. Biobehav. Rev.*, pii: S0149-7634(17)30972–7.

Chahrour, M., and Zoghbi, H.Y. (2007). The story of Rett syndrome: from clinic to neurobiology, *Neuron*, 56, 422–437.

Chen, T., Giri, M., Xia, Z., Subedi, Y.N., and Li, Y. (2017a). Genetic and epigenetic mechanisms of epilepsy: a review, *Neuropsychiatr. Dis. Treat.*, 13, 1841–1859.

Chen, X., Peng, X., Wang, L., Fu, X., Zhou, J.X., Zhu, B., Luo, J., Wang, X., and Xiao, Z. (2017b). Association of RASgrf1 methylation with epileptic seizures, *Oncotarget*, 8, 46286–46297.

Cheng, T.L., and Qiu, Z. (2014). MeCP2: multifaceted roles in gene regulation and neural development, *Neurosci. Bull.*, 30, 601–609.

Clark, R.S., Carcillo, J.A., Kochanek, P.M., Obrist, W.D., Jackson, E.K., Mi, Z., Wisneiwski, S.R., Bell, M.J., and Marion, D.W. (1997). Cerebrospinal fluid adenosine concentration and uncoupling of cerebral blood flow and oxidative metabolism after severe head injury in humans, *Neurosurgery*, 41, 1284–1292; discussion 1292–1293.

Colquitt, B.M., Allen, W.E., Barnea, G., and Lomvardas, S. (2013). Alteration of genic 5-hydroxymethylcytosine patterning in olfactory neurons correlates with changes in gene expression and cell identity, *Proc. Nat. Acad. Sci. U S A*, 110, 14682–14687.

Crosio, C., Heitz, E., Allis, C.D., Borrelli, E., and Sassone-Corsi, P. (2003). Chromatin remodeling and neuronal response: multiple signaling pathways induce specific histone H3 modifications and early gene expression in hippocampal neurons, *J. Cell Sci.*, 116, 4905–4914.

D'Alessandro, R., Klajn, A., and Meldolesi, J. (2009). Expression of dense-core vesicles and of their exocytosis are governed by the repressive transcription factor NRSF/REST, *Ann. N Y Acad Sci.*, 1152, 194–200.

Dash, P.K., Orsi, S.A., and Moore, A.N. (2009a). Histone deactylase inhibition combined with behavioral therapy enhances learning and memory following traumatic brain injury, *Neuroscience*, 163, 1–8.

Dash, P.K., Orsi, S.A., Zhang, M., Grill, R.J., Pati, S., Zhao, J., and Moore, A.N. (2010). Valproate administered after traumatic brain injury provides neuroprotection and improves cognitive function in rats, *PloS One*, 5, e11383.

Dash, P.K., Zhao, J., Orsi, S.A., Zhang, M., and Moore, A.N. (2009b). Sulforaphane improves cognitive function administered following traumatic brain injury, *Neurosci. Lett.*, 460, 103–107.

de Groot, M., Iyer, A., Zurolo, E., Anink, J., Heimans, J.J., Boison, D., Reijneveld, C.J., and Aronica, E. (2012). Overexpression of ADK in human astrocytic tumors and peritumoral tissue is related to tumor-associated epilepsy., *Epilepsia*, 53, 58–66.

Deutsch, S.I., Mastropaolo, J., Burket, J.A., and Rosse, R.B. (2009). An epigenetic intervention interacts with genetic strain differences to modulate the stress-induced reduction of flurazepam's antiseizure efficacy in the mouse, *Eur. Neuropsychopharmacol.*, 19, 398–401.

Deutsch, S.I., Rosse, R.B., Long, K.D., Gaskins, B.L., Burket, J.A., and Mastropaolo, J. (2008). Sodium butyrate, an epigenetic interventional strategy, attenuates a stress-induced alteration of MK-801's pharmacologic action, *Eur. Neuropsychopharmacol.*, 18, 565–568.

Eleuteri, S., Monti, B., Brignani, S., and Contestabile, A. (2009). Chronic dietary administration of valproic acid protects neurons of the rat nucleus basalis magnocellularis from ibotenic acid neurotoxicity, *Neurotox. Res.*, 15, 127–132.

Estes, M.L. and McAllister, A.K. (2016). Maternal immune activation: Implications for neuropsychiatric disorders, *Science*, 353, 772–777.

Fasolino, M. and Zhou, Z. (2017). The Crucial Role of DNA Methylation and MeCP2 in Neuronal Function, *Genes*, 8.

Fedele, D.E., Gouder, N., Güttinger, M., Gabernet, L., Scheurer, L., Rulicke, T., Crestani, F., and Boison, D. (2005). Astrogliosis in epilepsy leads to overexpression of adenosine kinase resulting in seizure aggravation, *Brain*, 128, 2383–2395.

Fedele, D.E., Koch, P., Brüstle, O., Scheurer, L., Simpson, E.M., Mohler, H., and Boison, D. (2004). Engineering embryonic stem cell derived glia for adenosine delivery, *Neurosci. Lett.*, 370, 160–165.

Freeman, J.M., Vining, E.P., Kossoff, E.H., Pyzik, P.L., Ye, X., and Goodman, S.N. (2009). A blinded, crossover study of the efficacy of the ketogenic diet, *Epilepsia*, 50, 322–325.

Gardener, H., Spiegelman, D., and Buka, S.L. (2011). Perinatal and neonatal risk factors for autism: a comprehensive meta-analysis, *Pediatrics*, 128, 344–355.

Garriga-Canut, M., Schoenike, B., Qazi, R., Bergendahl, K., Daley, T.J., Pfender, R.M., Morrison, J.F., Ockuly, J., Stafstrom, C., Sutula, T., and Roopra, A. (2006). 2-Deoxy-D-glucose reduces epilepsy progression by NRSF-CtBP-dependent metabolic regulation of chromatin structure, *Nat. Neurosci.*, 9, 1382–1387.

Gillies, S., Haddley, K., Vasiliou, S., Bubb, V.J., and Quinn, J.P. (2009). The human neurokinin B gene, TAC3, and its promoter are regulated by Neuron Restrictive Silencing Factor (NRSF) transcription factor family, *Neuropeptides*, 43, 333–340.

Gottlicher, M. (2004). Valproic acid: an old drug newly discovered as inhibitor of histone deacetylases, *Ann. Hematol.*, 83 Suppl 1, S91–92.

Gouder, N., Scheurer, L., Fritschy, J.-M., and Boison, D. (2004). Overexpression of adenosine kinase in epileptic hippocampus contributes to epileptogenesis, *J. Neurosci.*, 24, 692–701.

Grote, A., Schoch, S., and Becker, A.J. (2015). Temporal lobe epilepsy: a unique window into living human brain epigenetic gene regulation, *Brain*, 138, 509–511.

Gurkas, E., Serdaroglu, A., Hirfanoglu, T., Kartal, A., Yilmaz, U., and Bilir, E. (2016). Sleep-wake distribution and circadian patterns of epileptic seizures in children, *Eur. J. Paediatr. Neurol.*, 20, 549–554.

Hajkova, P., Jeffries, S.J., Lee, C., Miller, N., Jackson, S.P., and Surani, M.A. (2010). Genome-wide reprogramming in the mouse germ line entails the base excision repair pathway, *Science*, 329, 78–82.

Heinrich, C., Nitta, N., Flubacher, A., Muller, M., Fahrner, A., Kirsch, M., Freiman, T., Suzuki, F., Depaulis, A., Frotscher, M., and Haas, C.A. (2006). Reelin deficiency and displacement of mature neurons, but not neurogenesis, underlie the formation of granule cell dispersion in the epileptic hippocampus, *J. Neurosci.*, 26, 4701–4713.

Henshall, D.C. and Kobow, K. (2015). Epigenetics and epilepsy, *Cold Spring Harb. Perspect. Med.*, 5 pii: a022731. doi: 10.1101/cshperspect.a022731.

Howard, M.A. and Baraban, S.C. (2017). Catastrophic epilepsies of childhood, *Ann. Rev. Neurosci.*, 40, 149–166.

Hu, K., Xie, Y.Y., Zhang, C., Ouyang, D.S., Long, H.Y., Sun, D.N., Long, L.L., Feng, L., Li, Y., and Xiao, B. (2012). MicroRNA expression profile of the hippocampus in a rat model of temporal lobe epilepsy and miR-34a-targeted neuroprotection against hippocampal neurone cell apoptosis post-status epilepticus, *BMC Neurosci.*, 13, 115.

Hu, K., Zhang, C., Long, L., Long, X., Feng, L., Li, Y., and Xiao, B. (2011a). Expression profile of microRNAs in rat hippocampus following lithium-pilocarpine-induced status epilepticus, *Neurosci. Lett.*, 488, 252–257.

Hu, X.L., Cheng, X., Cai, L., Tan, G.H., Xu, L., Feng, X.Y., Lu, T.J., Xiong, H., Fei, J., and Xiong, Z.Q. (2011b). Conditional deletion of NRSF in forebrain neurons accelerates epileptogenesis in the kindling model, *Cereb. Cortex*, 21, 2158–2165.

Huang, Y., Doherty, J.J., and Dingledine, R. (2002). Altered histone acetylation at glutamate receptor 2 and brain-derived neurotrophic factor genes is an early event triggered by status epilepticus, *J. Neurosci.*, 22, 8422–8428.

Huang, Z.L., Urade, Y., and Hayaishi, O. (2011). The role of adenosine in the regulation of sleep, *Curr. Top. Med. Chem.*, 11, 1047–1057.

Hwang, J.Y., Aromolaran, K.A., and Zukin, R.S. (2013). Epigenetic mechanisms in stroke and epilepsy, *Neuropsychopharmacology*, 38, 167–182.

Jessberger, S., Nakashima, K., Clemenson, G.D., Jr., Mejia, E., Mathews, E., Ure, K., Ogawa, S., Sinton, C.M., Gage, F.H., and Hsieh, J. (2007). Epigenetic modulation of seizure-induced neurogenesis and cognitive decline, *J. Neurosci.*, 27, 5967–5975.

Jimenez-Mateos, E.M., Bray, I., Sanz-Rodriguez, A., Engel, T., McKiernan, R.C., Mouri, G., Tanaka, K., Sano, T., Saugstad, J.A., Simon, R.P.,

Stallings, R.L. and Henshall, D.C. (2011). miRNA Expression profile after status epilepticus and hippocampal neuroprotection by targeting miR-132, *Am. J. Pathol.*, 179, 2519–2532.
Jimenez-Mateos, E.M., Engel, T., Merino-Serrais, P., Fernaud-Espinosa, I., Rodriguez-Alvarez, N., Reynolds, J., Reschke, C.R., Conroy, R.M., McKiernan, R.C., deFelipe, J., and Henshall, D.C. (2015). Antagomirs targeting microRNA-134 increase hippocampal pyramidal neuron spine volume in vivo and protect against pilocarpine-induced status epilepticus, *Brain Struct. Funct.*, 220, 2387–2399.
Jimenez-Mateos, E.M., Engel, T., Merino-Serrais, P., McKiernan, R.C., Tanaka, K., Mouri, G., Sano, T., O'Tuathaigh, C., Waddington, J.L., Prenter, S., Delanty, N., Farrell, M.A., O'Brien, D.F., Conroy, R.M., Stallings, R.L., DeFelipe, J., and Henshall, D.C. (2012). Silencing microRNA-134 produces neuroprotective and prolonged seizure-suppressive effects, *Nat. Med.,* 18, 1087–1094.
Kaas, G.A., Zhong, C., Eason, D.E., Ross, D.L., Vachhani, R.V., Ming, G.L., King, J.R., Song, H., and Sweatt, J.D. (2013). TET1 controls CNS 5-methylcytosine hydroxylation, active DNA demethylation, gene transcription, and memory formation, *Neuron*, 79, 1086–1093.
Kaelin, W.G., Jr. and McKnight, S.L. (2013). Influence of metabolism on epigenetics and disease, *Cell*, 153, 56–69.
Kinnaird, A., Zhao, S., Wellen, K.E., and Michelakis, E.D. (2016). Metabolic control of epigenetics in cancer, *Nat. Rev. Cancer*, 16, 694–707.
Kobow, K. and Blumcke, I. (2011). The methylation hypothesis: do epigenetic chromatin modifications play a role in epileptogenesis?, *Epilepsia*, 52 Suppl 4, 15–19.
Kobow, K. and Blumcke, I. (2012). The emerging role of DNA methylation in epileptogenesis, *Epilepsia*, 53 Suppl 9, 11–20.
Kobow, K. and Blumcke, I. (2014). Epigenetic mechanisms in epilepsy, *Progress in brain research*, 213, 279–316.
Kobow, K., El-Osta, A., and Blumcke, I. (2013a). The methylation hypothesis of pharmacoresistance in epilepsy, *Epilepsia*, 54 Suppl 2, 41–47.
Kobow, K., Jeske, I., Hildebrandt, M., Hauke, J., Hahnen, E., Buslei, R., Buchfelder, M., Weigel, D., Stefan, H., Kasper, B., Pauli, E., and Blumcke, I. (2009). Increased reelin promoter methylation is associated with granule cell dispersion in human temporal lobe epilepsy, *J. Neuropathol. Exp. Neurol.*, 68, 356–364.
Kobow, K., Kaspi, A., Harikrishnan, K.N., Kiese, K., Ziemann, M., Khurana, I., Fritzsche, I., Hauke, J., Hahnen, E., Coras, R., Muhlebner, A., El-Osta,

A., and Blumcke, I. (2013b). Deep sequencing reveals increased DNA methylation in chronic rat epilepsy, *Acta Neuropathol.*, 126, 741–756.

Kolevzon, A., Gross, R., and Reichenberg, A. (2007). Prenatal and perinatal risk factors for autism: a review and integration of findings, *Arch. Pediatr. Adolesc. Med.*, 161, 326–333.

Kossoff, E.H. and Rho, J.M. (2009). Ketogenic diets: evidence for short- and long-term efficacy, *Neurotherapeutics*, 6, 406–414.

Kossoff, E.H., Zupec-Kania, B.A., and Rho, J.M. (2009). Ketogenic diets: an update for child neurologists, *J. Child Neurol.*, 24, 979–988.

Krajnc, N. (2015). Management of epilepsy in patients with Rett syndrome: perspectives and considerations, *Ther. Clin. Risk Manag.*, 11, 925–932.

Kriaucionis, S. and Bird, A. (2003). DNA methylation and Rett syndrome, *Hum. Mol. Genet.*, 12 Spec No 2, R221–227.

Levenson, J.M., Roth, T.L., Lubin, F.D., Miller, C.A., Huang, I.C., Desai, P., Malone, L.M., and Sweatt, J.D. (2006). Evidence that DNA (cytosine-5) methyltransferase regulates synaptic plasticity in the hippocampus, *J. Biol. Chem.*, 281, 15763–15773.

Li, T., Ren, G., Lusardi, T., Wilz, A., Lan, J.Q., Iwasato, T., Itohara, S., Simon, R.P., and Boison, D. (2008). Adenosine kinase is a target for the prediction and prevention of epileptogenesis in mice, *J. Clin. Inv.*, 118, 571–582.

Li, T., Steinbeck, J.A., Lusardi, T., Koch, P., Lan, J.Q., Wilz, A., Segschneider, M., Simon, R.P., Brustle, O., and Boison, D. (2007). Suppression of kindling epileptogenesis by adenosine releasing stem cell-derived brain implants, *Brain*, 130, 1276–1288.

Lopez-Ramirez, M.A., Wu, D., Pryce, G., Simpson, J.E., Reijerkerk, A., King-Robson, J., Kay, O., de Vries, H.E., Hirst, M.C., Sharrack, B., Baker, D., Male, D.K., Michael, G.J., and Romero, I.A. (2014). MicroRNA-155 negatively affects blood-brain barrier function during neuroinflammation, *FASEB J.*, 28, 2551–2565.

Lusardi, T.A., Akula, K.K., Coffman, S.Q., Ruskin, D.N., Masino, S.A., and Boison, D. (2015). Ketogenic diet prevents epileptogenesis and disease progression in adult mice and rats, *Neuropharmacology*, 99, 500–509.

Lusardi, T.A., Lytle, N.K., Szybala, C., and Boison, D. (2012). Caffeine prevents acute mortality after TBI in rats without increased morbidity, *Exp. Neurol.*, 234, 161–168.

Mabunga, D.F., Gonzales, E.L., Kim, J.W., Kim, K.C., and Shin, C.Y. (2015). Exploring the validity of valproic acid animal model of autism, *Exp. Neurobiol.*, 24, 285–300.

Masino, S.A., Li, T., Theofilas, P., Sandau, U.S., Ruskin, D.N., Fredholm, B.B., Geiger, J.D., Aronica, E., and Boison, D. (2011). A ketogenic diet suppresses seizures in mice through adenosine A1 receptors, *J. Clin. Inv.*, 121, 2679–2683.

Mayne, S.T., Playdon, M.C., and Rock, C.L. (2016). Diet, nutrition, and cancer: past, present and future, *Nature reviews. Clin. Oncol.*, 13, 504–515.

Mazarati, A.M., Lewis, M.L., and Pittman, Q.J. (2017). Neurobehavioral comorbidities of epilepsy: Role of inflammation, *Epilepsia*, 58 Suppl 3, 48–56.

McKiernan, R.C., Jimenez-Mateos, E.M., Sano, T., Bray, I., Stallings, R.L., Simon, R.P., and Henshall, D.C. (2012). Expression profiling the microRNA response to epileptic preconditioning identifies miR-184 as a modulator of seizure-induced neuronal death, *Exp. Neurol.*, 237, 346–354.

Meyer, U. (2014). Prenatal poly(i:C) exposure and other developmental immune activation models in rodent systems, *Biol. Psychiatry*, 75, 307–315.

Miller-Delaney, S.F., Bryan, K., Das, S., McKiernan, R.C., Bray, I.M., Reynolds, J.P., Gwinn, R., Stallings, R.L., and Henshall, D.C. (2015). Differential DNA methylation profiles of coding and non-coding genes define hippocampal sclerosis in human temporal lobe epilepsy, *Brain*, 138, 616–631.

Newby, A.C. (1984). Adenosine and the concept of 'retaliatory metabolites'. *Trends Biochem. Sci.*, 9, 42–44.

Palm, K., Belluardo, N., Metsis, M., and Timmusk, T. (1998). Neuronal expression of zinc finger transcription factor REST/NRSF/XBR gene, *J. Neurosci.*, 18, 1280–1296.

Park, J. and Gupta, R.S. (2013). Adenosine metabolism, adenosine kinase, and evolution. In Adenosine: a key link between metabolism and central nervous system activity, D. Boison, and M.A. Masino, eds. (New York: Springer), pp. 23–54.

Patterson, P.H. (2009). Immune involvement in schizophrenia and autism: etiology, pathology and animal models, *Behav. Brain Res.*, 204, 313–321.

Peng, J., Omran, A., Ashhab, M.U., Kong, H., Gan, N., He, F., and Yin, F. (2013). Expression patterns of miR-124, miR-134, miR-132, and miR-21 in an immature rat model and children with mesial temporal lobe epilepsy, *J. Mol. Neurosci.*, 50, 291–297.

Pineda, E., Shin, D., You, S.J., Auvin, S., Sankar, R., and Mazarati, A. (2013). Maternal immune activation promotes hippocampal kindling epileptogenesis in mice, *Ann. Neurol.*, 74, 11–19.

Pitkanen, A. and Lukasiuk, K. (2011). Mechanisms of epileptogenesis and potential treatment targets, *Lancet Neurol.*, 10, 173–186.

Porkka-Heiskanen, T. and Kalinchuk, A.V. (2011). Adenosine, energy metabolism and sleep homeostasis, *Sleep Med. Rev.*, 15, 123–135.

Qureshi, I.A., Gokhan, S., and Mehler, M.F. (2010). REST and CoREST are transcriptional and epigenetic regulators of seminal neural fate decisions, *Cell Cycle*, 9, 4477–4486.

Qureshi, I.A. and Mehler, M.F. (2009). Regulation of non-coding RNA networks in the nervous system — what's the REST of the story?, *Neurosci. Lett.*, 466, 73–80.

Qureshi, I.A. and Mehler, M.F. (2010a). Emerging role of epigenetics in stroke: part 1: DNA methylation and chromatin modifications, *Arch. Neurol.*, 67, 1316–1322.

Qureshi, I.A. and Mehler, M.F. (2010b). Epigenetic mechanisms underlying human epileptic disorders and the process of epileptogenesis, *Neurobiol. Dis.*, 39, 53–60.

Qureshi, I.A. and Mehler, M.F. (2014a). Epigenetic mechanisms underlying the pathogenesis of neurogenetic diseases, *Neurotherapeutics*, 11, 708–720.

Qureshi, I.A. and Mehler, M.F. (2014b). Epigenetics of sleep and chronobiology, *Cur. Neurol. Neurosci. Rep.* 14, 432.

Qureshi, I.A. and Mehler, M.F. (2014c). An evolving view of epigenetic complexity in the brain, *Philos. Trans. R. Soc. Lond. B Biol. Sci.*, 369, pii: 20130506, doi: 10.1098/rstb.2013.0506.

Qureshi, I.A. and Mehler, M.F. (2014d). Sex, epilepsy, and epigenetics, *Neurobiol Dis.*, 72 Pt B, 210–216.

Ramgopal, S., Powell, C., Zarowski, M., Alexopoulos, A.V., Kothare, S.V., and Loddenkemper, T. (2014). Predicting diurnal and sleep/wake seizure patterns in paediatric patients of different ages, *Epileptic Disord.*, 16, 56–66.

Ramgopal, S., Vendrame, M., Shah, A., Gregas, M., Zarowski, M., Rotenberg, A., Alexopoulos, A.V., Wyllie, E., Kothare, S.V., and Loddenkemper, T. (2012). Circadian patterns of generalized tonic-clonic evolutions in pediatric epilepsy patients, *Seizure*, 21, 535–539.

Rao, M.S., Hattiangady, B., Reddy, D.S., and Shetty, A.K. (2006). Hippocampal neurodegeneration, spontaneous seizures, and mossy fiber sprouting in the F344 rat model of temporal lobe epilepsy, *J. Neurosci. Res.*, 83, 1088–1105.

Ryley Parrish, R., Albertson, A.J., Buckingham, S.C., Hablitz, J.J., Mascia, K.L., Davis Haselden, W., and Lubin, F.D. (2013). Status epilepticus triggers early and late alterations in brain-derived neurotrophic factor and NMDA glutamate receptor Grin2b DNA methylation levels in the hippocampus, *Neuroscience*, 248C, 602–619.

Sano, T., Reynolds, J.P., Jimenez-Mateos, E.M., Matsushima, S., Taki, W., and Henshall, D.C. (2012). MicroRNA-34a upregulation during seizure-induced neuronal death, *Cell Death Dis.*, 3, e287.

Sato, F., Tsuchiya, S., Meltzer, S.J., and Shimizu, K. (2011). MicroRNAs and epigenetics, *FEBS J.*, 278, 1598–1609.

Selvamani, A., Sathyan, P., Miranda, R.C., and Sohrabji, F. (2012). An antagomir to microRNA Let7f promotes neuroprotection in an ischemic stroke model, *PloS One*, 7, e32662.

Shaked, I., Meerson, A., Wolf, Y., Avni, R., Greenberg, D., Gilboa-Geffen, A., and Soreq, H. (2009). MicroRNA-132 potentiates cholinergic anti-inflammatory signaling by targeting acetylcholinesterase, *Immunity*, 31, 965–973.

Shein, N.A., Grigoriadis, N., Alexandrovich, A.G., Simeonidou, C., Lourbopoulos, A., Polyzoidou, E., Trembovler, V., Mascagni, P., Dinarello, C.A., and Shohami, E. (2009). Histone deacetylase inhibitor ITF2357 is neuroprotective, improves functional recovery, and induces glial apoptosis following experimental traumatic brain injury, *FASEB J.*, 23, 4266–4275.

Shen, H.Y., van Vliet, E.A., Bright, K.A., Hanthorn, M., Lytle, N.K., Gorter, J., Aronica, E., and Boison, D. (2015). Glycine transporter 1 is a target for the treatment of epilepsy, *Neuropharmacology*, 99, 554–565.

Shimazu, T., Hirschey, M.D., Newman, J., He, W., Shirakawa, K., Le Moan, N., Grueter, C.A., Lim, H., Saunders, L.R., Stevens, R.D., Newgard, C.B., Farese, R.V., Jr., de Cabo, R., Ulrich, S., Akassoglou, K., and Verdin, E. (2013). Suppression of oxidative stress by beta-hydroxybutyrate, an endogenous histone deacetylase inhibitor, *Science*, 339, 211–214.

Simeone, K.A., Matthews, S.A., Rho, J.M., and Simeone, T.A. (2016). Ketogenic diet treatment increases longevity in Kcna1-null mice, a model of sudden unexpected death in epilepsy, *Epilepsia*, 57, e178–182.

Singh, V., Sharma, P., and Capalash, N. (2013). DNA methyltransferase-1 inhibitors as epigenetic therapy for cancer, *Curr. Cancer Drug Targets*, 13, 379–399.

Sng, J.C., Taniura, H., and Yoneda, Y. (2006). Histone modifications in kainate-induced status epilepticus, *Eur. J. Neurosci.*, 23, 1269–1282.

Song, Y.J., Tian, X.B., Zhang, S., Zhang, Y.X., Li, X., Li, D., Cheng, Y., Zhang, J.N., Kang, C.S., and Zhao, W. (2011). Temporal lobe epilepsy induces differential expression of hippocampal miRNAs including let-7e and miR-23a/b, *Brain Res.*, 1387, 134–140.

Stafstrom, C.E. (2004). Dietary approaches to epilepsy treatment: old and new options on the menu, *Epilepsy Curr.*, 4, 215–222.

Stafstrom, C.E. and Rho, J.M. (2012). The ketogenic diet as a treatment paradigm for diverse neurological disorders, *Front. Pharmacol.*, 3, 59.

Surani, M.A., Hayashi, K., and Hajkova, P. (2007). Genetic and epigenetic regulators of pluripotency, *Cell*, 128, 747–762.

Szybala, C., Pritchard, E.M., Wilz, A., Kaplan, D.L., and Boison, D. (2009). Antiepileptic effects of silk-polymer based adenosine release in kindled rats., *Exp. Neurol.*, 219, 126–135.

Tahiliani, M., Mei, P., Fang, R., Leonor, T., Rutenberg, M., Shimizu, F., Li, J., Rao, A., and Shi, Y. (2007). The histone H3K4 demethylase SMCX links REST target genes to X-linked mental retardation, *Nature*, 447, 601–605.

Tan, C.L., Plotkin, J.L., Veno, M.T., von Schimmelmann, M., Feinberg, P., Mann, S., Handler, A., Kjems, J., Surmeier, D.J., O'Carroll, D., Greengard, P., and Schaefer, A. (2013). MicroRNA-128 governs neuronal excitability and motor behavior in mice, *Science*, 342, 1254–1258.

Tanaka, H., Grooms, S.Y., Bennett, M.V., and Zukin, R.S. (2000). The AMPAR subunit GluR2: still front and center-stage, *Brain Res.*, 886, 190–207.

Tsankova, N.M., Kumar, A., and Nestler, E.J. (2004). Histone modifications at gene promoter regions in rat hippocampus after acute and chronic electroconvulsive seizures, *J. Neurosci.*, 24, 5603–5610.

Tuesta, L.M. and Zhang, Y. (2014). Mechanisms of epigenetic memory and addiction, *EMBO J.*, 33, 1091–1103.

Vezzani, A., French, J., Bartfai, T., and Baram, T.Z. (2011). The role of inflammation in epilepsy, *Nat. Rev. Neurol.*, 7, 31–40.

Virani, S., Colacino, J.A., Kim, J.H., and Rozek, L.S. (2012). Cancer epigenetics: a brief review, *ILAR J.*, 53, 359–369.

Vogel Ciernia, A., and LaSalle, J. (2016). The landscape of DNA methylation amid a perfect storm of autism aetiologies, *Nat. Rev. Neurosci.*, 17, 411–423.

Wan, M., Lee, S.S., Zhang, X., Houwink-Manville, I., Song, H.R., Amir, R.E., Budden, S., Naidu, S., Pereira, J.L., Lo, I.F., Zoghbi, H.Y., Schanen, N.C., and Francke, U. (1999). Rett syndrome and beyond: recurrent spontaneous and familial MECP2 mutations at CpG hotspots, *Am. J. Hum. Genet.*, 65, 1520–1529.

Washington, J., 3rd, Kumar, U., Medel-Matus, J.S., Shin, D., Sankar, R., and Mazarati, A. (2015). Cytokine-dependent bidirectional connection between impaired social behavior and susceptibility to seizures associated with maternal immune activation in mice, *Epilepsy Behav.*, 50, 40–45.

Weaver, I.C., Diorio, J., Seckl, J.R., Szyf, M., and Meaney, M.J. (2004). Early environmental regulation of hippocampal glucocorticoid receptor gene expression: characterization of intracellular mediators and potential genomic target sites, *Ann. N Y Acad. Sci.*, 1024, 182–212.

Weaver, I.C., Meaney, M.J., and Szyf, M. (2006). Maternal care effects on the hippocampal transcriptome and anxiety-mediated behaviors in the offspring that are reversible in adulthood, *Proc. Nat. Acad. Sci. U S A*, 103, 3480–3485.

Williams-Karnesky, R.L., Sandau, U.S., Lusardi, T.A., Lytle, N.K., Farrell, J.M., Pritchard, E.M., Kaplan, D.L., and Boison, D. (2013). Epigenetic changes induced by adenosine augmentation therapy prevent epileptogenesis, *J. Clin. Inv.*, 123, 3552–3563.

Yin, K.J., Hamblin, M., and Chen, Y.E. (2014). Non-coding RNAs in cerebral endothelial pathophysiology: emerging roles in stroke, *Neurochem. Int.*, 77, 9–16.

Younus, I. and Reddy, D.S. (2017). Epigenetic interventions for epileptogenesis: A new frontier for curing epilepsy, *Pharmacol. Ther.*, 177, 108–122.

Zhang, B., West, E.J., Van, K.C., Gurkoff, G.G., Zhou, J., Zhang, X.M., Kozikowski, A.P., and Lyeth, B.G. (2008). HDAC inhibitor increases histone H3 acetylation and reduces microglia inflammatory response following traumatic brain injury in rats, *Brain Res.*, 1226, 181–191.

Zhang, Y., Kim, J., Mueller, A.C., Dey, B., Yang, Y., Lee, D.H., Hachmann, J., Finderle, S., Park, D.M., Christensen, J., Schiff, D., Purow, B., Dutta, A., and Abounader, R. (2014). Multiple receptor tyrosine kinases converge on microRNA-134 to control KRAS, STAT5B, and glioblastoma, *Cell Death Differ.*, 21, 720–734.

Zhu, Q., Wang, L., Zhang, Y., Zhao, F.H., Luo, J., Xiao, Z., Chen, G.J., and Wang, X.F. (2012). Increased expression of DNA methyltransferase 1 and 3a in human temporal lobe epilepsy, *J. Mol. Neurosci.*, 46, 420–426.

Chapter 8
Models and Mechanisms of Epileptic Encephalopathies

Aristea S. Galanopoulou, MD, PhD

Saul R. Korey Department of Neurology,
Dominick P. Purpura Department of Neuroscience,
Isabelle Rapin Division of Child Neurology,
Laboratory of Developmental Epilepsy,
Albert Einstein College of Medicine, Bronx, NY 10461, USA

8.1 Introduction

Epileptic encephalopathies (EEs) are conditions whereby intense epileptic activity is thought to adversely impact the functioning of the brain, to a degree far beyond what is expected from the underlying etiology or pathology [Scheffer *et al.*, 2017]. EEs are often associated with cognitive, behavioral or psychiatric abnormalities. Based on the definition above, it is also expected that treating the underlying epileptic activities should ameliorate the cognitive and behavioral manifestations. EEs are more common during the early years of human life, including the neonatal, infantile and pediatric ages and they are often linked to epilepsies that are medically resistant. The etiologies can be diverse, including an increasing number of genetic variants (reviewed in [Epi4K Consortium *et al.*, 2013; Epilepsy Phenome/Genome *et al.*, 2017; Epilepsy Phenome/Genome Project Epi, 2015; Galanopoulou and Moshe, 2015]), malformations of brain development, structural or metabolic disorders, infectious or inflammatory or autoimmune processes. Each of these may independently have an effect on brain development.

However, there are situations when a distinction between the impact of etiology and/or underlying pathologies and the consequences of ongoing epileptic activity is difficult, generating discussion and debate about whether epilepsies with specific genetic etiologies should be considered as EEs rather than encephalopathies driven by the developmental and functional consequences of the genetic defect. Similar concerns can be raised for various types of EEs due to structural or metabolic etiologies. Increasing knowledge on the variability of the genotype-phenotype (and more broadly of the etiology/phenotype) associations, evidence that the genetic or other structural or metabolic defects may have various complex interactions with age, sex, region/cell type and environmental factors, as well as epilepsy and comorbidities, that may determine outcomes further complicate such definitions and terminologies. It is therefore likely that a variety of factors contribute to the cognitive/behavioral decline observed in EEs, with ongoing epilepsy contributing the major, or at least a significant, role.

In clinical practice, however, there is a significant merit in using this term "epileptic encephalopathy", since it helps focus the physicians into prioritizing the treatment of the epileptic conditions with the aim of improving outcomes, particularly at times when specific treatments targeting each of the etiologies are sparse or lacking. In this review, I discuss the recent literature that offers insights, largely driven by new animal models, on mechanisms and treatments for such conditions. I primarily cover some of the EEs that occur during early life (neonatal, infantile), which are more common and often difficult to treat.

8.2 EEs of neonatal/infantile age

8.2.1 *West syndrome or infantile spasms (IS)*

West syndrome [Pellock *et al.*, 2010; West, 1841] is an infantile EE that encompasses at least two of the three following features:

(a) infantile spasms (IS), which are characteristic flexion or extension or mixed flexion-extension tonic spasms of the body and limbs associated with a characteristic ictal pattern, the electrodecremental response (EDR);

(b) hypsarrhythmia, a chaotic, high amplitude, disorganized multifocal epileptic interictal EEG pattern that indicates bilateral, multifocal dysfunction and epileptogenicity, and

(c) intellectual disabilities, occurring in the majority of affected infants (~90%).

The characteristic diagnostic type of epileptic seizures in West syndrome is IS which is typically age-specific, manifesting during the first two years of life. Later-onset epileptic spasms are sometimes observed. Other types of seizures can be seen, which may precede or follow the onset of IS and often evolve into drug-resistant epilepsies that persist. Evolution to Lennox-Gastaut syndrome (LGS) is observed in a proportion of infants with IS. Etiologies of IS include structural/metabolic (~60% of infants with IS), or genetic causes [Epi4K Consortium *et al.*, 2013; Galanopoulou and Moshe, 2015], while in a significant number of patients the cause cannot be identified with the current diagnostic methods. Hypsarrhythmia occurs in most patients with IS, yet in certain patients EEG can be epileptic without necessarily being classified as hypsarrhythmic, as has been reported in individuals with IS due to tuberous sclerosis complex (TSC) [Dulac *et al.*, 2010]. The treatment of IS includes hormonal treatments (adrenocorticotropic hormone (ACTH) or glucocorticosteroids), vigabatrin (a GABA aminotransferase inhibitor), and the ketogenic diet, while other antiseizure drugs have a secondary role in patients that do not respond or also manifest other types of seizures.

Early theories attempting to explain the pathogenesis of IS proposed a key role for cortical or subcortical structures in the generation of IS; more recently network dysfunction at the level of cortical-subcortical structure interactions was also proposed [Lado *et al.*, 2000]. Following an NINDS/NIH (National Institute of Neurological Disorders and Stroke / National Institute of Health) sponsored workshop on models of pediatric epilepsies (Bethesda MD, May 2004) which outlined the need and criteria for a model of IS

[Stafstrom *et al.*, 2006], publications describing animal models that manifest features of this syndrome appeared.

The existing animal models of IS include (a) acute models that manifest epileptic spasms during the few hours following selected chemoconvulsants, and (b) chronic models that manifest spasms over a period of days to weeks at least but may also exhibit other features of the chronic course of the syndrome, such as other types of seizures or cognitive/behavioral deficits (reviewed in [Galanopoulou and Moshe, 2015; Galanopoulou and Moshé, 2017]). Acute models may give insight on mechanisms involved on ictogenesis, while chronic models may indicate pathologies important for the chronic phenotype of epilepsy and associated comorbidities. Some of these are reviewed in the sections below, highlighting their contribution on molecular aspects involved in the pathogenesis of IS and West syndrome.

8.2.1.1 *Acute models of IS and ictogenic pathways*

The glutamatergic drug N-methyl-D-aspartate (NMDA) may trigger spasms ("*emprosthotonus*") in postnatal day (PN) 7–18 naïve rodents [Mares and Velisek, 1992]. While originally this NMDA model was described as model of ACTH-resistant spasms in Sprague-Dawley rats [Velisek *et al.*, 2007], based on the lack of response to $ACTH_{1-24}$ or rat synthetic $ACTH_{1-39}$, independent studies showed that NMDA spasms in Wistar rats or C57 mice respond to porcine $ACTH_{1-39}$ [Shi *et al.*, 2015; Wang *et al.*, 2012b]. Although epilepsy has not been described, early exposure to NMDA-induced status epilepticus (SE) between PN12–20 has resulted in deficits in spatial memory in adulthood and increased susceptibility to pentylenetetrazole (PTZ) seizures [Stafstrom and Sasaki-Adams, 2003]. The model therefore supports the age-specific role of NMDA receptor pathway in the generation of IS-like tonic seizures, yet, the lack of a chronic epileptic state does not permit the study of the chronic epilepsy and EE.

A variety of approaches have been used to study how pre-existing conditions may alter the phenotype of NMDA spasms induced postnatally in rats PN12–15. These include: prenatal betamethasone given at gestational day (G) 15 [Velisek *et al.*, 2007], prenatal restraint stress at G15 [Yum *et al.*, 2012], postnatal adrenalectomy at PN10 [Wang *et al.*, 2012b], and prenatal methylazoxymethanol acetate (MAM) at G15 [Kim *et al.*, 2017]. These pre-existing conditions simulated either prenatal stress or perinatal disruption of hypothalamic-pituitary-adrenal axis (HPA) or induced pathologies such as dysplasias, showing that these exacerbate the NMDA-induced spasms frequency. Of interest, prenatal exposure to betamethasone renders ACTH spasms more sensitive to ACTH postnatally [Velisek *et al.*, 2007], whereas NMDA spasms in postnatally adrenalectomized rats were still sensitive to ACTH [Wang *et al.*, 2012b]. Although the prenatal MAM/postnatal NMDA model has been described as ACTH-resistant, it would be relevant to also test the ACTH treatment protocol previously reported to reduce NMDA spasms in other studies [Shi *et al.*, 2015; Wang *et al.*, 2012b]. In regards to long-term outcomes, no epilepsy has been reported in these models, suggesting that more elements are needed to generate the chronic epileptic phenotype and EE of West syndrome. With regard to the clinical relevance of the NMDA model, it is worth citing the genetic association data whereby NMDA receptor 2D (NR2D) genetic mutations have been associated with IS in some patients who improved partially with the NMDA receptor antagonist memantine [Li *et al.*, 2016]. In addition, association of NR2B (GRIN2B) or NR1 (GRIN1) genetic defects has been reported with IS [Epi4K Consortium *et al.*, 2013; Lemke *et al.*, 2014].

The relatively high incidence of IS in Down syndrome (0.6–13%) suggests some common precipitating factors in the two conditions. Using a mouse model of Down syndrome, the Ts(17^{16})65Dn (Ts65Dn) mouse model, Cortez *et al* showed that injection of gamma-butyrolactone (GBL; prodrug of gamma-hydroxybutyrate, weak $GABA_B$ receptor agonist) triggers acute extensor epileptic spasms (AEES) with facial myoclonias and bursts of EDRs on the EEG [Cortez *et al.*, 2009]. Such AEES were reduced by $ACTH_{1-24}$ but not by $ACTH_{1-39}$ and, unexpectedly, were sensitive to ethosuximide, a drug used to treat absence seizures. This model lacks the age-specificity of IS and no chronic epilepsy phenotype has been associated. It suggests a role for $GABA_B$ receptor over activation in spasms within the context of Down syndrome. Association of $GABA_B$ receptor genetic defects with a patient with IS has been reported [Euro Epinomics-RES Consortium *et al.*, 2014].

8.2.1.2 *Chronic models of spasms and epileptogenic pathways*

Several chronic models of IS or epileptic spasms have been proposed, modeling spasms of structural, genetic or other pre-existing etiologies, such as early chronic stress.

The multiple-hit rat model of IS was intended to model IS of structural etiology [Scantlebury *et al.*, 2010]. Induction consists of right intracerebroventricular (icv) injection of doxorubicin and right intraparietal injection of lipopolysaccharide on PN3 rats, followed by systemic administration of p-chlorophenylalanine (PCPA) on PN5. The combination of doxorubicin and lipopolysaccharide suffices to produce a predominantly right hemispheric structural lesion, including cortical, subcortical regions and white matter connections [Briggs *et al.*, 2014; Jequier Gygax *et al.*, 2014; Scantlebury *et al.*, 2010] due to cytotoxic and proinflammatory triggers. The model exhibits a period of clusters of spasms (PN4–13), emergence of other seizure types from PN9 and on, including adulthood, as well as deficits in visuospatial learning and memory and sociability [Briggs *et al.*, 2014; Raffo *et al.*, 2011; Scantlebury *et al.*, 2010]. Although the underlying structural lesion contributes to these deficits, the visuospatial learning deficits can be partially improved by a pulse, 3-day high-dose treatment with the mTOR inhibitor rapamycin, given after spasms onset, between PN4–6 [Raffo *et al.*, 2011]. The same treatment also stops spasms earlier than expected. These findings suggest that these cognitive deficits are due in part to the underlying epileptogenic pathology, which includes dysregulation and overactivation of the mTOR pathway. In the multiple-hit model of IS, spasms are refractory to synthetic $ACTH_{1-24}$ doses that were half the lethal dose, but partially sensitive to vigabatrin; it has therefore been used as a model of refractory spasms to identify new therapies. This model has revealed a role for mTOR pathway dysregulation in IS and associated cognitive deficits in a model that is not due to genetic deficits in components of the mTOR pathway, provided evidence for interneuronal cortical deficits (acquired interneuronopathy) [Katsarou *et al.*, 2017], as well as inflammatory pathway activation. Several drugs have been studied as potential new candidate treatments for IS. CPP-115, a new high affinity vigabatrin analog with less risk for retinal toxicity compared to vigabatrin, has shown better efficacy and tolerability properties in this model [Briggs *et al.*, 2014], and effectiveness has also recently been demonstrated in a case report of a human infant with IS [Doumlele *et al.*, 2016]. Furthermore, candidate treatments that could offer an advantage by earlier cessation of spasms have been investigated in this model, such as carisbamate (currently assigned as orphan drug for IS), which suppresses spasms within the first hours of administration.

Another model of epileptic spasms with a structural etiology is the tetrodotoxin (TTX) model [Lee *et al.*, 2008], in which chronic infusion of TTX intracerebrally (right cortex and/or hippocampus) between PN10–40 results in spasms seen as early as PN16–20 and lasting through adulthood. Although spasms in the TTX model lack the age-specificity of IS, the observance of spasms in older rats allowed the flexibility of multi-electrode recordings that provided evidence for hypsarrhythmic patterns in the EEG. Of note, hypsarrhythmia cannot be recorded in younger rodents (first two weeks of life) due to the limitations of the small size and fragility of the skull, which limits the number of electrodes that can be placed. Spasms in this TTX model are responsive to vigabatrin [Frost *et al.*, 2015].

An older theory of the pathogenesis of IS proposed that aberrant and exaggerated stress responses may subject immature animals to the proconvulsant effects of hormones like corticotropin releasing hormone (CRH) [Baram, 1993; Baram and Schultz, 1991]. Even though the CRH-induced seizures in these early studies did not have the features of IS, subsequent studies investigated the effect of chronic early stress [Dube *et al.*, 2015]. Restriction in nesting and bedding, and altered, elevated mesh floors led to low-frequency behaviors described as spasms associated with spikes, followed by a low voltage background resembling an EDR. Increased CRH expression was found in the amygdala of PN45 early stressed rats. The pharmacosensitivity and behavioral phenotype of the stressed rats with spasms are not yet known.

Genetic models of IS include two models of *Arx* (aristaless X-linked homeobox gene) [Marsh *et al.*, 2009; Price *et al.*, 2009], a gene associated with various early life epilepsies, including IS or Ohtahara syndrome, which demonstrate interneuronopathy, i.e. defective migration of interneuron progenitors. There are several genetic mouse models of *Arx* (reviewed in [Katsarou *et al.*, 2017]) but spasms have only been described in the $Arx^{(GCG)10+7}$ (*Arx* plus 7) knockin (KI) mouse model [Price *et al.*, 2009] and a conditional *Arx* knockout mouse (cKO) model [Marsh *et al.*, 2009]. The *Arx* plus 7 KI also manifests spasms between PN7–11. Events that resemble EDR have been recorded by EEG between PN16–20, while behavioral tests show less anxiety and more retreats in the social dominance test, interpreted as autism-like behaviors. Neonatal estradiol given between PN3–10, but not later, restored the interneuronopathy reported in this model and prevented epilepsy [Olivetti *et al.*, 2014]. This neonatal estradiol treatment could be promising for further investigation as a candidate treatment for epilepsy and interneuronopathy due to *Arx* genetic defect, since these patients could be identified early with appropriate genetic testing. However, other models of spasms from different etiologies have not extended these observations in non-*Arx* models [Chachua *et al.*, 2016; Galanopoulou *et al.*, 2017].

The *Arx* cKO model also demonstrates epileptic spasms, but in adulthood, whereas limbic seizures occur in the second week of life. Both *Arx* models are useful tools to advocate for the concept of interneuronopathy in the pathogenesis of IS of genetic etiology, albeit there are some differences in the type of interneuron deficits observed [Katsarou *et al.*, 2017; Marsh *et al.*, 2009, 2016; Price *et al.*, 2009]. The concept of interneuronopathies, first proposed by Kato *et al.* [Kato and Dobyns, 2005] and supported in both genetic [Marsh *et al.*, 2016; Price *et al.*, 2009] and acquired [Katsarou *et al.*, 2017] models of IS aligns with the beneficial effects that vigabatrin may have in treating IS. However, as discussed by Katsarou and colleagues [Katsarou *et al.*, 2017] a strict and specific pathology-phenotype association between interneuronopathies (or certain types of it) and IS cannot be made, since more widespread dysfunction may occur, in epilepsy or behavioral/cognitive domains, which may interact and can be hard to dissociate. They do offer an interesting mechanism to explore and determine whether specific treatments can be provided that could be implemented in specific patient populations.

Unlike *Arx*, which is well known in human patients with EEs, a less known gene, adenomatous polyposis colon (*Apc*) has been recently linked with IS in a new mouse model, the *Apc* cKO model of IS where *Apc* KO is done in excitatory forebrain neurons [Pirone *et al.*, 2017]. APC is a known tumor suppressor gene that interferes with the ubiquitination of certain proteins, including beta-catenin and other epilepsy-related proteins. Spasms have been reported in PN9 *Apc* cKO mice and adult mice manifest spontaneous seizures. No data have been reported as yet on comorbidities or treatment response. The model poses a role for beta-catenin accumulation in IS pathogenesis.

Although TSC is one of the leading genetic causes of IS, the available models of TSC have not been associated with IS. Recently acute recordings from a mouse model of $Tsc1^{+/-}$ demonstrated electrographic patterns that resembled those seen in spasms in PN12–16 mice, described as high amplitude spikes followed by fast activity [Gataullina *et al.*, 2016]. Further characterization of the model with in vivo vEEG studies for better electroclinical characterization would be useful to more accurately describe the phenotype.

8.2.2 *Dravet syndrome or severe myoclonic epilepsy of infancy (SMEI) and Genetic epilepsy with febrile seizures plus (GEFS+)*

Dravet syndrome is an infantile onset epilepsy syndrome with typically drug resistant seizures, cognitive disabilities and high incidence of sudden death [Dravet and Oguni, 2013]. Seizures may start as prolonged febrile seizures but they evolve into afebrile seizures that may include focal or generalized clonic, tonic-clonic, or atypical absence. The association of Dravet syndrome with certain genetic defects in sodium channels or, less frequently, $GABA_A$ receptors (reviewed in

[Galanopoulou and Moshe, 2015; Katsarou *et al.*, 2017]) led to several animal models that have provided insight into various aspects of the genotype-phenotype association and molecular mechanisms underlying them. The observation that similar genes, albeit different mutations, have been linked with genetic epilepsy with febrile seizures plus syndrome (GEFS+) often results in these syndromes being discussed together (reviewed in [Galanopoulou and Moshe, 2015; Katsarou *et al.*, 2017]).

There are several models of Dravet syndrome, including cKO deletion of exon 25 of the *Scn1a* gene in forebrain GABAergic neurons [Cheah *et al.*, 2012], cKO *Scn1a* exon 7 deletion models from global inhibitory neurons, forebrain excitatory neurons or parvalbumin GABAergic interneurons [Ogiwara *et al.*, 2007], and an R1407X mutation in *Scn1a* gene [Ito *et al.*, 2013; Ogiwara *et al.*, 2013]. Most of these models have been tested in hyperthermia settings and for spontaneous seizures. Epilepsy and sudden death have been observed in models carrying *Scn1a* deletions in GABAergic interneurons, such as parvalbumin interneurons. Interestingly, selective *Scn1a* deletions in excitatory neurons ameliorated the epilepsy phenotype, underlying the important contribution of interneuron dysfunction in this epileptic phenotype [Cheah *et al.*, 2012].

A genetic model of GEFS+ (the mouse model of the R43Q KI mutation of the $GABA_A$ receptor γ2 subunit) raises the following important considerations. The developmental window during which a mutation is expressed may influence outcome, while early developmental expression of a mutation may have lasting effects [Chiu *et al.*, 2008]. Furthermore, the genetic background is critical for the final genotype-phenotype correlation, as recently demonstrated for the same mutation by Reid and colleagues [Reid *et al.*, 2013].

8.2.3 *KCNQ2 and KCNQ3 early onset epilepsies*

Mutations in *KCNQ2* or *KCNQ3* potassium channel genes have been linked with self-limited neonatal convulsions although more severe conditions manifesting with encephalopathy can be seen [Serino *et al.*, 2013]. Mouse models of $Kcnq2^{A306T/+}$ or $Kcnq3^{G311V/+}$ mutations have been developed that demonstrate epilepsy and increased risk of early death, usually associated with generalized seizures [Singh *et al.*, 2008]. Generalized tonic-clonic seizures start early in life and continue through adulthood, although the classic hippocampal pathology of hippocampal sclerosis was not seen in pathology studies of these mice, prompting their classification as representative of the more benign form of the human condition. It is interesting, however, that the genetic substrate of the mouse strains used is also critical determining factor of the severity of the epilepsy [Singh *et al.*, 2008], which may also reflect the variability in genotype-phenotype associations in humans. In a different mouse model with a $Kcnq2^{Y284C}$ mutation, blockade of $GABA_A$ receptors with bicuculline decreased the abnormal bursting from neonatal hippocampal CA1 neurons, attributed to excessive GABA release, which mediates excitatory effects on CA1 neurons [Uchida *et al.*, 2017]. This study attributes the age-specific expression of these self-limited seizures to the presence of depolarizing $GABA_A$ receptor signaling in neonatal neurons (for review see [Galanopoulou, 2008]). However, age-specific expression of *KCNQ2* and *KCNQ3*, which increases during late fetal and infantile life in humans, has also been implicated [Kanaumi *et al.*, 2008].

8.2.4 *Other early onset infantile epileptic encephalopathies (EIEE)*

A growing number of EIEE genes has been discovered and some of these have been studied in mouse models (reviewed in [Galanopoulou and Moshe, 2015]). Some of these genes have reproduced cognitive or developmental deficits, without definite evidence of epilepsy. For example, *Cdkl5* KO mice [Amendola *et al.*, 2014; Wang *et al.*, 2012a] have autistic symptoms and motor deficits without seizures, which are also different in mice with cKO deletions of *Cdkl5* in excitatory vs inhibitory neurons. Similarly, haploinsufficiency of *Stxbp1* (syntaxin binding protein 1, or *Munc18-1*) in mice produces anxiety behavior but no seizures [Hager *et al.*, 2014], unlike humans in whom the gene generates EIEE including IS [Epi4K Consortium *et al.*, 2013]. Other mouse models of gene variants seen in EIEE do manifest seizures. For example, mutations of sodium channel 8A (*Scn8A*), as in *Scn8A*^{N1768D} mice, result in ataxia, generalized tonic-clonic seizures and perhaps death [Wagnon *et al.*, 2015]. The age-specific symptomatology in such mice was partially attributed to compensatory expression of genes (i.e., *Scn2a*) that complement the functional deficits triggered by the *Scn8a* defect. Overall, the increasing number of animal models developed to help understand the pathogenic mechanisms of genetic defects associated with EIEEs will eventually lead to the understanding of the age-specific mechanisms underlying the pathogenesis of epilepsy vs neurodevelopmental deficits, compensatory and modifying factors, and development of syndrome-specific treatments.

8.3 Other EEs

There is still a need to develop animal models for other EEs of the pediatric age range. There is currently no clearly described model of Lennox-Gastaut syndrome, Landau-Kleffner syndrome or continuous spike waves of slow wave sleep (CSWS). A report of a neonatal cortical freeze mouse model of cortical dysplasia was recently proposed as a CSWS model, in which ethosuximide improved the EEG findings [Sun *et al.*, 2016]. Yet, further validation and replication of these findings and better characterization of the pharmacosensitivity profile and behavioral phenotype is warranted.

8.4 Conclusions

Significant progress has been made towards developing animal models that have features that replicate the etiology, phenotype, and treatment of EE in humans. Such models have provided evidence for a possible etiopathogenic role of certain early life insults and genes, modifiers or compensatory factors as well as age-specific features that shape the phenotype. Complete replication of the human phenotype in animal models is not possible and it is important to define the limitations and opportunities each model can offer so as to best utilize and integrate the knowledge derived from such studies. Technological improvements in our ability to monitor very young animals with vEEG is critical to better characterize the onset and phenotype of early onset epilepsies, particularly in very young mice. However, the recent progress made in understanding mechanisms, identifying possible novel therapy targets and developing new candidate treatments offer promise that more can be offered in the future to help children with these devastating syndromes and conditions.

Acknowledgments

ASG has been supported by research grants from NINDS-NS91170, NINDS-1U54NS100064, Department of Defense (W81XWH-13-1-0180), and the Infantile Spasms Initiative from CURE (Citizens United for Research in Epilepsy), and acknowledges also research funding from the Heffer Family and the Segal Family Foundations and the Abbe Goldstein/Joshua Lurie and Laurie Marsh/Dan Levitz families.

References

Amendola, E., Zhan, Y., Mattucci, C., Castroflorio, E., Calcagno, E., Fuchs, C., Lonetti, G., Silingardi, D., Vyssotski, A.L., Farley, D., Ciani, E., Pizzorusso, T., Giustetto, M., and Gross, C.T. (2014). Mapping pathological phenotypes in a mouse model of CDKL5 disorder, *PLoS One*, 9, e91613.

Baram, T.Z. (1993). Pathophysiology of massive infantile spasms: perspective on the putative role of the brain adrenal axis, *Ann. Neurol.*, 33, 231–236.

Baram, T.Z. and Schultz, L. (1991). Corticotropin-releasing hormone is a rapid and potent convulsant in the infant rat, *Brain Res. Dev. Brain Res.*, 61, 97–101.

Briggs, S.W., Mowrey, W., Hall, C.B., and Galanopoulou, A.S. (2014). CPP-115, a vigabatrin analogue, decreases spasms in the multiple-hit rat model of infantile spasms, *Epilepsia*, 55, 94–102.

Chachua, T., Di Grazia, P., Chern, C.R., Johnkutty, M., Hellman, B., Lau, H.A., Shakil, F., Daniel, M., Goletiani, C., Veliskova, J., and Velisek, L. (2016). Estradiol does not affect spasms in the betamethasone-NMDA rat model of infantile spasms, *Epilepsia*, 57, 1326–1336.

Cheah, C.S., Yu, F.H., Westenbroek, R.E., Kalume, F.K., Oakley, J.C., Potter, G.B., Rubenstein, J.L., and Catterall, W.A. (2012). Specific deletion of NaV1.1 sodium channels in inhibitory interneurons causes seizures and premature death in a mouse model of Dravet syndrome, *Proc. Natl. Acad. Sci. U.S.A.*, 109, 14646–14651.

Chiu, C., Reid, C.A., Tan, H.O., Davies, P.J., Single, F.N., Koukoulas, I., Berkovic, S.F., Tan, S.S., Sprengel, R., Jones, M.V., and Petrou, S. (2008). Developmental impact of a familial GABAA receptor epilepsy mutation, *Ann. Neurol.*, 64, 284–293.

Cortez, M.A., Shen, L., Wu, Y., Aleem, I.S., Trepanier, C.H., Sadeghnia, H.R., Ashraf, A., Kanawaty, A., Liu, C.C., Stewart, L., and Snead, O.C., 3rd (2009). Infantile spasms and Down syndrome: a new animal model, *Pediatr. Res.*, 65, 499–503.

Doumlele, K., Conway, E., Hedlund, J., Tolete, P., and Devinsky, O. (2016). A case report on the efficacy of vigabatrin analogue (1S, 3S)-3-amino-4-difluoromethylenyl-1-cyclopentanoic acid (CPP-115) in a patient with infantile spasms, *Epilepsy Behav. Case Rep.*, 6, 67–69.

Dravet, C. and Oguni, H. (2013). Dravet syndrome (severe myoclonic epilepsy in infancy), *Handb. Clin. Neurol.*, 111, 627–633.

Dube, C.M., Molet, J., Singh-Taylor, A., Ivy, A., Maras, P.M., and Baram, T.Z. (2015). Hyper-excitability and epilepsy generated by chronic early-life stress, *Neurobiol. Stress*, 2, 10–19.

Dulac, O., Bast, T., Dalla Bernardina, B., Gaily, E., and Neville, B. (2010). Infantile spasms: towards a selective diagnostic and therapeutic approach., *Epilepsia*, 51, 2218–2219.

Epi4K Consortium, Epilepsy Phenome/Genome, P., Allen, A.S., Berkovic, S.F., Cossette, P., Delanty, N., Dlugos, D., Eichler, E.E., Epstein, M.P., Glauser, T., Goldstein, D.B., Han, Y., Heinzen, E.L., Hitomi, Y., Howell, K.B., Johnson, M.R., Kuzniecky, R., Lowenstein, D.H., Lu, Y.F., Madou, M.R., Marson, A.G., Mefford, H.C., Esmaeeli Nieh, S., O'Brien, T.J., Ottman, R., Petrovski, S., Poduri, A., Ruzzo, E.K., Scheffer, I.E., Sherr, E.H., Yuskaitis, C.J., Abou-Khalil, B., Alldredge, B.K., Bautista, J.F., Berkovic, S.F., Boro, A., Cascino, G.D., Consalvo, D., Crumrine, P., Devinsky, O., Dlugos, D., Epstein, M.P., Fiol, M., Fountain, N.B., French, J., Friedman, D., Geller, E.B., Glauser, T., Glynn, S., Haut, S.R., Hayward, J., Helmers, S.L., Joshi, S., Kanner, A., Kirsch, H.E., Knowlton, R.C., Kossoff, E.H., Kuperman, R., Kuzniecky, R., Lowenstein, D.H., McGuire, S.M., Motika, P.V., Novotny, E.J., Ottman, R., Paolicchi, J.M., Parent, J.M., Park, K., Poduri, A., Scheffer, I.E.,

Shellhaas, R.A., Sherr, E.H., Shih, J.J., Singh, R., Sirven, J., Smith, M.C., Sullivan, J., Lin Thio, L., Venkat, A., Vining, E.P., Von Allmen, G.K., Weisenberg, J.L., Widdess-Walsh, P., and Winawer, M.R. (2013). De novo mutations in epileptic encephalopathies, *Nature*, 501, 217–221.

Epilepsy Phenome/Genome, P., Epi, K.C., and Euro, E.-R.E.S.C. (2017). De novo mutations in synaptic transmission genes including DNM1 cause epileptic encephalopathies, *Am. J. Hum. Genet.*, 100, 179.

Epilepsy Phenome/Genome Project Epi, K.C. (2015). Copy number variant analysis from exome data in 349 patients with epileptic encephalopathy, *Ann. Neurol.*, 78, 323–328.

Euro Epinomics-RES Consortium, Epilepsy Phenome/Genome Project, and Epi4K Consortium (2014). De novo mutations in synaptic transmission genes including DNM1 cause epileptic encephalopathies, *Am. J. Hum. Genet.*, 95, 360–370.

Frost, J.D., Jr., Le, J.T., Lee, C.L., Ballester-Rosado, C., Hrachovy, R.A., and Swann, J.W. (2015). Vigabatrin therapy implicates neocortical high frequency oscillations in an animal model of infantile spasms, *Neurobiol. Dis.*, 82, 1–11.

Galanopoulou, A.S. (2008). GABA(A) receptors in normal development and seizures: friends or foes?, *Curr. Neuropharmacol.*, 6, 1–20.

Galanopoulou, A.S., and Moshe, S.L. (2015). Pathogenesis and new candidate treatments for infantile spasms and early life epileptic encephalopathies: A view from preclinical studies, *Neurobiol. Dis.*, 79, 135–149.

Galanopoulou, A.S., and Moshé, S.L. (2017). Infantile spasms. In Models of seizures and epilepsy, A. Pitkanen, P. Buckmaster, A.S. Galanopoulou, and S.L. Moshe, eds. (London, U.K.: Elsevier, Inc.), pp. 977–993.

Galanopoulou, A.S., Mowrey, W.B., Liu, W., Li, Q., Shandra, O., and Moshe, S.L. (2017). Preclinical screening for treatments for infantile spasms in the multiple hit rat model of infantile spasms: An update, *Neurochem. Res.*, 42, 1949–1961.

Gataullina, S., Lemaire, E., Wendling, F., Kaminska, A., Watrin, F., Riquet, A., Ville, D., Moutard, M.L., de Saint Martin, A., Napuri, S., Pedespan, J.M., Eisermann, M., Bahi-Buisson, N., Nabbout, R., Chiron, C., Dulac, O., and Huberfeld, G. (2016). Epilepsy in young Tsc1(+/–) mice exhibits age-dependent expression that mimics that of human tuberous sclerosis complex, *Epilepsia*, 57, 648–659.

Hager, T., Maroteaux, G., Pont, P., Julsing, J., van Vliet, R., and Stiedl, O. (2014). Munc18-1 haploinsufficiency results in enhanced anxiety-like behavior as determined by heart rate responses in mice, *Behav. Brain Res.*, 260, 44–52.

Ito, S., Ogiwara, I., Yamada, K., Miyamoto, H., Hensch, T.K., Osawa, M., and Yamakawa, K. (2013). Mouse with Nav1.1 haploinsufficiency, a model for Dravet syndrome, exhibits lowered sociability and learning impairment, *Neurobiol. Dis.*, 49, 29–40.

Jequier Gygax, M., Klein, B.D., White, H.S., Kim, M., and Galanopoulou, A.S. (2014). Efficacy and tolerability of the galanin analog NAX 5055 in the multiple-hit rat model of symptomatic infantile spasms, *Epilepsy Res.*, 108, 98–108.

Kanaumi, T., Takashima, S., Iwasaki, H., Itoh, M., Mitsudome, A., and Hirose, S. (2008). Developmental changes in KCNQ2 and KCNQ3 expression in human brain: possible contribution to the age-dependent etiology of benign familial neonatal convulsions, *Brain Dev.*, 30, 362–369.

Kato, M., and Dobyns, W.B. (2005). X-linked lissencephaly with abnormal genitalia as a tangential migration disorder causing intractable epilepsy: proposal for a new term, "interneuronopathy", *J. Child Neurol.*, 20, 392–397.

Katsarou, A.-M., Moshé, S.L., and Galanopoulou, A.S. (2017). Interneuronopathies and their role in early life epilepsies and neurodevelopmental disorders, *Epilepsia Open*, 2, 284–306.

Kim, E.H., Yum, M.S., Lee, M., Kim, E.J., Shim, W.H., and Ko, T.S. (2017). A new rat model of epileptic spasms based on methylazoxymethanol-induced malformations of cortical development, *Front. Neurol.*, 8, 271.

Lado, F.A., Sankar, R., Lowenstein, D., and Moshe, S.L. (2000). Age-dependent consequences of seizures: relationship to seizure frequency, brain damage, and circuitry reorganization, *Ment. Retard. Dev. Disabil. Res. Rev.*, 6, 242–252.

Lee, C.L., Frost, J.D., Jr., Swann, J.W., and Hrachovy, R.A. (2008). A new animal model of infantile spasms with unprovoked persistent seizures, *Epilepsia*, 49, 298–307.

Lemke, J.R., Hendrickx, R., Geider, K., Laube, B., Schwake, M., Harvey, R.J., James, V.M., Pepler, A., Steiner, I., Hortnagel, K., Neidhardt, J., Ruf, S., Wolff, M., Bartholdi, D., Caraballo, R., Platzer, K., Suls, A., De Jonghe, P., Biskup, S., and Weckhuysen, S. (2014). GRIN2B mutations in West syndrome and intellectual disability with focal epilepsy, *Ann. Neurol.*, 75, 147–154.

Li, D., Yuan, H., Ortiz-Gonzalez, X.R., Marsh, E.D., Tian, L., McCormick, E.M., Kosobucki, G.J., Chen, W., Schulien, A.J., Chiavacci, R., Tankovic, A., Naase, C., Brueckner, F., von Stulpnagel-Steinbeis, C., Hu, C., Kusumoto, H., Hedrich, U.B., Elsen, G., Hortnagel, K., Aizenman, E., Lemke, J.R., Hakonarson, H., Traynelis, S.F., and Falk, M.J. (2016). GRIN2D Recurrent de novo dominant mutation causes a severe epileptic encephalopathy treatable with NMDA receptor channel blockers, *Am. J. Hum. Genet.*, 99, 802–816.

Mareš, P., and Velíšek, L. (1992). N-methyl-D-aspartate (NMDA)-induced seizures in developing rats, *Brain Res. Dev. Brain Res.* 65, 185–189.

Marsh, E., Fulp, C., Gomez, E., Nasrallah, I., Minarcik, J., Sudi, J., Christian, S.L., Mancini, G., Labosky, P., Dobyns, W., Brooks-Kayal, A., and Golden, J.A. (2009). Targeted loss of Arx results in a developmental epilepsy mouse model and recapitulates the human phenotype in heterozygous females, *Brain*, 132, 1563–1576.

Marsh, E.D., Nasrallah, M.P., Walsh, C., Murray, K.A., Nicole Sunnen, C., McCoy, A., and Golden, J.A. (2016). Developmental interneuron subtype deficits after targeted loss of Arx, *BMC Neurosci.*, 17, 35.

Ogiwara, I., Iwasato, T., Miyamoto, H., Iwata, R., Yamagata, T., Mazaki, E., Yanagawa, Y., Tamamaki, N., Hensch, T.K., Itohara, S., and Yamakawa, K. (2013). Nav1.1 haploinsufficiency in excitatory neurons ameliorates seizure-associated sudden death in a mouse model of Dravet syndrome, *Hum. Mol. Genet.*, 22, 4784–4804.

Ogiwara, I., Miyamoto, H., Morita, N., Atapour, N., Mazaki, E., Inoue, I., Takeuchi, T., Itohara, S., Yanagawa, Y., Obata, K., Furuichi, T., Hensch, T.K., and Yamakawa, K. (2007). Nav1.1 localizes to axons of parvalbumin-positive inhibitory interneurons: a circuit basis for epileptic seizures in mice carrying an Scn1a gene mutation, *J. Neurosci.*, 27, 5903–5914.

Olivetti, P.R., Maheshwari, A., and Noebels, J.L. (2014). Neonatal estradiol stimulation prevents epilepsy in Arx model of X-linked infantile spasms syndrome, *Sci. Transl. Med.*, 6, 220ra212.

Pellock, J.M., Hrachovy, R., Shinnar, S., Baram, T.Z., Bettis, D., Dlugos, D.J., Gaillard, W.D., Gibson, P.A., Holmes, G.L., Nordl, D.R., O'Dell, C., Shields, W.D., Trevathan, E., and Wheless, J.W. (2010). Infantile spasms: a U.S. consensus report, *Epilepsia*, 51, 2175–2189.

Pirone, A., Alexander, J., Lau, L.A., Hampton, D., Zayachkivsky, A., Yee, A., Yee, A., Jacob, M.H., and Dulla, C.G. (2017). APC conditional knock-out mouse is a model of infantile spasms with elevated neuronal beta-catenin levels, neonatal spasms, and chronic seizures, *Neurobiol Dis.*, 98, 149–157.

Price, M.G., Yoo, J.W., Burgess, D.L., Deng, F., Hrachovy, R.A., Frost, J.D., Jr., and Noebels, J.L. (2009). A triplet repeat expansion genetic mouse model of infantile spasms syndrome, Arx(GCG)10+7, with interneuronopathy, spasms in infancy, persistent seizures, and adult cognitive and behavioral impairment, *J. Neurosci.*, 29, 8752–8763.

Raffo, E., Coppola, A., Ono, T., Briggs, S.W., and Galanopoulou, A.S. (2011). A pulse rapamycin therapy for infantile spasms and associated cognitive decline, *Neurobiol. Dis.*, 43, 322–329.

Reid, C.A., Kim, T., Phillips, A.M., Low, J., Berkovic, S.F., Luscher, B., and Petrou, S. (2013). Multiple molecular mechanisms for a single GABAA mutation in epilepsy, *Neurology*, 80, 1003–1008.

Scantlebury, M.H., Galanopoulou, A.S., Chudomelova, L., Raffo, E., Betancourth, D., and Moshe, S.L. (2010). A model of symptomatic infantile spasms syndrome, *Neurobiol. Dis.*, 37, 604–612.

Scheffer, I.E., Berkovic, S., Capovilla, G., Connolly, M.B., French, J., Guilhoto, L., Hirsch, E., Jain, S., Mathern, G.W., Moshe, S.L., Nordli, D.R., Perucca, E., Tomson, T., Wiebe, S., Zhang, Y.H., and Zuberi, S.M. (2017). ILAE classification of the epilepsies: Position paper of the ILAE Commission for Classification and Terminology, *Epilepsia*, 58, 512–521.

Serino, D., Specchio, N., Pontrelli, G., Vigevano, F., and Fusco, L. (2013). Video/EEG findings in a KCNQ2 epileptic encephalopathy: a case report and revision of literature data, *Epileptic Disord.*, 15, 158–165.

Shi, X.Y., Yang, X.F., Tomonoh, Y., Hu, L.Y., Ju, J., Hirose, S., and Zou, L.P. (2015). Development of a mouse model of infantile spasms induced by N-methyl-D-aspartate, *Epilepsy Res.*, 118, 29–33.

Singh, N.A., Otto, J.F., Dahle, E.J., Pappas, C., Leslie, J.D., Vilaythong, A., Noebels, J.L., White, H.S., Wilcox, K.S., and Leppert, M.F. (2008). Mouse models of human KCNQ2 and KCNQ3 mutations for benign familial neonatal convulsions show seizures and neuronal plasticity without synaptic reorganization, *J. Physiol.*, 586, 3405–3423.

Stafstrom, C.E., Moshe, S.L., Swann, J.W., Nehlig, A., Jacobs, M.P., and Schwartzkroin, P.A. (2006). Models of pediatric epilepsies: strategies and opportunities, *Epilepsia*, 47, 1407–1414.

Stafstrom, C.E., and Sasaki-Adams, D.M. (2003). NMDA-induced seizures in developing rats cause long-term learning impairment and increased seizure susceptibility, *Epilepsy Res.*, 53, 129–137.

Sun, Q.Q., Zhou, C., Yang, W., and Petrus, D. (2016). Continuous spike-waves during slow-wave sleep in a mouse model of focal cortical dysplasia, *Epilepsia*, 57, 1581–1593.

Uchida, T., Lossin, C., Ihara, Y., Deshimaru, M., Yanagawa, Y., Koyama, S., and Hirose, S. (2017). Abnormal gamma-aminobutyric acid neurotransmission in a Kcnq2 model of early onset epilepsy, *Epilepsia*, 58, 1430–1439.

Velíšek, L., Jehle, K., Asche, S., and Velíšková, J. (2007). Model of infantile spasms induced by N-methyl-D-aspartic acid in prenatally impaired brain, *Ann. Neurol.*, 61, 109–119.

Wagnon, J.L., Korn, M.J., Parent, R., Tarpey, T.A., Jones, J.M., Hammer, M.F., Murphy, G.G., Parent, J.M., and Meisler, M.H. (2015). Convulsive seizures and SUDEP in a mouse model of SCN8A epileptic encephalopathy, *Hum. Mol. Genet.*, 24, 506–515.

Wang, I.T., Allen, M., Goffin, D., Zhu, X., Fairless, A.H., Brodkin, E.S., Siegel, S.J., Marsh, E.D., Blendy, J.A., and Zhou, Z. (2012a). Loss of CDKL5 disrupts kinome profile and event-related potentials leading to autistic-like phenotypes in mice, *Proc. Natl. Acad. Sci. U.S.A.*, 109, 21516–21521.

Wang, Y.J., Zhang, Y., Liang, X.H., Yang, G., and Zou, L.P. (2012b). Effects of adrenal dysfunction and high-dose adrenocorticotropic hormone on NMDA-induced spasm seizures in young Wistar rats, *Epilepsy Res.*, 100, 125–131.

West, W.J. (1841). On a peculiar form of infantile convulsions, *Lancet*, 35, 724–725.

Yum, M.S., Chachua, T., Velíšková, J., and Velíšek, L. (2012). Prenatal stress promotes development of spasms in infant rats, *Epilepsia*, 53, e46–49.

Chapter 9

Prenatal/Perinatal Stress and Developmental Epilepsy: Lessons from Life and Experiment

Libor Velíšek, MD, PhD

Departments of Cell Biology & Anatomy, Pediatrics, and Neurology, New York Medical College, Valhalla, NY 10595, USA

9.1 Introduction

There is significant evidence from both the human condition and animal experiments that adversities during pregnancy or early postnatal life can significantly affect physiology of the offspring. Stress is a common component of our lives and indeed can be one of those pre- or perinatal adversities. Elevated levels of endogenous glucocorticoids mediate the effects of stress. This notion is important in obstetrics; synthetic glucocorticoid analogues are frequently used in pregnancies in imminent danger of premature delivery between gestational weeks 24–35 [Korosi and Baram, 2008; McGowan and Matthews, 2018].

The stress and associated enhanced glucocorticoid levels can also alter susceptibility to seizures and seizure recurrence. Studies investigating the relationship of stress and seizures/epilepsy in humans are still inconclusive as will be discussed below. Stress plays a role in epilepsy in the adult brain. The purpose of this chapter is to extend the important findings of stress, seizures and epilepsy to the developing brain. The model used here to illustrate the relationship is the developing brain preconditioned by stress and affected by epilepsy.

The chapter is no replacement for outstanding authoritative reviews that exhaustively cover the topics of hypothalamo-pituitary-adrenal (HPA) axis [Ishimoto and Jaffe, 2011; Wood and Walker, 2016] and its development [Bedont *et al.*, 2015; Lee *et al.*, 2014; Shimogori *et al.*, 2010], stress and seizures [Bale *et al.*, 2010], prenatal stress [Weinstock, 2008, 2017] or programming effects of prenatal steroids [Moisiadis *et al.*, 2017; Moisiadis and Matthews, 2014a, b], or developmental seizures in great detail.

9.2 HPA axis in stress response

The substrate for the stress effect is the elevation of glucocorticoid levels. These raised levels of hormones affect the HPA axis (Figure 9.1) and represent a final common pathway in the stress response. The stress response in the adult HPA system is well described and involves (through hippocampal and amygdala mediation of adverse events) triggering the endocrine cascade, starting in the hypothalamic paraventricular nucleus. Here the corticotropin releasing factor/hormone (CRF/CRH) is liberated (as well as arginine vasopressin, AVP) and these events lead to synthesis of a precursor of adrenocorticotropin (ACTH), the pro-opiomelanocortin (POMC) molecule. ACTH and additional peptides are cleaved from POMC and ACTH is released into the circulation from the adenohypophysis (anterior pituitary). ACTH effectors (for the purpose of the straightforward HPA axis response) are localized in the adrenal cortex, and the immediate effect is a release of a major glucocorticoid. In humans, this glucocorticoid is cortisol and in rats it is corticosterone. Adrenal glucocorticoids engage a variety of tissues *via* their own glucocorticoid (GR) and also mineralocorticoid (MR) receptors, which provide specific feedback at all levels of the HPA axis, including the highest regulatory centers. Thus, activation of these receptors in the hippocampus would attenuate the HPA response, while activation of amygdala GR would potentiate this response. This is a crude simplification of how the fully developed system should work under an acute stress load in adults.

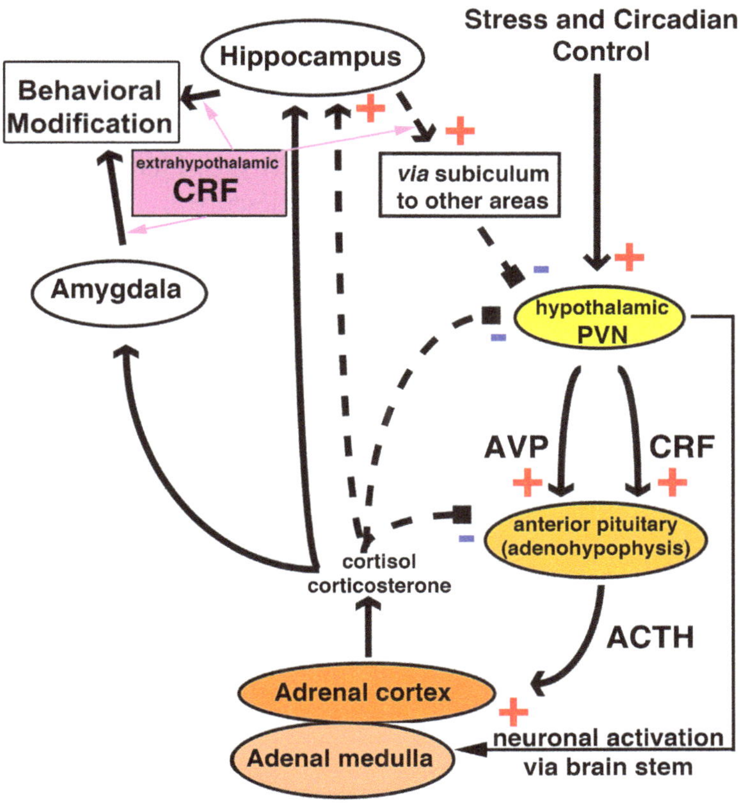

Figure 9.1. A simplified cartoon depicting important elements of the HPA axis contributing to the stress response, their mutual relationship and effects on behavior. (+) indicates activation, (–) indicates suppression.

However, in the developing brain, the stress load may not be acute but if repeated or even chronic, may respond differently from that of the adult. Also, the timing of the stress may critically influence the response. During pregnancy, even small timing differences may have differential effects on outcome. For example, stress during the first trimester of pregnancy (organogenesis) increases risk for fetal birth defects affecting heart development, neurulation (see Chapter 1), and palate development. Stress of a similar intensity during the third trimester carries fewer risks, with subtler effects on behavior [Bale,

2005; Glynn *et al.*, 2001]. Yet, the affected behavioral paradigms may still represent a function of exposure timing within this trimester.

The initial assumption here is that the specific responses of the HPA axis depend on the presence of fully developed effectors encompassing the individual components of HPA axis. First, the ontogeny of the components of the HPA system is described.

9.3 Ontogeny of HPA axis components

9.3.1 *CRF/CRH and its receptor systems (Figure 9.2)*

9.3.1.1 *Rodents*

The CRF system has at least two different components: First is the CRF peptide itself. In both rats and humans, the CRF is homologous, a 41-amino acid peptide. The gene in the rat (*Crh*) encodes a 187 amino acid precursor (pre-prohormone). During rat ontogeny, CRF peptide is first found only after the embryonic=gestational day 18 (E=G18) in the neurons of the paraventricular hypothalamic nucleus (PVN) [Bugnon *et al.*, 1982]. In the hippocampus, early signs of the CRF protein appear at postnatal day (P) 1 [Chen *et al.*, 2001] and in the amygdala at P6 [Vazquez *et al.*, 2006]. Similarly, in the PVN, CRF mRNA expression is strong during E18–19 and decreases perinatally (E20–21). After the early postnatal rise, CRF mRNA expression reaches adult levels at the end of the first postnatal week [Baram and Lerner, 1991; Grino *et al.*, 1989]. Interestingly, CRF mRNA in PVN in mice first appears at E13.5 [Keegan *et al.*, 1994], about five days earlier than in rats [Murray *et al.*, 2010].[1] This finding indicates that any (adverse) events involving the embryonic HPA axis happening prior to those developmental milestones will avoid activation or action of CRF, unless specific developmental programming is induced.

---

[1]Gestational period in rats and mice is very constant. However, there is a strong dependence on the rodent strain. Sprague-Dawley rats have gestational period of 23 days. In contrast, Wistar rats regularly gestate 21–22 days (21.5 days). Mice have shorter gestation, likely determined genetically. Specifically the C57BL6/J strain has gestational period of 19.25 days. Thus CRF mRNA appears disproportionally earlier in the mouse PVN compared to the rat.

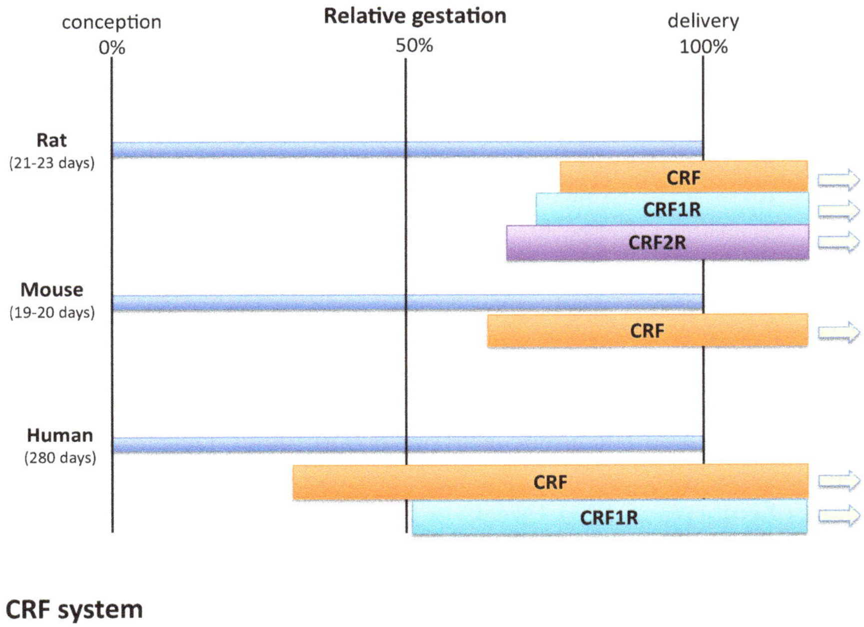

Figure 9.2. Developmental origins of the CRF system effectors in the CNS of the rat, mouse and human. Timing is relative to the duration of pregnancy (mentioned in parentheses) of each species. Green arrows indicate continuation of development postnatally. For many effectors the information is not available. CRF: corticotropin releasing factor (hormone; also CRH). CRF1R, CRF2R: CRF receptors subtype 1 and 2.

CRF mediates its action through two subtypes of G-protein linked receptors, the CRF1 receptor (CRF1R) and the CRF2R [Lovenberg *et al.*, 1995]. In rat brain tissue, CRFR1R is detected around E17 with total levels at about 40% of those found in adulthood. In the hippocampus by P6, the density of CRF1R overshoots adult values several times, in the amygdala about twice by P9. By E16–19, CRF2R can be detected in the ventromedial hypothalamus and in the amygdala, and by P1 also in the hippocampus. These findings are consistent with the previous binding and cAMP activation study indicating early occurrence of brain binding sites for CRF already at G17 [Insel *et al.*, 1988].

Thus, despite presence of the ligand (CRF), there may be brain tissue-specific deficiencies in the effectors (CRF receptors) that may preclude developmental action of CRF. Alternatively, occurrence of CRF2R in the ventromedial hypothalamus preceding the occurrence of the CRF peptide may indicate another functional role of CRF2R, or they may be activated by different ligands such as urocortin 1, which might be specific for the CRF2R and might affect the receptors independent of stress [Korosi and Baram, 2008].

9.3.1.2 *Humans*

While much is known about the ontogeny and developmental distribution of the CRF peptide and its receptor system in experimental animals, little is known about its ontogeny in humans. The CRF gene in humans encodes a 196 amino-acid pre-prohormone. Developmentally, the presence and activity of the CRF system has been shown in brain tissue of embryos at 12–13 weeks of gestational age. Further investigation of the CRF immunoreactivity as well as the CRF bioactivity (using stimulation of ACTH release) showed a positive correlation with gestational age [Ackland *et al.*, 1986]. These findings were confirmed by immunohistochemical study with anti-rat CRF antibody (human CRF molecule is homologous with rat) showing CRF immunopositivity in the human hypothalamus at gestational age of 12 weeks [Bresson *et al.*, 1987]. In human adrenal tissue, CRF1R appears at about mid-gestation [Smith *et al.*, 1998], while exact information on CRF2R developmental appearance in humans is not yet available.

9.3.1.3 *Additional remarks*

CRF production occurs not only in the hypothalamic parvocellular PVN-producing neurons; there is also a significant extrahypothalamic production of CRF in those brain regions that may have significance for origin and control of seizures, namely the hippocampus and amygdala [Maras and Baram, 2012]. This is even more important since in developing animals (rats), CRF is a potent convulsant in the range of picomolar concentrations [Baram and Schultz, 1991]. Hence the early developmental boosts in CRF peptide may contribute to the enhanced propensity of the immature brain to develop seizures.

In many parvocellular neurons within the PVN, CRF is produced together with arginine-vasopressin (AVP). Co-release of CRF and AVP potentiates CRF activity. Since the neuronal populations (producing only CRF and both CRF and AVP) occupy different PVN compartments, it is probably also important for the magnitude of the CRF and the HPA stress response, as to which of those compartments gets activated. AVP by itself can modify seizures in a biphasic manner (lower concentrations are proconvulsant, higher concentrations are anticonvulsant) [Javadian *et al.*, 2016]. This biphasic seizure modulation of AVP may add a significant confounder to studies investigating relationship between endogenous CRF release and seizure susceptibility.

The CRF-producing neurons in the anterior PVN project mostly to the portal vasculature supplying the pituitary. However, the CRF-producing neurons in the posterior PVN compartments project to brainstem areas, particularly to the locus coeruleus, to participate in the sympato-adrenergic component of the stress response. Hence, mutual interaction between CRF and the norepinephrine system may be also important for seizure control.

Interestingly, human placenta also produces CRF (placental CRF, pCRF) as early as the seventh week of gestation and this pCRF is released to both maternal and fetal circulation [Power and Schulkin, 2006]. This feature suggests that pCRF may regulate fetal ACTH production as well as development of the fetal nervous system and likely is a part of the feto-placental stress machinery [Ishimoto and Jaffe, 2011; Smith *et al.*, 1998]. By exponential increase in levels during advancing pregnancy, pCRF also modifies maternal stress responses [Sandman, 2015]. Thus, in humans, pCRF production corresponds to gestational age as well to the initiation of parturition. Human pCRF expression can be stimulated by circulating corticosteroids, an opposite feedback compared to the suppression of hypothalamic CRF production by corticosteroids [Robinson *et al.*, 1988].

Pre- or peri-natal stress also augments hypothalamic CRF expression [Hatalski *et al.*, 1998; Korgan *et al.*, 2015]). This finding is very important because it indicates (together with CRF-related seizure information shown below) that pre- and peri-natal stress may affect seizure susceptibility in the affected offspring [Dube *et al.*, 2015; Velíšek *et al.*, 2007; Yum *et al.*, 2012]. Second, the results clearly indicate that the HPA system can already autoregulate pre- and peri-natally [Wood and Walker, 2016], with consequences for developmental disorders [Harris and Seckl, 2011; Reynolds, 2013].

9.3.2 *ACTH and the melanocortin receptor system*

The next component in the HPA chain consists of pituitary ACTH and its receptor systems (Figure. 9.3). The receptors for ACTH (and melanocortins in general) represent a quite complex system.

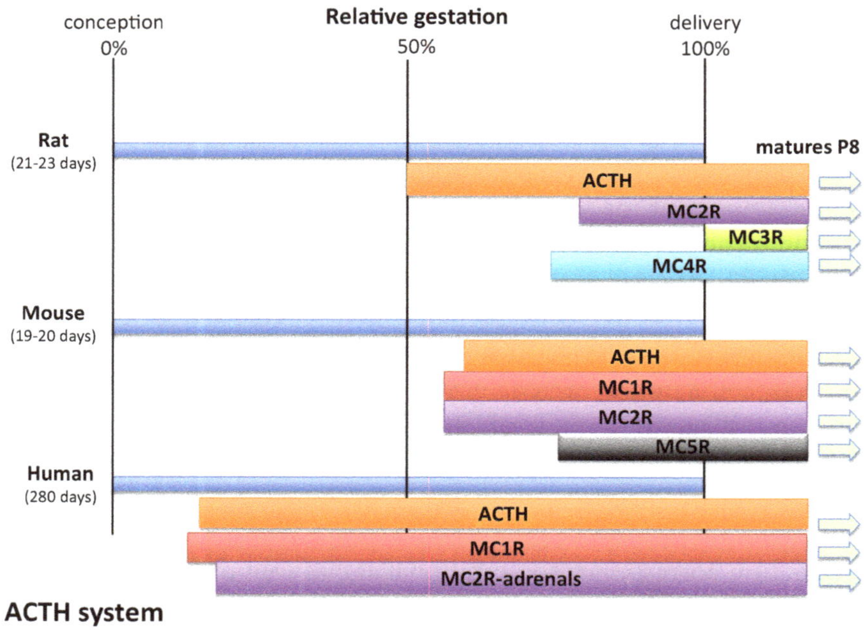

Figure 9.3. Developmental origins of the ACTH system effectors in the CNS of the rat, mouse and human. Timing is relative to the duration of pregnancy (mentioned in parentheses) of each species. Green arrows indicate continuation of development postnatally. For many effectors the information is not available. ACTH: adrenocorticotropin. MC1R–MC5R: melanocortin receptors subtype 1–5. ACTH production and release in the rat matures at 8 postnatal days (P8).

9.3.2.1 *Rodents*

In rats, mRNA encoding the ACTH precursor pro-opiomelanocortin (POMC) is detected already on E12.5 in hypothalamic neurons and on E13 in the anterior lobe of pituitary [Kistler-Heer *et al.*, 1998]. However, according to a newer study, CNS presence of POMC transcripts is detected already at E11.5 [Thomas *et al.*, 2018]. There still may not be transcription of the message between E11.5–12.5. Adult levels of POMC mRNA in the anterior pituitary lobe are reached by P8. This indicates that in the fetus, ACTH can be cleaved from POMC well before the CRF system is developed and likely, CRF of a different origin controls ACTH production. This observation strongly suggests that during this period of prenatal development, maternal pCRF communicates with fetal pituitary and plays a role in triggering its responses. Interestingly, in mice the embryonic period of the first POMC mRNA occurrence is very close to that of rats, at E12.5. Some ACTH forms produced during fetal development are polymorphic and may not be biologically active. Yet at E18, the pituitary system is capable of producing ACTH as a response to maternal stress [Cohen *et al.*, 1983].

ACTH exerts its effect through the melanocortin receptor system (MCR). ACTH is an agonist at all five MCR isoforms (MC1R-MC5R). MC2R represents the major ACTH receptor system in the adrenal cortex, i.e., the receptor system mediating HPA axis function. Interestingly, rat MC2R in the adrenals first occurs on E17, rising rapidly in concentration though E19 and decreasing to low levels during the first postnatal week in the rat. In the mouse adrenals, MC2R is first observed already on E11.5 [Schulte *et al.*, 2007], again peaking around E19. Other MCRs have also interesting developmental patterns. MC3R and MC4R are abundant in the central nervous system and thus can mediate effects of ACTH or it analogues (such as α-MSH) on seizure activity. In the rat nervous system, mRNA for MC4R is detectable since E14 in the sympathetic ganglia and epithalamus, later (E16) in the brainstem and the striatum and even later (E18) in the cerebellum and inferior olive. MC3R transcript was detected only beginning at P1 in the ventromedial hypothalamus and hypothalamic arcuate nucleus. Postnatally, MC4R is widely distributed in more than 100 brain nuclei, while MC3R is more restricted to the hypothalamus and limbic structures [Girardet and Butler, 2014]. In the mouse, MC2R is also transiently present in the brain and spinal cord but only between E11.5–13.5, while MC5R appears in the telencephalon from E16.5 on (or at least through E18.5) [Nimura *et al.*, 2006]. MC1R in the mouse is present at E11.5 in the dorsal root and cranial ganglia and in the ventricular zone, significant presence of the MC1R protein is seen in the CNS at E13.5 [Thomas *et al.*, 2018].

9.3.2.2 *Humans*

ACTH in humans develops early. Its first appearance in pituitary was initially estimated at 16 weeks of embryonic development [Taylor *et al.*, 1953]. However, more detailed study of ACTH ontogeny determined that in the pituitary, trace amounts of ACTH are already detectable in 9 week old embryos. This low concentration of ACTH continues to be observed through weeks 10–19 of embryonic life [Pavlova *et al.*, 1968]. More recent study specifies even earlier occurrence of ACTH in the fetal pituitary, at 52 days post conception (dpc) increasing through 56 dpc (this development follows expression of glucocorticoid receptors in the hypothalamus, see below). After 20 weeks of embryonic life (140 dpc), ACTH in the pituitary sharply rises about 3-fold and continues to rise with peaks through weeks 26–27 of gestation. In a full term baby, ACTH concentration slightly decreases compared to the pre-delivery period [Pavlova *et al.*, 1968].

Melanocortin receptors, the effectors (or targets) of ACTH, also develop very early. MC2R, the adrenal targets of ACTH are detected as early as 8 weeks (56 dpc) post conception [Goto *et al.*, 2006]. Interestingly, MC1R transcripts are present in the adrenal cortex at 8 weeks of gestation (56 dpc) as well. MC1R protein is expressed in the ventricular zone and floor plate at the age at 6–7 weeks of gestation (43–49 dpc) [Thomas *et al.*, 2018]. MC1R cDNA was present in the brain at 18 weeks of gestation (126 dpc). In humans, there is no available information on fetal brain development of MC2R,

MC3R, and MC4R despite the significant role that MC4R plays in childhood obesity [Kohlsdorf *et al.*, 2018].

9.3.2.3 *Additional remarks*

The condition of familial glucocorticoid deficiency (FGD) helped to characterize a new protein in the melanocortin receptor response to ACTH. This component is MC2R accessory protein (MRAP), a novel interacting partner of the ACTH receptors that is essential in the trafficking of MC2R to the cell surface [Chan *et al.*, 2008]. Mutations of the MRAP gene are responsible for 15–20% FGD cases. The syndrome of FGD presents with glucocorticoid deficiency in the absence of mineralocorticoid deficiency. Patients with FGD typically have hypoglycemic seizures, hyperpigmentation, recurrent infections, failure to thrive, collapse, and coma during the neonatal period or childhood [Chan *et al.*, 2008].

9.3.3 *Glucocorticoids, mineralocorticoids and their receptor systems (Figure 9.4)*

In rodents, corticosterone is the major bioactive glucocorticoid while in humans it is cortisol. Cortisone represents biologically inactive form that can be metabolized to the active form or *vice versa*. Receptor systems include glucocorticoid receptors (GR, encoded by the *Nr3c1* gene) and mineralocorticoid receptors (MR, encoded by the *Nr3c2* gene). In contrast to CRF and MCR, MR and GR in their classic forms are cytosolic receptors forming a complex with membrane permeable ligands. After ligand-dependent nuclear translocation occurs, the dimerized receptor-ligand binds specific hormone-responsive elements leading to transactivation of numerous genes. There is also a non-genomic pathway of action of corticosteroids, which involves multiple tissue-specific pathways and is much less understood than the genomic action.

9.3.3.1 *Rodents*

Adrenal secretion in rats occurs already at E16 and peaks at E18–19. Around this developmental period, corticosteroids also initiate their

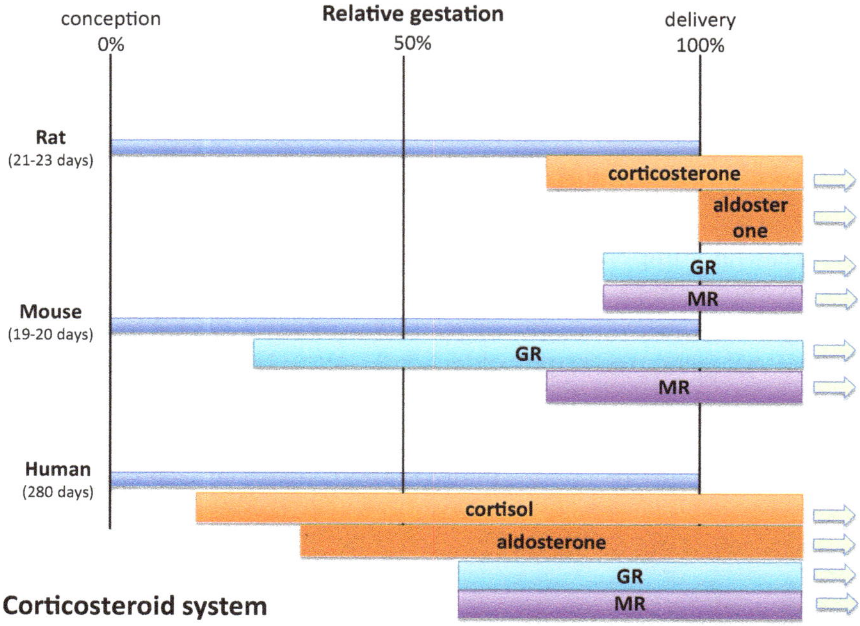

Figure 9.4. Developmental origins of the corticosteroid system effectors in the periphery (adrenal cortex) and CNS of the rat, mouse and human. Timing is relative to the duration of pregnancy (mentioned in parentheses) of each species. Green arrows indicate continuation of development postnatally. For some effectors information is not available. GR: glucocorticoid receptor. MR: mineralocorticoid receptor.

peripheral and central control of ACTH production and release. Fetal secretion of plasma corticosterone decreases after E19 at the end of rat gestation. Maternal corticosterone continues to rise during this period. Production of aldosterone is evident in neonates. Mouse GR mRNA occurs first at E9.5 [Cole *et al.*, 1993]. In the rat however, there is evidence for a parallel increase in the GR protein and transcript only from E18 to P11, with majority of development occurring during postnatal life [Bohn *et al.*, 1994]. More recent studies even indicate the presence of GR transcript from P5 on [Noorlander *et al.*, 2006]. At least in the hippocampus this parallel GR and MR development is accompanied by increasing expression of the protein [Bohn *et al.*, 1994; Meaney *et al.*, 1985a, b]. In the mouse, hippocampal MR transcript appears between E14–15.5 and then, slightly decreases through P10 followed by an additional increase between P10–20.

9.3.3.2 *Humans*

In humans (primates, some mouse strains and lately found also in the rats) during fetal development, a "fetal" zone (also called zone-X) exists in the adrenal cortex as well as a smaller definitive zone. The fetal zone disappears by 6 months of age while the definitive zone fully differentiates by 3 years of age. Cells in the fetal zone produce large amounts of an androgen, dehydroepiandrosterone (DHEA) as well as cortisol (corticosterone). Its mass in human development rapidly increases during the third trimester of gestation (so at birth the adrenals weigh twice as much as in the adult) and regresses after birth [Kempna and Fluck, 2008]. Both zone X and definitive zone in the adrenal cortex are responsive to ACTH and capable of synthesizing and releasing corticosteroids (not only cortisol, but also cortisone and corticosterone). Fine balancing of these three products with differential biological activity may help to explain differences in adrenal sensitivity in premature infants. In humans, *de novo* cortisol synthesis requires presence and activity of type 2,3beta-hydroxysteroid dehydrogenase/DELTA$^{4-5}$ isomerase, which is positive in adrenals at 50–52 dpc. Peak activity of this enzyme is detected at dpc 56–64 dpc, declining towards zero at dpc 100 [Goto *et al.*, 2006]. However, during late gestation it again rises significantly [Lockwood *et al.*, 1996]. CYP11B2 (an enzyme producing primary mineralocorticoid aldosterone) is detected a little later, at 13 weeks post conception (91 dpc) together with fetal aldosterone production and secretion. Aldosterone synthesis is also suppressed by mid gestation but increases around delivery [Bayard *et al.*, 1970], In human hippocampus, both MR and GR are expressed at 24 weeks of gestation with concentrations unchanged through 34 weeks of gestation.

9.3.3.3 *Additional remarks*

The fetus is protected from high maternal glucocorticoid levels by the enzyme 11β-hydroxysteroid dehydrogenase type 2 (HSD11β2). This enzyme forms the "placental glucocorticoid barrier", by converting biologically active glucocorticoids to inactive forms (cortisol in humans to cortisone; and corticosterone in rodents to 11-dehydro-corticosterone) during transplacental passage [Waddell *et al.*, 2010]. It is worth mentioning the three different approaches that can be used to overcome this placental barrier: (1) Overloading maternal circulation by such amount of natural corticosteroids (be it by excess stress or exogenous delivery) that causes saturation of the enzyme and the unmetabolized hormone will eventually pass to the fetus. (2) An inhibitor of this enzyme (carbenoxolone) can be used to permit passage of biologically active maternal corticosteroids to the fetus. (3) A synthetic corticosteroid can be administered to the mother, as it does not represent substrate for this enzyme. All these approaches are utilized experimentally and in human treatment to deliver corticosteroids to the fetus if necessary.

Major mineralocorticoid aldosterone and corticosteroids are capable of binding to MR with the same affinity. As corticosteroid concentrations in tissues are at least 100x higher than aldosterone concentrations, mineralocorticoid selectivity of MR is achieved by presence of tissue enzyme HSD11β2 again converting biologically active corticosteroid species (see above) to inactive. The net result is specific selection of aldosterone for activation of MR. While this enzyme is present already early in gestation, its deletion in both rodents and humans does not affect embryonic or fetal development. Developmentally in rat, mouse, and human fetal brain, there are high levels of HSD11β2. Thus, HSD11β2 may protect brain during fetal development from overactivation of GR or MR by circulating glucocorticoids or shifting the preference to aldosterone activation of MR [Varga *et al.*, 2013]. Neonatally, HSD11β2 gene expression is more restricted and in the adult brain, there is no expression of HSD11β2. Furthermore, there are two MR isoforms (α and β). While isoform α and total expression of MR transcripts are stable during development, isoform β is essentially expressed during the first two weeks of life in rodents.

While natural (endogenous) glucocorticoids bind to both GR and MR, synthetic glucocorticoids (betamethasone or dexamethasone) bind with high affinity only to GR. Finally, mineralocorticoids (aldosterone) bind with high affinity to MR. This pattern indicates that binding of endogenous corticosteroids to GR triggering HPA negative feedback with suppressed synthesis of natural glucocorticoids may affect MR by starving them of ligand. This situation may eventually lead to MR upregulation.

9.4 HPA components in developmental seizures

Similar to previous subheadings, excellent reviews have been published on the topic of stress and seizures and should be sought for broader and more detailed information [Gelisse *et al.*, 2015; Gunn and Baram, 2017; Maguire and Salpekar, 2013; McKee and Privitera, 2017; van Campen *et al.*, 2014; Wulsin *et al.*, 2016].

9.4.1 *CRF system*

9.4.1.1 *Basic and translational research*

Since late seventies and early eighties, there has been much interest in the CNS effects of small peptides including CRF. CRF was investigated after microiontophoretic administration to the vicinity of neurons in various parts of the brain. Interestingly, while CRF activated (increased firing) of neurons in the neocortex and hypothalamus, in other parts of the brain such as thalamus and lateral septum, CRF inhibited neuronal activity [Eberly *et al.*, 1983]. Intracerebroventricular (icv) CRF administration usually had activating effects on behavior with increases in locomotor activity, and also produced arousal or attenuated food intake [Zadina *et al.*, 1986].

One of the first observations about a convulsant action of CRF in adult rats comes from a 1983 study [Ehlers *et al.*, 1983]. After a few-hour delay following the icv administration of low concentrations of CRF (0.15–3.75 nM), paroxysmal EEG activity started in the amygdala and spread to the dorsal hippocampus and neocortex.

Electrographic seizures in the amygdala and hippocampus were associated with behavioral arrest and wet dog shakes and reappeared every 5–60 minutes. Once the electrographic discharges involved neocortex (3–7 hours after the icv CRF), chewing, rearing, forelimb clonus and falling appeared in the behavioral spectrum. These delayed seizures were very similar to those seen in electrical amygdala kindling [McIntyre and Racine, 1986].

Developmentally, there has been much research on CRF effects in the CNS by Dr. Tallie Baram and her team that should be acknowledged here. In her primary study [Baram and Schultz, 1991], she determined convulsant effects of CRF after icv administration in P5–18 rats. The lowest effective CRF concentration capable of inducing jaw myoclonus (25% occurrence in P8 animals) was 15 pM. Additional motor seizures (tonic extension, leg clonus) were limited to P5 and P10 animals and did not occur later in development (e.g., P18 rats) despite CRF concentrations as high as 300–500 pM. This study also determined that the seizures are likely not due to the stress response; they are epileptiform in nature (responded to phenytoin) and mediated by specific CRF-operated system. α-helical CRF_{9-41} molecule, an inactive CRF analogue, blocked the convulsant effects of the icv CRF. The massive convulsant effect of CRF in the immature brain is mediated through CRF1R as the specific CRF1R blocker (NBI27914) had dose-dependent effects in terms of CRF seizure suppression if applied intraperitoneally (ip) [Baram *et al.*, 1997]. Effects of this CRF1R blocker after oral administration were inconsistent probably because of incomplete bioavailability. Seizure suppression was confirmed with additional CRF antagonists (α-helical CRF_{9-41} and D-Phe-CRF_{12-41}), which suppressed CRF-induced seizures as well as with CRF1R agonist urocortin, which produced seizures similar to those induced by CRF itself.

Thus, this extensive body of work clearly determined strong convulsant features of CRF in the developing brain, an effect mediated by brain CRF1R. A search for the detailed mechanisms of these effects revealed additional functions of CRF that may have important roles in developmental susceptibility to seizures. First, developmentally, CRF1R appears to be important for control of dendritic spine density. In mouse hippocampus, exposure to CRF results in dendritic spine loss by an active spine elimination process, which can be prevented by a selective blockade by the CRF1R antagonist, NBI30775. Mice deficient in CRF1R have increased spine density [Chen *et al.*, 2008]. Interestingly, selective augmentation of CRF in the amygdala is found after chronic early life stress induced by providing limited nesting material to the dam between pup ages P2–P9 [Hatalski *et al.*, 1998; Ivy *et al.*, 2010]. This CRF increase is associated with occurrence of spontaneous seizures of spastic character in developing rats of the offspring (P17–35) [Dube *et al.*, 2015]. Another group used prenatal (predator) stress in pregnant rat dams and found increases in hypothalamic expression of the CRF immunoreactivity in a sex-dependent manner. Further, in females only, the CRF increase was dampened by enhanced home cage environment (enriched environment). Extension of this finding may have importance for the occurrence of febrile seizures in a subset of children with fever [Korgan *et al.*, 2014, 2015]. However, the effects of prenatal stress exposure on seizure susceptibility were very variable in this experiment [Boersma and Tamashiro, 2015]. Additionally, this group also found increases in anxiety and depressive behaviors (both of which represent comorbidities of epilepsy) after prenatal predator stress. Our studies also indicate profound changes in susceptibility to develop N-methyl-D-aspartate (NMDA)-induced spasms in the terrain of the prenatally stressed brain (or by prenatal corticosteroid administration) [Velíšek *et al.*, 2007; Yum *et al.*, 2012]. While we have not determined CRF brain levels *per se*, our prenatal stress timing (G15) is very close to the previously mentioned study [Korgan *et al.*, 2015].

There is also a reversed relationship between seizures and CRF. Both pilocarpine- and kainic acid-induced seizures in mice are capable of altering features of KCC2 (potassium-chloride co-transporter responsible for chloride extrusion from neurons) in hypothalamic PVN neurons producing CRF. After seizures, KCC2 is dephosphorylated and downregulated. These actions of seizures impair KCC2 function and increase intraneuronal chloride concentration. As neurons utilize their chloride gradient to determine the polarity of GABA function (inhibitory vs excitatory), this change results in diminished inhibition of CRF-producing neurons, increasing their firing and increasing release of proconvulsant CRF [O'Toole *et al.*, 2014]. This may be one of the mechanisms by which "seizures beget seizures".

9.4.1.2 *Clinical correlation — infantile spasms*

In humans, stress or a perception of stress is often reported before seizure occurrence [Nakken *et al.*, 2005]. Children with generalized epilepsy show increased levels of CRF1R, CRF, and CRF-binding protein (CRF-BP) but not CRF2R [Wang *et al.*, 2001], consistent with animal research on proconvulsant and even convulsant features of the CRF, which include CRF1R but not CRF2R [Baram *et al.*, 1997; Baram and Schultz, 1991].

Much more attention has been paid on the relationship of CRF with infantile spasms, a devastating generalized epilepsy syndrome of infancy. In infantile spasms, the involvement of the HPA axis appears to be prominent irrespective of the etiopathogenesis of this syndrome. This notion is supported by the treatment efficacy of ACTH and oral corticosteroids [Knupp *et al.*, 2016a], both elements of the HPA axis. The theory has anticipated elevation of endogenous CRF levels (due to any unknown reason) in infants with infantile spasms [Baram and Hatalski, 1998] consistent with profound effects of the CRF on neuronal excitability and even neurotoxicity of CRF in the immature brain [Baram and Ribak, 1995]. Thus, based on the finding of (chronically) decreased levels of ACTH [Baram *et al.*, 1992, 1995; Heiskala, 1997; Nalin *et al.*, 1985; Riikonen, 1996], the assumption has been made that this decrease in endogenous ACTH is responsible for elevations of endogenous CRF, resulting in increased excitability and possibly spasms during infancy. Elevated CRF through CRF1R increases seizure susceptibility and may lead to occurrence of infantile spasms. Accordingly, administration of CRF receptor antagonist could reduce seizures in children with infantile spasms [Baram *et al.*, 1999]. One such antagonist [α-helical CRF9–41] has been already used in an FDA-approved human study, which showed no adverse effects [Baram *et al.*, 1996b]. This antagonist was then used in six children with infantile spasms in a two-day treatment paradigm (50 μg/kg in the iv infusion on day 1 and 100 μg/kg on day 2) [Baram *et al.*, 1999]. Interestingly, plasma hormone measurements revealed ACTH downregulation after the iv infusion of this CRF antagonist on day 1 but a robust ACTH increase on day 2 suggesting rapid development of tolerance. No significant change was seen in the number of spasms clusters in the patients in this study. This lack of effect was ascribed to the failure to penetrate the blood-brain barrier because of the helix-shaped three-dimensional structure of this CRF antagonist, as previously demonstrated in infant rats [Baram *et al.*, 1996a].

There is another explanation for the failure of the CRF receptor antagonist in infantile spasms in humans and many other CRF receptor antagonists in animal models of seizures and spasms. Several human studies looking at genetic profiles of patients with infantile spasms and childhood seizures demonstrated association of 17q21.31 microdeletion with seizures and infantile spasms [Bernardo *et al.*, 2016; Wray, 2013]. Interestingly, polymorphism in the CRF1R gene was not associated with infantile spasms, maybe because of relatively small number of individuals enrolled in the case controlled study [Yang *et al.*, 2015]. Thus it appears that deficits in the CRF1R may be responsible for lower levels of ACTH in patients with infantile spasms; there still may be a compensatory rise in proconvulsant CRF but its proconvulsant effects may be mediated differently than previously thought [Baram *et al.*, 1997]. Indeed, CRF1R antagonists would not work properly in the environment of deficient or altered CRF1R. These findings are consistent with the data showing that CRF downregulates its own CRF1R [Brunson *et al.*, 2002b].

CRF may still participate in seizures and spasms during childhood. However, it seems that its effects are quite complex, possibly requiring additional effector systems. Alternatively, a mere disruption of HPA axis signaling may result in CRF upregulation and convulsant effects, yet this outcome cannot easily account for the loss of efficacy of the CRF receptor antagonists.

9.4.2 *ACTH system*

9.4.2.1 *Basic and translational research*

ACTH has been tested in several seizure models, including developmental seizures. One of the first reports in rats indicates that ACTH can delay progress of kindling epileptogenesis if administered early after kindling stimulus [Rose and Bridger, 1982]. Holmes extensively examined effects of ACTH on immature brain, showing that in 15, 22 and 30 day old developing rats, acute (2 day) or chronic (14 day) pretreatment with ACTH prior to kindling significantly delayed kindling rate [Holmes and Weber, 1986]. However, once the 16 day old rats were fully kindled, ACTH did not prevent transfer of kindling from the originally stimulated amygdala to the contralateral amygdala [Thompson and Holmes, 1987]. ACTH was also tested in other developmental seizure models in 15 day old rats [Edwards *et al.*, 2002c] such as minimal (clonic) and maximal (tonic-clonic) pentylenetetrazole (PTZ)-induced seizures, maximal electroshock-induced seizures and hippocampal kindled seizures. ACTH had no effect in any of these models. Others found ACTH effective in a developmental model of infantile spasms with prenatally impaired brain, with the impairment targeted specifically towards the HPA axis, but not in the spasms induced without prior prenatal brain impairment [Mareš and Velíšek, 1992; Velíšek *et al.*, 2007]. Similarly, ACTH was unable to control seizures induced by exogenous CRF [Baram and Schultz, 1995], which indicates that ACTH might not be able to counteract convulsant effects of exogenous CRF, which does not activate (in this treatment paradigm) the HPA axis. However, ACTH may be effective in those conditions with elevations in endogenous CRF activating the HPA axis [Baram and Schultz, 1995]. In rat amygdala, exogenous ACTH was able to reduce CRF mRNA expression in the central nucleus without concurrent activation of glucocorticoid release from adrenals (as the effect was identical in adrenalectomized rats). Interestingly, adrenalectomy boosted endogenous ACTH levels and reduced expression of amygdala CRF mRNA. Additionally, if only the centrally acting ACTH fragment (ACTH4-10) was used, the effect was identical, indicating that ACTH suppresses amygdala (but not hippocampal) expression of CRF mRNA central effects [Brunson *et al.*, 2001]. These effects are most likely mediated via melanocortin receptors (MC3R and MC4R).

9.4.2.2 *Clinical correlation*

In clinical setting, ACTH (as initially described already in 1958 [Sorel and Dusaucy — Bauloye, 1958]) has a prime role in management of infantile spasms (West syndrome). There are several studies indicating that ACTH in several forms (full molecule, or synthetic 1–24 fragment tetracosactide, high doses or low doses) is very effective thought other treatments are used including glucocorticoids (that in high dose may be as effective as ACTH [Kossoff *et al.*, 2009]), and vigabatrin closely follows [Go *et al.*, 2012; Knupp *et al.*, 2016a,b; Lux *et al.*, 2004, 2005; Mackay *et al.*, 2004; Pellock *et al.*, 2010; Stafstrom *et al.*, 2011; Vigevano and Cilio, 1997; Yanagaki *et al.*, 1999]. ACTH is used also for treatment of additional developmental seizures and syndromes, but in comparison to its use in infantile spasms, these other applications are quite rare [Gobbi *et al.*, 2014; Mikati and Shamseddine, 2005; Shimakawa *et al.*, 2015].

Regarding mechanisms of action of ACTH in these developmental epilepsy syndromes, and especially spasms, there is still much debate [Rho, 2004]. Several studies have found that in children with infantile spasms, CSF levels of ACTH are decreased [Baram *et al.*, 1995; Nagamitsu *et al.*, 2001; Nalin *et al.*, 1985]. Then, the expected effect of the exogenous ACTH would be replacement of deficient endogenous peptide with all associated effects (such as suppression of proconvulsant CRF). Another possibility of how ACTH mediates its effects is through the enhanced release of adrenal glucocorticoids. This hypothesis makes sense, as ACTH is directly responsible for this effect and glucocorticoids are also effective in treatment of pediatric epilepsy syndromes including infantile spasms [Baram *et al.*, 1996c]. Two reasons argue against this. First, ACTH is effective against infantile spasms also in patients with ablated adrenal function and second, the efficacy of glucocorticoids *per se* originally appeared to be lower than that of high doses of ACTH indicating an additional effect of ACTH [Brunson *et al.*, 2002a]. It should be noted here that high doses of oral prednisolone may be as effective as ACTH [Kossoff *et al.*, 2009]. This suggests that ACTH works independently of MC2R-mediated rise in adrenal corticosteroids and likely action at other MCR (such as MC3R and MC4R) is involved [Brunson *et al.*, 2002a].

9.4.3 *Corticosteroid system*

9.4.3.1 *Basic and translational research*

Corticosteroids (glucocorticoids) may sensitize brain regions to the damaging effects of seizures by *e.g.* dendritic atrophy in some regions (hippocampus, medial prefrontal cortex) or dendritic growth in other (amygdala) [Vyas *et al.*, 2002]. These effects are dependent on the concentration and composition of the corticosteroid receptor system *in situ* as well as on the magnitude and duration of the excess glucocorticoid exposure. Hyperactivity of the HPA may therefore contribute to deleterious effects of subsequent seizures or may exacerbate the damage afforded by preceding seizures [Duffy *et al.*, 2014]. In some models (e.g., WAG/Rij rat model of absence seizures), stress-induced raise in corticosteroids may have biphasic effects from initial suppression to delayed facilitation of seizures [Tolmacheva *et al.*, 2012]. Similarly, chronic glucocorticoid treatment may even enhance convulsant activity of CRF [Rosen *et al.*, 1994]. Also glucocorticoids potentiate kainic acid-induced seizures [Lee *et al.*, 1989]. Accordingly, adrenalectomy suppresses hippocampal damage afforded by kainic acid [Stein and Sapolsky, 1988]. On the other hand, in a model of focal epileptiform activity (neocortical penicillin focus in rats), there was a suppression of activity with dexamethasone [Yilmaz *et al.*, 2014]. Thus, the variety of available data indicates that exposure, timing, dose, duration and even corticosteroid species may significantly affect the final outcome of seizure susceptibility.

These examples illustrate complexity of a relationship between corticosteroids and seizure occurrence. Once the ontogeny or even fetal development is added to the equation, the situation becomes even more complicated. Our studies have demonstrated that prenatal corticosteroid exposure (two injections of synthetic betamethasone on gestational day G,15) is capable of enhancing susceptibility to NMDA-triggered spasms in developing rats. However in infant rats, flurothyl-induced seizures were suppressed and there was suppression of developmental kindling (P15–16), while kainic acid-induced seizures were not affected (tested at P15; [Velíšek, 2011]). These findings were corroborated by Young and colleagues, who, after prenatal dexamethasone, also found reduced susceptibility to kindling and maximal electroshock seizures in 2 week old rats [Fujii *et al.*, 1993; Young *et al.*, 2006]. Prenatal hydrocortisone (two injections on G15) did not affect either flurothyl or kainic acid-induced seizures in developing rats. Fujii and co-workers, using a three-day single injection hydrocortisone exposure (G9–11 or G13–15) also found a decreased response to developmental kainic acid-induced seizures [Fujii *et al.*, 1993]. However, when prenatal stress was used (employing different corticosteroid species), there was acceleration of developmental kindling [Edwards *et al.*, 2002a]. If corticosterone was used postnatally, it suppressed minimal PTZ-induced seizures (forelimb clonus) and had no effect on maximal PTZ-induced seizures (tonic-clonic), maximal electroshock (transaural trigger of tonic-clonic seizures), or hippocampal kindling [Edwards *et al.*, 2002b]. Interestingly, a precursor of adrenal steroids, deoxycorticosterone, had suppressive effects on seizures induced in immature rats (maximal electroshock and maximal PTZ-induced seizures) but its efficacy was lost with puberty [Edwards *et al.*, 2002c].

It has been also shown that corticosteroids may be linked to depression, a common comorbidity of epilepsy [Pineda *et al.*, 2010]. Accordingly, models of depression have been developed in rodents based on the administration of corticosterone [Sterner and Kalynchuk, 2010; Zhao *et al.*, 2008].

These results further illustrate the complexity of the effects of corticosteroids on developmental seizures. Factors involve prenatal vs. postnatal exposure, acute vs. chronic exposure, low vs. high dose, exact prenatal timing of prenatal corticosteroid exposure as well as particular model of seizures, epilepsy, or associated comorbidities to those investigated. Last but not least, the sex of the subjects modifies the outcome [Braun *et al.*, 2017]. There are likely more factors involved, including all possible permutations that might result in quite unexpected outcome twists.

9.4.3.2 *Clinical correlations*

There is a fine line between corticosteroids promoting seizures in epilepsy patients and use of corticosteroids as treatment for some special seizure syndromes. Stress and the associated increase in corticosteroids are considered precipitants of seizures in patients with epilepsy [Haut *et al.*, 2007; Sperling *et al.*, 2008; Temkin and Davis, 1984]. In some patients with epilepsy, basal cortisol levels are increased compared to the normal population, or cortisol levels rise during postictal period [Culebras *et al.*, 1987]. Steroids have also role in management of infantile spasms as already mentioned above [Kossoff *et al.*, 2009]. The precipitating effect of stress has been studied in a controlled study after Netherlands flooding of 1995 [Swinkels *et al.*, 1998], suggesting increased seizure rate in patients with epilepsy. However, this was a retrospective study that did not take into account lapses in medication during evacuation as well as sleep disturbances. A population study of parents (using the Danish patient registry) after a loss of a child determined that there is a moderate increase in risk of being diagnosed with epilepsy after this stressful event compared to unaffected population [Christensen *et al.*, 2007]. On the other hand, risk of epilepsy in children (again assessed from the Danish patient registry) exposed to severe stress (due to loss of another child to their mothers) during prenatal life was not higher than what was seen among the unexposed children [Li *et al.*, 2008]. This outcome indicates that even severe prenatal stress is not likely to provoke epilepsy later in life. However, there are some drawbacks. The major one is that epilepsy was classified by numerical diagnosis (ICD 8 code 345, ICD 10 code G40), which indicates that individual epilepsy types and syndromes were not distinguished. Thus a significant rise in occurrence of a particular syndrome might have been compensated by decline in occurrence in one or rather several other syndromes. Along this line of minimal effects of prenatal/perinatal stress on epilepsy postnatally, follow up studies of children with antenatal corticosteroid exposure did not show an increase in epilepsy diagnoses [Asztalos *et al.*, 2013; Crowther *et al.*, 2007, 2013, 2015].

In humans, GR antagonists have already been successfully tested for management of depression, the most frequently occurring epilepsy comorbidity [Young, 2006], suggesting intertwining of the corticoid system with depression [Kanner, 2009].

Steroid treatments are also used in special cases of seizures and seizure syndromes such as Landau-Kleffner syndrome, Rasmussen encephalitis and some cases of Lennox-Gastaut syndrome [Dang and Silverstein, 2017; Mikati and Shamseddine, 2005]. Also, seizures associated with Hashimoto disease or thyroiditis associated with encephalopathy [Gul Mert *et al.*, 2014; Patnaik *et al.*, 2014] respond to corticosteroids. Administration of corticosteroids has also its place in patients with brain tumors (with or without associated seizures), i.e., in secondary epilepsies, though their administration may further complicate management of these seizures [Sperling and Ko, 2006]. This notion further supports seizure-promoting effects of corticosteroids, limiting their use for the management of specific childhood epilepsy syndromes. One can only speculate whether the beneficial effects of corticosteroids on seizures occurring during early brain development are related to incomplete development of their receptor system — once the receptor system matures, the beneficial effects are lost.

Preclinical as well as clinical data therefore suggest that HPA hyperactivity associated with increases in glucocorticoid release and stimulation of their receptors may play a role in the expression and exacerbation of comorbid psychopathologies of epilepsy [Wulsin *et al.*, 2016].

9.5 HPA impairment precedes developmental seizures

A different situation may occur when the stress of corticosteroid exposure primes brain development for seizures/epilepsy to occur in the future. This issue was already discussed above. However, there are some key findings and excellent reviews on the topic that are recommended [Cottrell and Seckl, 2009; Kapoor *et al.*, 2006; Matthews, 2002; Moisiadis and Matthews, 2014a, b; Seckl and Holmes, 2007; Weinstock, 2017].

9.5.1 *Stress*

Prenatal or perinatal stress is associated with increased levels of endogenous corticosteroids. If the situation happens prenatally, the stress is mediated from maternal adverse events. However, as mentioned above, the placenta is equipped with the enzyme HSD11β2, which serves as a placental protective barrier [Waddell *et al.*, 2010].

Hence, the maternal adverse events projecting to the fetus by means of maternal corticosteroids must be severe, associated with significant increase in endogenous corticosteroid levels. Only these high corticosteroid levels can saturate HSD11β2 enzymatic capacity and cross the placental barrier.

In animal models, effects of various prenatal and perinatal stressors on behavior have been investigated and reviewed extensively [Cottrell and Seckl, 2009; Kapoor *et al.*, 2006; Matthews, 2002; Moisiadis and Matthews, 2014a, b; Seckl and Holmes, 2007; Weinstock, 2017]. The studies emphasize a variety of outcomes, depending on the variety of input factors (duration of stress, timing during pregnancy, sex of the offspring, single vs. repeated exposure, etc.) as well as significant permanence of the effects afforded by prenatal stress (stress steroids), exposure termed "prenatal programming." Prenatal programming should be considered for well-being during pregnancy as these effects, once acquired, are not only retained but may be also propagated through generations by means of epigenetic modifications (see below and Chapter 7), mostly DNA methylations [Cao-Lei *et al.*, 2017; Moisiadis and Matthews, 2014b].

For example, early maternal stress in rats (day 5–12 gestation) did not have any effect on kindling afterdischarge threshold in adult offspring. However, late gestational stress (days 12–20 of gestation) significantly decreased afterdischarge thresholds for hippocampal kindling in male offspring but not in females [Edwards *et al.*, 2002a]. Behavioral changes in the offspring are likely due to permanent reprogramming of multiple systems in the brain, *e.g.*, the NMDA receptor system [Son *et al.*, 2006; Yaka *et al.*, 2007].

In humans, studies investigating prenatal stress and its effect on postnatal outcomes, including seizures and epilepsy, evaluate significant stressful events. These stressful conditions may include events during aftermath of World Trade Center destruction in 2001, earthquakes [Berkowitz *et al.*, 2003; Glynn *et al.*, 2001], Canadian ice storm, flooding in Netherlands, the Chernobyl disaster, or personal disasters such as loss of a child or a spouse during pregnancy. These events raise corticosteroids and have a significant effect on the development of nervous and endocrine systems (HPA axis), and result in behavioral changes in affected children [Buss *et al.*, 2012; Howland *et al.*, 2017; Li *et al.*, 2008; Martini *et al.*, 2017; O'Donnell and Meaney, 2017; Sandman and Davis, 2012; Van den Bergh *et al.*, 2017; Zijlmans *et al.*, 2015].

Interestingly, it seems that the effects of severe prenatal/perinatal stress on behaviors (with relevance for seizures and epilepsy) are more congruent between experimental animals (rodents) and humans compared to the effects of administration of synthetic corticosteroids (see below).

9.5.2 *Corticosteroids*

In animal models, prenatal or perinatal administration of corticosteroids may have varying effects on offspring depending on many factors such as corticosteroids species (specifically naturally occurring vs. synthetic), dose, duration (pulse vs. long-term), and timing. Different prenatal periods reflect differential sensitivity to circulating corticosteroids (see Chapter 1 and the text above on development of corticosteroid effectors). In addition, prenatal exposure of rodents to corticosteroids a few prenatal days apart may have completely different behavioral outcomes in offspring, and these differences may be also reflected in seizure susceptibility. As an example in mice, a single exposure to prenatal betamethasone altered performance in a battery of behavioral tests while multiple prenatal exposures to betamethasone had no behavioral effects in the offspring [Rayburn *et al.*, 1997, 1998]. Similar to prenatal stress, prenatal corticosteroids also affect hippocampal plasticity [Noorlander *et al.*, 2008].

In humans, antenatal or perinatal administration of corticosteroids may have similar effects as prenatal or perinatal exposure to stress. However, there are some differences that may be important for modification of early seizure susceptibility. First, if synthetic corticosteroids are used for antenatal exposure (imminent delivery before gestational week 34 in humans or adrenogenital syndrome) they are more potent than naturally-occurring corticosteroids. Second, synthetic corticosteroids do not represent a substrate for placental HSD11β2 and therefore, they cross placental barrier without limitations even in low doses. A study in children exposed to synthetic corticosteroids during pregnancy revealed that multiple courses had behavioral effects compared to a single course of antenatal corticosteroid treatment [French *et al.*, 2004]. More recent prospective studies in children after multiple antenatal corticosteroid treatments suggest attention problems at age of 2 years [Crowther *et al.*, 2007], though at age 6–8 years, no deficits were found [Crowther *et al.*, 2016]. A single antenatal betamethasone treatment had no effect on behavioral and cognitive outcome at 31 years of age in offspring [Dalziel *et al.*, 2005]. Another prospective study did not find any nervous system dysfunction in children at 5 years of age exposed prenatally to a single or multiple corticosteroid courses [Asztalos *et al.*, 2013]. These prospective studies also did not record any increase in seizures/epilepsy in the offspring.

In conclusion, there is a gap between significant effects of prenatal synthetic corticosteroids in rodents and minor reported effects in humans. This needs to be further investigated in transgenerational human studies (see below).

9.5.3 *Notes on developmental and transgenerational programming of the brain*

The issue of developmental programming by prenatal corticosteroids has been raised for years (comprehensively reviewed in [Cao-Lei *et al.*, 2017; Charil *et al.*, 2010; Cottrell and Seckl, 2009; Graignic-Philippe *et al.*, 2014; Harris *et al.*, 2013; McGowan and Matthews, 2018]) including programming of the stress pathways [Constantinof *et al.*, 2016]. However, in guinea pigs, there is maternal transmission of the prenatal exposure to synthetic glucocorticoids [Iqbal *et al.*, 2012]. Thus, F_0 generation mothers were injected with betamethasone, F_1 pregnancy was not manipulated, and the behavior and HPA function were affected in both males and females of the F_2 generation compared to F_2 offspring raised from F_0 mothers receiving saline injections. Specifically, in F_2 males, total activity in the open field was significantly reduced. On the other hand, F_2 females had no cortisol response after swim stress and F_2 males had this response significantly reduced in comparisons to control F_2 males. These findings have been recently expanded to the F_3 generation [Moisiadis *et al.*, 2017]. Both maternal and paternal transmission is involved in the generational transfer through epigenetics (DNA methylation) involving genes in the PVN and prefrontal cortex [Constantinof *et al.*, 2016; McGowan and Matthews, 2018].

9.5.4 *Conclusions*

Data indicate that prenatal and perinatal stress may significantly affect seizures and epilepsy in offspring. The mechanisms are complex and likely involve both genomic effects of the corticosteroid species involved, their direct receptor effects, as well as effects mediated by other molecules affected by corticosteroids (such as BDNF) and epigenetics. Severe stressors may contribute to increased occurrence of epilepsy in offspring (both in rodents and humans). Still, the outcome may vary based on the input conditions. Prenatal and perinatal administration of corticosteroids, while having significant effects on rodent behavior, has only minor effects on behaviors and neurodevelopment of exposed children. Regarding seizures and epilepsy, in experimental animals prenatally exposed to synthetic corticosteroids, the outcome is inconsistent, affected by multiple factors and reports indicate few increases in seizure susceptibility and many “no changes” or decreases, again depending on the inputs. Uneven development of the individual components of the HPA axis in the widest terms likely contributes to the varying outcomes. Finally, trans-generational effects of prenatal stress or prenatal corticosteroids described in details in experimental animals need to be followed in humans to determine whether we are not causing our own genetic drift.

References

Ackland, J.F., Ratter, S.J., Bourne, G.L., and Rees, L.H. (1986). Corticotrophin-releasing factor-like immunoreactivity and bioactivity of human fetal and adult hypothalami, *J. Endocrinol.*, 108, 171–180.

Asztalos, E.V., Murphy, K.E., Willan, A.R., Matthews, S.G., Ohlsson, A., Saigal, S., Armson, B.A., Kelly, E.N., Delisle, M.F., Gafni, A., Lee, S.K., Sananes, R., Rovet, J., Guselle, P., Amankwah, K., Saleem, M., Sanchez, J., and Group, M.-C. (2013). Multiple courses of antenatal corticosteroids for preterm birth study: outcomes in children at 5 years of age (MACS-5), *JAMA Pediatr.*, 167, 1102–1110.

Bale, T.L. (2005). Is mom too sensitive? Impact of maternal stress during gestation, *Front. Neuroendocrinol.*, 26, 41–49.

Bale, T.L., Baram, T.Z., Brown, A.S., Goldstein, J.M., Insel, T.R., McCarthy, M.M., Nemeroff, C.B., Reyes, T.M., Simerly, R.B., Susser, E.S., and Nestler, E.J. (2010). Early life programming and neurodevelopmental disorders, *Biol. Psychiatry*, 68, 314–319.

Baram, T.Z., Chalmers, D.T., Chen, C., Koutsoukos, Y., and De Souza, E.B. (1997). The CRF1 receptor mediates the excitatory actions of corticotropin releasing factor (CRF) in the developing rat brain: in vivo evidence using a novel, selective, non-peptide CRF receptor antagonist, *Brain Res.*, 770, 89–95.

Baram, T.Z. and Hatalski, C.G. (1998). Neuropeptide-mediated excitability: a key triggering mechanism for seizure generation in the developing brain, *Trends Neurosci.*, 21, 471–476.

Baram, T.Z., Koutsoukos, Y., Schultz, L., and Rivier, J. (1996a). The effect of 'Astressin', a novel antagonist of corticotropin releasing hormone (CRH), on CRH-induced seizures in the infant rat: comparison with two other antagonists, *Mol. Psychiatry*, 1, 223–226.

Baram, T.Z. and Lerner, S.P. (1991). Ontogeny of corticotropin releasing hormone gene expression in rat hypothalamus — comparison with somatostatin, *Int. J. Dev. Neurosci.*, 9, 473–478.

Baram, T.Z., Mitchell, W.G., Brunson, K., and Haden, E. (1999). Infantile spasms: hypothesis-driven therapy and pilot human infant experiments using corticotropin-releasing hormone receptor antagonists, *Dev. Neurosci.*, 21, 281–289.

Baram, T.Z., Mitchell, W.G., and Haden, E. (1996b). Inhibition of pituitary-adrenal secretion by a corticotropin releasing hormone antagonist in humans, *Mol. Psychiatry*, 1, 320–324.

Baram, T.Z., Mitchell, W.G., Hanson, R.A., Snead, O.C., and Horton, E.J. (1995). Cerebrospinal fluid corticotropin and cortisol are reduced in infantile spasms, *Pediatr. Neurol.*, 13, 108–110.

Baram, T.Z., Mitchell, W.G., Snead, O.C., Horton, E.J., and Saito, M. (1992). Brain-adrenal axis hormones are altered in the CSF of infants with massive infantile spasms, *Neurology*, 42, 1171–1175.

Baram, T.Z., Mitchell, W.G., Tournay, A., Snead, O.C., Hanson, R.A., and Horton, E.J. (1996c). High-dose corticotropin (ACTH) versus prednisone for infantile spasms: a prospective, randomized, blinded study, *Pediatrics*, 97, 375–379.

Baram, T.Z. and Ribak, C.E. (1995). Peptide-induced infant status epilepticus causes neuronal death and synaptic reorganization, *Neuroreport*, 6, 277–280.

Baram, T.Z. and Schultz, L. (1991). Corticotropin-releasing hormone is a rapid and potent convulsant in the infant rat, *Dev. Brain Res.*, 61, 97–101.

Baram, T.Z. and Schultz, L. (1995). ACTH does not control neonatal seizures induced by administration of exogenous corticotropin-releasing hormone, *Epilepsia*, 36, 174–178.

Bayard, F., Ances, I.G., Tapper, A.J., Weldon, V.V., Kowarski, A., and Migeon, C.J. (1970). Transplacental passage and fetal secretion of aldosterone, *J. Clin. Invest*, 49, 1389–1393.

Bedont, J.L., Newman, E.A., and Blackshaw, S. (2015). Patterning, specification, and differentiation in the developing hypothalamus, *Wiley Interdiscip. Rev. Dev. Biol.*, 4, 445–468.

Berkowitz, G.S., Wolff, M.S., Janevic, T.M., Holzman, I.R., Yehuda, R., and Landrigan, P.J. (2003). The World Trade Center disaster and intrauterine growth restriction, *JAMA*, 290, 595–596.

Bernardo, P., Madia, F., Santulli, L., Del Gaudio, L., Caccavale, C., Zara, F., Traverso, M., Cirillo, M., Striano, S., and Coppola, A. (2016). 17q21.31 microdeletion syndrome: Description of a case further contributing to the delineation of Koolen-de Vries syndrome, *Brain Dev.*, 38, 663–668.

Boersma, G.J. and Tamashiro, K.L. (2015). Individual differences in the effects of prenatal stress exposure in rodents, *Neurobiol. Stress*, 1, 100–108.

Bohn, M.C., Dean, D., Hussain, S., and Giuliano, R. (1994). Development of mRNAs for glucocorticoid and mineralocorticoid receptors in rat hippocampus, *Brain Res. Dev. Brain Res.*, 77, 157–162.

Braun, K., Bock, J., Wainstock, T., Matas, E., Gaisler-Salomon, I., Fegert, J., Ziegenhain, U., and Segal, M. (2017). Experience-induced transgenerational (re)-programming of neuronal structure and functions: Impact of stress prior and during pregnancy, *Neurosci. Biobehav. Rev.* https://doi.org/10.1016/j.neubiorev.2017.05.021

Bresson, J.L., Clavequin, M.C., Fellmann, D., and Bugnon, C. (1987). Human corticoliberin hypothalamic neuroglandular system: comparative immunocytochemical study with anti-rat and anti-ovine corticotropin-releasing factor sera in the early stages of development, *Brain Res.*, 429, 241–246.

Brunson, K.L., Avishai-Eliner, S., and Baram, T.Z. (2002a). ACTH treatment of infantile spasms: mechanisms of its effects in modulation of neuronal excitability, *Int. Rev. Neurobiol.*, 49, 185–197.

Brunson, K.L., Grigoriadis, D.E., Lorang, M.T., and Baram, T.Z. (2002b). Corticotropin-releasing hormone (CRH) downregulates the function of its receptor (CRF1) and induces CRF1 expression in hippocampal and cortical regions of the immature rat brain, *Exp. Neurol.*, 176, 75–86.

Brunson, K.L., Khan, N., Eghbal-Ahmadi, M., and Baram, T.Z. (2001). Corticotropin (ACTH) acts directly on amygdala neurons to down-regulate corticotropin-releasing hormone gene expression, *Ann. Neurol.*, 49, 304–312.

Bugnon, C., Fellmann, D., Gouget, A., and Cardot, J. (1982). Ontogeny of the corticoliberin neuroglandular system in rat brain, *Nature*, 298, 159–161.

Buss, C., Davis, E.P., Shahbaba, B., Pruessner, J.C., Head, K., and Sandman, C.A. (2012). Maternal cortisol over the course of pregnancy and subsequent child amygdala and hippocampus volumes and affective problems, *Proc. Natl. Acad. Sci. USA*, 109, E1312–1319.

Cao-Lei, L., de Rooij, S.R., King, S., Matthews, S.G., Metz, G.A.S., Roseboom, T.J., and Szyf, M. (2017). Prenatal stress and epigenetics, *Neurosci. Biobehav. Rev.* https://doi.org/10.1016/j.neubiorev.2017.05.016

Chan, L.F., Clark, A.J., and Metherell, L.A. (2008). Familial glucocorticoid deficiency: advances in the molecular understanding of ACTH action, *Horm. Res.*, 69, 75–82.

Charil, A., Laplante, D.P., Vaillancourt, C., and King, S. (2010). Prenatal stress and brain development, *Brain Res. Rev.*, 65, 56–79.

Chen, Y., Bender, R.A., Frotscher, M., and Baram, T.Z. (2001). Novel and transient populations of corticotropin-releasing hormone- expressing neurons in developing hippocampus suggest unique functional roles: a quantitative spatiotemporal analysis, *J. Neurosci.*, 21, 7171–7181.

Chen, Y., Dube, C.M., Rice, C.J., and Baram, T.Z. (2008). Rapid loss of dendritic spines after stress involves derangement of spine dynamics by corticotropin-releasing hormone, *J. Neurosci.*, 28, 2903–2911.

Christensen, J., Li, J., Vestergaard, M., and Olsen, J. (2007). Stress and epilepsy: a population-based cohort study of epilepsy in parents who lost a child, *Epilepsy Behav.*, 11, 324–328.

Cohen, A., Chatelain, A., and Dupouy, J.P. (1983). Late pregnancy maternal and fetal time-course of plasma ACTH and corticosterone after continuous ether inhalation by pregnant rats. Cytoimmunological study of fetal hypophyseal cells, *Biol. Neonate*, 43, 220–228.

Cole, T.J., Blendy, J.A., Schmid, W., Strahle, U., and Schutz, G. (1993). Expression of the mouse glucocorticoid receptor and its role during development, *J. Steroid Biochem. Mol. Biol.*, 47, 49–53.

Constantinof, A., Moisiadis, V.G., and Matthews, S.G. (2016). Programming of stress pathways: A transgenerational perspective, *J. Steroid Biochem. Mol. Biol.*, 160, 175–180.

Cottrell, E.C. and Seckl, J.R. (2009). Prenatal stress, glucocorticoids and the programming of adult disease, *Front. Behav. Neurosci.*, 3, 19.

Crowther, C.A., Anderson, P.J., McKinlay, C.J., Harding, J.E., Ashwood, P.J., Haslam, R.R., Robinson, J.S., Doyle, L.W., and Group, A.F.-u. (2016). Mid-childhood outcomes of repeat antenatal corticosteroids: A randomized controlled trial, *Pediatrics*, 138.

Crowther, C.A., Doyle, L.W., Haslam, R.R., Hiller, J.E., Harding, J.E., and Robinson, J.S. (2007). Outcomes at 2 years of age after repeat doses of antenatal corticosteroids, *N. Engl. J. Med.*, 357, 1179–1189.

Crowther, C.A., Harding, J.E., Middleton, P.F., Andersen, C.C., Ashwood, P., Robinson, J.S., and Group, A.S.S. (2013). Australasian randomised trial to evaluate the role of maternal intramuscular dexamethasone versus betamethasone prior to preterm birth to increase survival free of childhood neurosensory disability (A*STEROID): study protocol, *BMC Pregnancy Childbirth*, 13, 104.

Crowther, C.A., McKinlay, C.J., Middleton, P., and Harding, J.E. (2015). Repeat doses of prenatal corticosteroids for women at risk of preterm birth for improving neonatal health outcomes, *Cochrane Database Syst. Rev.*, CD003935.

Culebras, A., Miller, M., Bertram, L., and Koch, J. (1987). Differential response of growth hormone, cortisol, and prolactin to seizures and to stress, *Epilepsia*, 28, 564–570.

Dalziel, S.R., Lim, V.K., Lambert, A., McCarthy, D., Parag, V., Rodgers, A., and Harding, J.E. (2005). Antenatal exposure to betamethasone: psychological functioning and health related quality of life 31 years after inclusion in randomised controlled trial, *BMJ*, 331, 665.

Dang, L.T. and Silverstein, F.S. (2017). Drug treatment of seizures and epilepsy in newborns and children, *Pediatr. Clin. North Am.*, 64, 1291–1308.

Dube, C.M., Molet, J., Singh-Taylor, A., Ivy, A., Maras, P.M., and Baram, T.Z. (2015). Hyper-excitability and epilepsy generated by chronic early-life stress, *Neurobiol. Stress*, 2, 10–19.

Duffy, B.A., Chun, K.P., Ma, D., Lythgoe, M.F., and Scott, R.C. (2014). Dexamethasone exacerbates cerebral edema and brain injury following lithium-pilocarpine induced status epilepticus, *Neurobiol. Dis.*, 63, 229–236.

Eberly, L.B., Dudley, C.A., and Moss, R.L. (1983). Iontophoretic mapping of corticotropin-releasing factor (CRF) sensitive neurons in the rat forebrain, *Peptides*, 4, 837–841.

Edwards, H.E., Dortok, D., Tam, J., Won, D., and Burnham, W.M. (2002a). Prenatal stress alters seizure thresholds and the development of kindled seizures in infant and adult rats, *Horm. Behav.*, 42, 437–447.

Edwards, H.E., Vimal, S., and Burnham, W.M. (2002b). Dose-, time-, age-, and sex-response profiles for the anticonvulsant effects of deoxycorticosterone in 15-day-old rats, *Exp. Neurol.*, 176, 364–370.

Edwards, H.E., Vimal, S., and Burnham, W.M. (2002c). The effects of ACTH and adrenocorticosteroids on seizure susceptibility in 15-day-old male rats, *Exp. Neurol.*, 175, 182–190.

Ehlers, C.L., Henriksen, S.J., Wang, M., Rivier, J., Vale, W., and Bloom, F.E. (1983). Corticotropin releasing factor produces increases in brain excitability and convulsive seizures in rats, *Brain Res.*, 278, 332–336.

French, N.P., Hagan, R., Evans, S.F., Mullan, A., and Newnham, J.P. (2004). Repeated antenatal corticosteroids: effects on cerebral palsy and childhood behavior, *Am. J. Obstet. Gynecol.*, 190, 588–595.

Fujii, T., Horinaka, M., and Hata, M. (1993). Functional effects of glucocorticoid exposure during fetal life, *Prog. Neuropsychopharmacol. Biol. Psychiatry*, 17, 279–293.

Gelisse, P., Genton, P., Coubes, P., Tang, N.P., and Crespel, A. (2015). Can emotional stress trigger the onset of epilepsy?, *Epilepsy Behav.*, 48, 15–20.

Girardet, C. and Butler, A.A. (2014). Neural melanocortin receptors in obesity and related metabolic disorders, *Biochim. Biophys. Acta*, 1842, 482–494.

Glynn, L.M., Wadhwa, P.D., Dunkel-Schetter, C., Chicz-Demet, A., and Sandman, C.A. (2001). When stress happens matters: effects of earthquake timing on stress responsivity in pregnancy, *Am. J. Obstet. Gynecol.*, 184, 637–642.

Go, C.Y., Mackay, M.T., Weiss, S.K., Stephens, D., Adams-Webber, T., Ashwal, S., Snead, O.C., 3rd, Child Neurology Society, and American Academy of Neurology. (2012). Evidence-based guideline update: medical treatment of infantile spasms. Report of the Guideline Development Subcommittee of the American Academy of Neurology and the Practice Committee of the Child Neurology Society, *Neurology*, 78, 1974–1980.

Gobbi, G., Loiacono, G., Boni, A., Marangio, L., and Verrotti, A. (2014). Can ACTH therapy improve the long-term outcome of drug-resistant frontal lobe epilepsy?, *Epileptic Disord.*, 16, 185–190.

Goto, M., Piper Hanley, K., Marcos, J., Wood, P.J., Wright, S., Postle, A.D., Cameron, I.T., Mason, J.I., Wilson, D.I., and Hanley, N.A. (2006). In humans, early cortisol biosynthesis provides a mechanism to safeguard female sexual development, *J. Clin. Invest.*, 116, 953–960.

Graignic-Philippe, R., Dayan, J., Chokron, S., Jacquet, A.Y., and Tordjman, S. (2014). Effects of prenatal stress on fetal and child development: a critical literature review, *Neurosci. Biobehav. Rev.*, 43, 137–162.

Grino, M., Young, W.S., 3rd, and Burgunder, J.M. (1989). Ontogeny of expression of the corticotropin-releasing factor gene in the hypothalamic paraventricular nucleus and of the proopiomelanocortin gene in rat pituitary, *Endocrinology*, 124, 60–68.

Gul Mert, G., Horoz, O.O., Herguner, M.O., Incecik, F., Yildizdas, R.D., Onenli Mungan, N., Yuksel, B., and Altunbasak, S. (2014). Hashimoto's encephalopathy: four cases and review of literature, *Int. J. Neurosci.*, 124, 302–306.

Gunn, B.G., and Baram, T.Z. (2017). Stress and seizures: space, time and hippocampal circuits, *Trends Neurosci.*, 40, 667–679.

Harris, A., and Seckl, J. (2011). Glucocorticoids, prenatal stress and the programming of disease, *Horm. Behav.*, 59, 279–289.

Harris, A.P., Holmes, M.C., de Kloet, E.R., Chapman, K.E., and Seckl, J.R. (2013). Mineralocorticoid and glucocorticoid receptor balance in control of HPA axis and behaviour, *Psychoneuroendocrinology*, 38, 648–658.

Hatalski, C.G., Guirguis, C., and Baram, T.Z. (1998). Corticotropin releasing factor mRNA expression in the hypothalamic paraventricular nucleus and the central nucleus of the amygdala is modulated by repeated acute stress in the immature rat, *J. Neuroendocrinol.*, 10, 663–669.

Haut, S.R., Hall, C.B., Masur, J., and Lipton, R.B. (2007). Seizure occurrence: precipitants and prediction, *Neurology*, 69, 1905–1910.

Heiskala, H. (1997). CSF ACTH and beta-endorphin in infants with West syndrome and ACTH therapy, *Brain Dev.*, 19, 339–342.

Holmes, G.L. and Weber, D.A. (1986). Effects of ACTH on seizure susceptibility in the developing brain, *Ann. Neurol.*, 20, 82–88.

Howland, M.A., Sandman, C.A., and Glynn, L.M. (2017). Developmental origins of the human hypothalamic-pituitary-adrenal axis, *Expert Rev. Endocrinol. Metab.*, 12, 321–339.

Insel, T.R., Battaglia, G., Fairbanks, D.W., and De Souza, E.B. (1988). The ontogeny of brain receptors for corticotropin-releasing factor and the development of their functional association with adenylate cyclase, *J. Neurosci.*, 8, 4151–4158.

Iqbal, M., Moisiadis, V.G., Kostaki, A., and Matthews, S.G. (2012). Transgenerational effects of prenatal synthetic glucocorticoids on hypothalamic-pituitary-adrenal function, *Endocrinology*, 153, 3295–3307.

Ishimoto, H. and Jaffe, R.B. (2011). Development and function of the human fetal adrenal cortex: a key component in the feto-placental unit, *Endocr. Rev.*, 32, 317–355.

Ivy, A.S., Rex, C.S., Chen, Y., Dube, C., Maras, P.M., Grigoriadis, D.E., Gall, C.M., Lynch, G., and Baram, T.Z. (2010). Hippocampal dysfunction and cognitive impairments provoked by chronic early-life stress involve excessive activation of CRH receptors, *J. Neurosci.*, 30, 13005–13015.

Javadian, N., Rahimi, N., Javadi-Paydar, M., Doustimotlagh, A.H., and Dehpour, A.R. (2016). The modulatory effect of nitric oxide in pro- and anti-convulsive effects of vasopressin in PTZ-induced seizures threshold in mice, *Epilepsy Res.*, 126, 134–140.

Kanner, A.M. (2009). Depression and epilepsy: do glucocorticoids and glutamate explain their relationship?, *Curr. Neurol. Neurosci. Rep.*, 9, 307–312.

Kapoor, A., Dunn, E., Kostaki, A., Andrews, M.H., and Matthews, S.G. (2006). Fetal programming of hypothalamo-pituitary-adrenal function: prenatal stress and glucocorticoids, *J. Physiol.*, 572, 31–44.

Keegan, C.E., Herman, J.P., Karolyi, I.J., O'Shea, K.S., Camper, S.A., and Seasholtz, A.F. (1994). Differential expression of corticotropin-releasing hormone in developing mouse embryos and adult brain, *Endocrinology*, 134, 2547–2555.

Kempna, P. and Fluck, C.E. (2008). Adrenal gland development and defects, *Best Pract. Res. Clin. Endocrinol. Metab.*, 22, 77–93.

Kistler-Heer, V., Lauber, M.E., and Lichtensteiger, W. (1998). Different developmental patterns of melanocortin MC3 and MC4 receptor mRNA: predominance of Mc4 in fetal rat nervous system, *J. Neuroendocrinol.*, 10, 133–146.

Knupp, K.G., Coryell, J., Nickels, K.C., Ryan, N., Leister, E., Loddenkemper, T., Grinspan, Z., Hartman, A.L., Kossoff, E.H., Gaillard, W.D., Mytinger, J.R., Joshi, S., Shellhaas, R.A., Sullivan, J., Dlugos, D., Hamikawa, L., Berg, A.T., Millichap, J., Nordli, D.R., Jr., Wirrell, E., and Pediatric Epilepsy Research, C. (2016a). Response to treatment in a prospective national infantile spasms cohort, *Ann. Neurol.*, 79, 475–484.

Knupp, K.G., Leister, E., Coryell, J., Nickels, K.C., Ryan, N., Juarez-Colunga, E., Gaillard, W.D., Mytinger, J.R., Berg, A.T., Millichap, J., Nordli, D.R., Jr., Joshi, S., Shellhaas, R.A., Loddenkemper, T., Dlugos, D., Wirrell, E., Sullivan, J., Hartman, A.L., Kossoff, E.H., Grinspan, Z.M., Hamikawa, L., and Pediatric Epilepsy Research, C. (2016b). Response to second treatment after initial failed treatment in a multi-center prospective infantile spasms cohort, *Epilepsia*, 57, 1834–1842.

Kohlsdorf, K., Nunziata, A., Funcke, J.B., Brandt, S., von Schnurbein, J., Vollbach, H., Lennerz, B., Fritsch, M., Greber-Platzer, S., Frohlich-Reiterer, E., Luedeke, M., Borck, G., Debatin, K.M., Fischer-Posovszky, P., and Wabitsch, M. (2018). Early childhood BMI trajectories in monogenic obesity due to leptin, leptin receptor, and melanocortin 4 receptor deficiency, *Int. J. Obesity* https://doi.org/10.1038/s41366-018-0049-6.

Korgan, A.C., Green, A.D., Perrot, T.S., and Esser, M.J. (2014). Limbic system activation is affected by prenatal predator exposure and postnatal environmental enrichment and further moderated by dam and sex, *Behav. Brain Res.*, 259, 106–118.

Korgan, A.C., Vonkeman, J., Esser, M.J., and Perrot, T.S. (2015). An enhanced home cage modulates hypothalamic CRH-ir labeling in juvenile rats, with and without sub-threshold febrile convulsions, *Dev. Psychobiol.*, 57, 374–381.

Korosi, A. and Baram, T.Z. (2008). The central corticotropin releasing factor system during development and adulthood, *Eur. J. Pharmacol.*, 583, 204–214.

Kossoff, E.H., Hartman, A.L., Rubenstein, J.E., and Vining, E.P. (2009). High-dose oral prednisolone for infantile spasms: an effective and less expensive alternative to ACTH, *Epilepsy Behav.*, 14, 674–676.

Lee, D.A., Yoo, S., Pak, T., Salvatierra, J., Velarde, E., Aja, S., and Blackshaw, S. (2014). Dietary and sex-specific factors regulate hypothalamic neurogenesis in young adult mice, *Front. Neurosci.*, 8, 157.

Lee, P.H., Grimes, L., and Hong, J.S. (1989). Glucocorticoids potentiate kainic acid-induced seizures and wet dog shakes, *Brain Res.*, 480, 322–325.

Li, J., Vestergaard, M., Obel, C., Precht, D.H., Christensen, J., Lu, M., and Olsen, J. (2008). Prenatal stress and epilepsy in later life: a nationwide follow-up study in Denmark, *Epilepsy Res.*, 81, 52–57.

Lockwood, C.J., Radunovic, N., Nastic, D., Petkovic, S., Aigner, S., and Berkowitz, G.S. (1996). Corticotropin-releasing hormone and related pituitary-adrenal axis hormones in fetal and maternal blood during the second half of pregnancy, *J. Perinat. Med.*, 24, 243–251.

Lovenberg, T.W., Liaw, C.W., Grigoriadis, D.E., Clevenger, W., Chalmers, D.T., De Souza, E.B., and Oltersdorf, T. (1995). Cloning and characterization of a functionally distinct corticotropin-releasing factor receptor subtype from rat brain, *Proc. Natl. Acad. Sci. U.S.A.*, 92, 836–840.

Lux, A.L., Edwards, S.W., Hancock, E., Johnson, A.L., Kennedy, C.R., Newton, R.W., O'Callaghan, F.J., Verity, C.M., and Osborne, J.P. (2004). The United Kingdom Infantile Spasms Study comparing vigabatrin with prednisolone or tetracosactide at 14 days: a multicentre, randomised controlled trial, *Lancet*, 364, 1773–1778.

Lux, A.L., Edwards, S.W., Hancock, E., Johnson, A.L., Kennedy, C.R., Newton, R.W., O'Callaghan, F.J., Verity, C.M., and Osborne, J.P. (2005). The United Kingdom Infantile Spasms Study (UKISS) comparing hormone treatment with vigabatrin on developmental and epilepsy outcomes to age 14 months: a multicentre randomised trial, *Lancet Neurol.*, 4, 712–717.

Mackay, M.T., Weiss, S.K., Adams-Webber, T., Ashwal, S., Stephens, D., Ballaban-Gill, K., Baram, T.Z., Duchowny, M., Hirtz, D., Pellock, J.M., Shields, W.D., Shinnar, S., Wyllie, E., and Snead, O.C., 3rd (2004). Practice parameter: medical treatment of infantile spasms: report of the American Academy of Neurology and the Child Neurology Society, *Neurology*, 62, 1668–1681.

Maguire, J. and Salpekar, J.A. (2013). Stress, seizures, and hypothalamic-pituitary-adrenal axis targets for the treatment of epilepsy, *Epilepsy Behav.*, 26, 352–362.

Maras, P.M. and Baram, T.Z. (2012). Sculpting the hippocampus from within: stress, spines, and CRH, *Trends Neurosci.*, 35, 315–324.

Mareš, P. and Velíšek, L. (1992). N-methyl-D-aspartate (NMDA)-induced seizures in developing rats, *Brain Res. Dev. Brain Res.*, 65, 185–189.

Martini, J., Petzoldt, J., Knappe, S., Garthus-Niegel, S., Asselmann, E., and Wittchen, H.U. (2017). Infant, maternal, and familial predictors and correlates of regulatory problems in early infancy: The differential role of infant temperament and maternal anxiety and depression, *Early Hum. Dev.*, 115, 23–31.

Matthews, S.G. (2002). Early programming of the hypothalamo-pituitary-adrenal axis, *Trends Endocrinol. Metab.*, 13, 373–380.

McGowan, P.O. and Matthews, S.G. (2018). Prenatal stress, glucocorticoids, and developmental programming of the stress response, *Endocrinology*, 159, 69–82.

McIntyre, D.C. and Racine, R.J. (1986). Kindling mechanisms: Current progress on an experimental epilepsy model, *Progr. Neurobiol.*, 27, 1–12.

McKee, H.R. and Privitera, M.D. (2017). Stress as a seizure precipitant: Identification, associated factors, and treatment options, *Seizure*, 44, 21–26.

Meaney, M.J., Sapolsky, R.M., and McEwen, B.S. (1985a). The development of the glucocorticoid receptor system in the rat limbic brain. I. Ontogeny and autoregulation, *Brain Res.*, 350, 159–164.

Meaney, M.J., Sapolsky, R.M., and McEwen, B.S. (1985b). The development of the glucocorticoid receptor system in the rat limbic brain. II. An autoradiographic study, *Brain Res.*, 350, 165–168.

Mikati, M.A. and Shamseddine, A.N. (2005). Management of Landau-Kleffner syndrome, *Paediatr. Drugs*, 7, 377–389.

Moisiadis, V.G., Constantinof, A., Kostaki, A., Szyf, M., and Matthews, S.G. (2017). Prenatal glucocorticoid exposure modifies endocrine function and behaviour for 3 generations following maternal and paternal transmission, *Sci. Rep.*, 7, 11814.

Moisiadis, V.G. and Matthews, S.G. (2014a). Glucocorticoids and fetal programming part 1: Outcomes, *Nat. Rev. Endocrinol.*, 10, 391–402.

Moisiadis, V.G. and Matthews, S.G. (2014b). Glucocorticoids and fetal programming part 2: Mechanisms, *Nat. Rev. Endocrinol.*, 10, 403–411.

Murray, S.A., Morgan, J.L., Kane, C., Sharma, Y., Heffner, C.S., Lake, J., and Donahue, L.R. (2010). Mouse gestation length is genetically determined, *PLoS One*, 5, e12418.

Nagamitsu, S., Matsuishi, T., Yamashita, Y., Shimizu, T., Iwanaga, R., Murakami, Y., Miyazaki, M., Hashimoto, T., and Kato, H. (2001).

Decreased cerebrospinal fluid levels of beta-endorphin and ACTH in children with infantile spasms, *J. Neural. Transm.*, 108, 363–371.

Nakken, K.O., Solaas, M.H., Kjeldsen, M.J., Friis, M.L., Pellock, J.M., and Corey, L.A. (2005). Which seizure-precipitating factors do patients with epilepsy most frequently report?, *Epilepsy Behav.*, 6, 85–89.

Nalin, A., Facchinetti, F., Galli, V., Petraglia, F., Storchi, R., and Genazzani, A.R. (1985). Reduced ACTH content in cerebrospinal fluid of children affected by cryptogenic infantile spasms with hypsarrhythmia, *Epilepsia*, 26, 446–449.

Nimura, M., Udagawa, J., Hatta, T., Hashimoto, R., and Otani, H. (2006). Spatial and temporal patterns of expression of melanocortin type 2 and 5 receptors in the fetal mouse tissues and organs, *Anat. Embryol. (Berl)*, 211, 109–117.

Noorlander, C.W., De Graan, P.N., Middeldorp, J., Van Beers, J.J., and Visser, G.H. (2006). Ontogeny of hippocampal corticosteroid receptors: effects of antenatal glucocorticoids in human and mouse, *J. Comp. Neurol.*, 499, 924–932.

Noorlander, C.W., Visser, G.H., Ramakers, G.M., Nikkels, P.G., and de Graan, P.N. (2008). Prenatal corticosteroid exposure affects hippocampal plasticity and reduces lifespan, *Dev. Neurobiol.*, 68, 237–246.

O'Donnell, K.J., and Meaney, M.J. (2017). Fetal origins of mental health: The developmental origins of health and disease hypothesis, *Am. J. Psychiatry*, 174, 319–328.

O'Toole, K.K., Hooper, A., Wakefield, S., and Maguire, J. (2014). Seizure-induced disinhibition of the HPA axis increases seizure susceptibility, *Epilepsy Res.*, 108, 29–43.

Patnaik, S.K., Upreti, V., and Dhull, P. (2014). Steroid responsive encephalopathy associated with autoimmune thyroiditis (SREAT) in childhood, *J. Pediatr. Endocrinol. Metab.*, 27, 737–744.

Pavlova, E.B., Pronina, T.S., and Skebelskaya, Y.B. (1968). Histostructure of adenohypophysis of human fetuses and contents of somatotropic and adrenocorticotropic hormones, *Gen. Comp. Endocrinol.*, 10, 269–276.

Pellock, J.M., Hrachovy, R., Shinnar, S., Baram, T.Z., Bettis, D., Dlugos, D.J., Gaillard, W.D., Gibson, P.A., Holmes, G.L., Nordl, D.R., O'Dell, C., Shields, W.D., Trevathan, E., and Wheless, J.W. (2010). Infantile spasms: a U.S. consensus report, *Epilepsia*, 51, 2175–2189.

Pineda, E., Shin, D., Sankar, R., and Mazarati, A.M. (2010). Comorbidity between epilepsy and depression: experimental evidence for the involvement of serotonergic, glucocorticoid, and neuroinflammatory mechanisms, *Epilepsia*, 51 Suppl 3, 110–114.

Power, M.L. and Schulkin, J. (2006). Functions of corticotropin-releasing hormone in anthropoid primates: from brain to placenta, *Am. J. Hum. Biol.*, 18, 431–447.

Rayburn, W.F., Christensen, H.D., and Gonzalez, C.L. (1997). A placebo-controlled comparison between betamethasone and dexamethasone for fetal maturation: differences in neurobehavioral development of mice offspring, *Am. J. Obstet. Gynecol.*, 176, 842–850; discussion 850–841.

Rayburn, W.F., Christensen, H.D., Gonzalez, C.L., Rayburn, L.A., and Stewart, J.D. (1998). Effect of in utero exposure to betamethasone on motivation/anxiety testing in mice offspring, *Neurotoxicol. Teratol.*, 20, 475–481.

Reynolds, R.M. (2013). Glucocorticoid excess and the developmental origins of disease: two decades of testing the hypothesis--2012 Curt Richter Award Winner, *Psychoneuroendocrinology*, 38, 1–11.

Rho, J.M. (2004). Basic science behind the catastrophic epilepsies, *Epilepsia*, 45 Suppl 5, 5–11.

Riikonen, R.S. (1996). How do cryptogenic and symptomatic infantile spasms differ? Review of biochemical studies in Finnish patients, *J. Child. Neurol.*, 11, 383–388.

Robinson, B.G., Emanuel, R.L., Frim, D.M., and Majzoub, J.A. (1988). Glucocorticoid stimulates expression of corticotropin-releasing hormone gene in human placenta, *Proc. Natl. Acad. Sci. U.S.A.*, 85, 5244–5248.

Rose, R.P. and Bridger, W.H. (1982). Hormonal influences on seizure kindling: the effects of post-stimulation ACTH or cortisone injections, *Brain Res.*, 231, 75–84.

Rosen, J.B., Pishevar, S.K., Weiss, S.R., Smith, M.A., Kling, M.A., Gold, P.W., and Schulkin, J. (1994). Glucocorticoid treatment increases the ability of CRH to induce seizures, *Neurosci Lett.*, 174, 113–116.

Sandman, C.A. (2015). Fetal exposure to placental corticotropin-releasing hormone (pCRH) programs developmental trajectories, *Peptides*, 72, 145–153.

Sandman, C.A. and Davis, E.P. (2012). Neurobehavioral risk is associated with gestational exposure to stress hormones, *Expert Rev Endocrinol. Metab.*, 7, 445–459.

Schulte, D.M., Shapiro, I., Reincke, M., and Beuschlein, F. (2007). Expression and spatio-temporal distribution of differentiation and proliferation markers during mouse adrenal development, *Gene Expr. Patterns*, 7, 72–81.

Seckl, J.R. and Holmes, M.C. (2007). Mechanisms of disease: glucocorticoids, their placental metabolism and fetal 'programming' of adult pathophysiology, *Na. Clin. Pract.. Endocrinol. Metab.*, 3, 479–488.

Shimakawa, S., Nomura, S., Ogino, M., Fukui, M., Kashiwagi, M., Tanabe, T., and Tamai, H. (2015). ACTH therapy on intractable epilepsy in Hemiconvulsion-Hemiplegia-Epilepsy syndrome, *Brain Dev.*, 37, 733–737.

Shimogori, T., Lee, D.A., Miranda-Angulo, A., Yang, Y., Wang, H., Jiang, L., Yoshida, A.C., Kataoka, A., Mashiko, H., Avetisyan, M., Qi, L., Qian, J., and Blackshaw, S. (2010). A genomic atlas of mouse hypothalamic development, *Nat. Neurosci.*, 13, 767–775.

Smith, R., Mesiano, S., Chan, E.C., Brown, S., and Jaffe, R.B. (1998). Corticotropin-releasing hormone directly and preferentially stimulates dehydroepiandrosterone sulfate secretion by human fetal adrenal cortical cells, *J. Clin. Endocrinol. Metab.*, 83, 2916–2920.

Son, G.H., Geum, D., Chung, S., Kim, E.J., Jo, J.H., Kim, C.M., Lee, K.H., Kim, H., Choi, S., Kim, H.T., Lee, C.J., and Kim, K. (2006). Maternal stress produces learning deficits associated with impairment of NMDA receptor-mediated synaptic plasticity, *J. Neurosci.*, 26, 3309–3318.

Sorel, L., and Dusaucy - Bauloye, A. (1958). A propos de 21 cas d'hypsarythmie de Gibbs. Son traitement spectaculaire par l'ACTH, *Acta Neurol. Belg.*, 58, 130–141.

Sperling, M.R. and Ko, J. (2006). Seizures and brain tumors, *Semin. Oncol.*, 33, 333–341.

Sperling, M.R., Schilling, C.A., Glosser, D., Tracy, J.I., and Asadi-Pooya, A.A. (2008). Self-perception of seizure precipitants and their relation to anxiety level, depression, and health locus of control in epilepsy, *Seizure*, 17, 302–307.

Stafstrom, C.E., Arnason, B.G., Baram, T.Z., Catania, A., Cortez, M.A., Glauser, T.A., Pranzatelli, M.R., Riikonen, R., Rogawski, M.A., Shinnar, S., and Swann, J.W. (2011). Treatment of infantile spasms: emerging insights from clinical and basic science perspectives, *J. Child. Neurol.*, 26, 1411–1421.

Stein, B.A. and Sapolsky, R.M. (1988). Chemical adrenalectomy reduces hippocampal damage induced by kainic acid, *Brain Res.*, 473, 175–180.

Sterner, E.Y. and Kalynchuk, L.E. (2010). Behavioral and neurobiological consequences of prolonged glucocorticoid exposure in rats: relevance to depression, *Prog. Neuropsychopharmacol. Biol. Psychiatry*, 34, 777–790.

Swinkels, W.A., Engelsman, M., Kasteleijn-Nolst Trenite, D.G., Baal, M.G., de Haan, G.J., and Oosting, J. (1998). Influence of an evacuation in February 1995 in The Netherlands on the seizure frequency in patients with epilepsy: a controlled study, *Epilepsia*, 39, 1203–1207.

Taylor, N.R., Loraine, J.A., and Robertson, H.A. (1953). The estimation of ACTH in human pituitary tissue, *J. Endocrinol.*, 9, 334–341.

Temkin, N.R. and Davis, G.R. (1984). Stress as a risk factor for seizures among adults with epilepsy, *Epilepsia*, 25, 450–456.

Thomas, A.C., Heux, P., Santos, C., Arulvasan, W., Solanky, N., Carey, M.E., Gerrelli, D., Kinsler, V.A., and Etchevers, H.C. (2018). Widespread dynamic and pleiotropic expression of the melanocortin-1-receptor (MC1R) system is conserved across chick, mouse and human embryonic development, *Birth Defects Res.*, 110, 443–455.

Thompson, J.L. and Holmes, G.L. (1987). Failure of ACTH to alter transfer kindling in the immature brain, *Epilepsia*, 28, 17–19.

Tolmacheva, E.A., Oitzl, M.S., and van Luijtelaar, G. (2012). Stress, glucocorticoids and absences in a genetic epilepsy model, *Horm. Behav.*, 61, 706–710.

van Campen, J.S., Jansen, F.E., de Graan, P.N., Braun, K.P., and Joels, M. (2014). Early life stress in epilepsy: a seizure precipitant and risk factor for epileptogenesis, *Epilepsy Behav.*, 38, 160–171.

Van den Bergh, B.R.H., van den Heuvel, M.I., Lahti, M., Braeken, M., de Rooij, S.R., Entringer, S., Hoyer, D., Roseboom, T., Raikkonen, K., King, S., and Schwab, M. (2017). Prenatal developmental origins of behavior and mental health: The influence of maternal stress in pregnancy, *Neurosci. Biobehav. Rev.*, https://doi.org/10.1016/j.neubiorev.2017.07.003

Varga, J., Ferenczi, S., Kovacs, K.J., Garafova, A., Jezova, D., and Zelena, D. (2013). Comparison of stress-induced changes in adults and pups: is aldosterone the main adrenocortical stress hormone during the perinatal period in rats?, *PLoS One*, 8, e72313.

Vazquez, D.M., Bailey, C., Dent, G.W., Okimoto, D.K., Steffek, A., Lopez, J.F., and Levine, S. (2006). Brain corticotropin-releasing hormone (CRH) circuits in the developing rat: effect of maternal deprivation, *Brain Res.*, 1121, 83–94.

Velíšek, L. (2011). Prenatal corticosteroid exposure alters early developmental seizures and behavior, *Epilepsy Res.*, 95, 9–19.

Velíšek, L., Jehle, K., Asche, S., and Velíšková, J. (2007). Model of infantile spasms induced by N-methyl-D-aspartic acid in prenatally impaired brain, *Ann. Neurol.*, 61, 109–119.

Vigevano, F. and Cilio, M.R. (1997). Vigabatrin versus ACTH as first-line treatment for infantile spasms: a randomized, prospective study, *Epilepsia*, 38, 1270–1274.

Vyas, A., Mitra, R., Shankaranarayana Rao, B.S., and Chattarji, S. (2002). Chronic stress induces contrasting patterns of dendritic remodeling in hippocampal and amygdaloid neurons, *J. Neurosci.*, 22, 6810–6818.

Waddell, B.J., Bollen, M., Wyrwoll, C.S., Mori, T.A., and Mark, P.J. (2010). Developmental programming of adult adrenal structure and steroidogenesis: effects of fetal glucocorticoid excess and postnatal dietary omega-3 fatty acids, *J. Endocrinol.*, 205, 171–178.

Wang, W., Dow, K.E., and Fraser, D.D. (2001). Elevated corticotropin releasing hormone/corticotropin releasing hormone-R1 expression in postmortem brain obtained from children with generalized epilepsy, *Ann. Neurol.*, 50, 404–409.

Weinstock, M. (2008). The long-term behavioural consequences of prenatal stress, *Neurosci. Biobehav. Rev.*, 32, 1073–1086.

Weinstock, M. (2017). Prenatal stressors in rodents: Effects on behavior, *Neurobiol. Stress*, 6, 3–13.

Wood, C.E. and Walker, C.D. (2016). Fetal and neonatal HPA axis, *Compr. Physiol.*, 6, 33–62.

Wray, C.D. (2013). 17q21.31 microdeletion associated with infantile spasms, *Eur. J. Med. Genet.*, 56, 59–61.

Wulsin, A.C., Solomon, M.B., Privitera, M.D., Danzer, S.C., and Herman, J.P. (2016). Hypothalamic-pituitary-adrenocortical axis dysfunction in epilepsy, *Physiol. Behav.*, 166, 22–31.

Yaka, R., Salomon, S., Matzner, H., and Weinstock, M. (2007). Effect of varied gestational stress on acquisition of spatial memory, hippocampal LTP and synaptic proteins in juvenile male rats, *Behav. Brain Res.*, 179, 126–132.

Yanagaki, S., Oguni, H., Hayashi, K., Imai, K., Funatuka, M., Tanaka, T., Yanagaki, M., and Osawa, M. (1999). A comparative study of high-dose and low-dose ACTH therapy for West syndrome, *Brain Dev.*, 21, 461–467.

Yang, G., Zou, L.P., Wang, J., Shi, X.Y., Yang, X.F., Wang, B., Liu, Y.J., Sun, Y.H., and Jia, F.Y. (2015). Association analysis of polymorphisms of the CRHR1 gene with infantile spasms, *Mol. Med. Rep.*, 12, 2539–2546.

Yilmaz, T., Akca, M., Turan, Y., Ocak, H., Kamasak, K., and Yildirim, M. (2014). Efficacy of dexamethasone on penicillin-induced epileptiform activity in rats: an electrophysiological study, *Brain Res.*, 1554, 67–72.

Young, A.H. (2006). Antiglucocoticoid treatments for depression, *Aust. N. Z. J. Psychiatry*, 40, 402–405.

Young, N.A., Teskey, G.C., Henry, L.C., and Edwards, H.E. (2006). Exogenous antenatal glucocorticoid treatment reduces susceptibility for hippocampal kindled and maximal electroconvulsive seizures in infant rats, *Exp. Neurol.*, 198, 303–312.

Yum, M.S., Chachua, T., Velíšková, J., and Velíšek, L. (2012). Prenatal stress promotes development of spasms in infant rats, *Epilepsia*, 53, e46–49.

Zadina, J.E., Banks, W.A., and Kastin, A.J. (1986). Central nervous system effects of peptides, 1980–1985: a cross-listing of peptides and their central actions from the first six years of the journal Peptides, *Peptides*, 7, 497–537.

Zhao, Y., Ma, R., Shen, J., Su, H., Xing, D., and Du, L. (2008). A mouse model of depression induced by repeated corticosterone injections, *Eur. J. Pharmacol.*, 581, 113–120.

Zijlmans, M.A., Riksen-Walraven, J.M., and de Weerth, C. (2015). Associations between maternal prenatal cortisol concentrations and child outcomes: A systematic review, *Neurosci. Biobehav. Rev.*, 53, 1–24.

Chapter 10

Immunity, Inflammation and Epileptogenesis in the Developing Brain

Sookyong Koh, MD, PhD

Department of Neurology, Emory University, Atlanta, Georgia, USA

10.1 Introduction

The central nervous system (CNS) used to be considered an "immune-privileged" site due to a lack of conventional lymphatic drainage, graft acceptance and the presence of a vascular brain barrier that tightly regulates infiltration of blood monocytes and lymphocytes. More recently, it has become clear that immune and inflammatory reactions do occur in the CNS, either intrinsically from the brain itself or in conjunction with systemic circulation through a damaged blood-brain barrier (BBB). The critical roles of brain-resident immune mediators and of brain-infiltrating peripheral leukocytes in the evolution of drug-resistant childhood epilepsy are increasingly recognized. Novel immunomodulatory drugs against the key constituents in immune pathways may thus represent a new therapeutic approach against childhood epilepsy.

For many decades, the functional roles of inflammation and the immune system in childhood epilepsy have been suspected because various common pediatric infectious or autoimmune diseases are often heralded by seizures at the onset or accompanied by seizures during the course of the illness. Also, immunotherapy effectively treats refractory seizures in select pediatric epilepsy syndromes [Kelley and Kossoff, 2010; Veggiotti *et al.*, 2012]. Active inflammation occurs not only in prototypical inflammatory epilepsies such as Rasmussen encephalitis or limbic encephalitis, but also in patients with drug-resistant epilepsy of diverse causes and in many animal models of seizures [Ravizza *et al.*, 2008; Vezzani *et al.*, 2013].

10.2 Emerging role of innate and adaptive immunity in childhood epilepsy

Epilepsy research has focused mainly on alterations of neuronal activities and excitability for centuries. Such a neuro-centric emphasis has neglected the role of glia and involvement of inflammation in the pathogenesis of epilepsy. After all, neurons are the excitable element in the brain, and epilepsy is a condition characterized by enduring changes in neuronal excitability. Yet, in the brain, neurons are vastly outnumbered by glia, which strongly influence neurons and their ability to process information. The brain exhibits a robust innate immune response mediated by CNS-resident immune cells, microglia and astrocytes [Turrin and Rivest, 2004]. Such neuroinflammation was viewed as an epiphenomenon, a passive bystander effect that occurs when damaged neurons elicit a response from glia. Recently, however, it has become clear that dysregulation of the normally reparative innate immune responses of glia may instead cause exacerbation of pathology and neuronal dysfunction [Crespel *et al.*, 2002; Ravizza *et al.*, 2008].

Aberrant or uncontrolled neuroinflammation that persists beyond elimination of the initial provoking stimulus — seizures in the epileptic brain, for example — can have a profound detrimental impact on neuron function, including a hyperexcitable state, encephalopathy and cognitive decline. Largely due to the BBB, the brain appears to exhibit dampened adaptive immunity in response to injury or infection. This notion has recently been challenged; breakdown of the BBB has been implicated in the initiation, progression and perpetuation of seizures in animal models [Fabene *et al.*, 2008; Khalili *et al.*, 2007; Kim *et al.*, 2009]. In addition, it is now well established that activated mononuclear leukocytes (T cells, macrophages and dendritic cells) can traverse the BBB using homing molecules such as VLA-4, the target of the multiple sclerosis drug, natalizumab [Khalili *et al.*, 2007]. The potential causative roles of innate and adaptive immunity in the development of chronic epilepsy that starts in childhood are being investigated actively.

10.2.1 *Damaged BBB in CNS injury and delayed onset of epilepsy*

The BBB consists of morphologically non-fenestrated endothelial cells with inter-endothelial tight junctions. Its maintenance depends on normal functioning of pericytes, perivascular microglia, astrocytes, and the basal lamina. Astrocytes act as important regulators of the balance between endothelial stability and permeability of the BBB. Under normal conditions, the BBB protects the CNS by regulating the entry of plasma-born substances and immune cells. Transient changes have been demonstrated in the physiology and structures of the BBB in various CNS injuries such as status epilepticus, infections, and traumatic and ischemic events [Ballabh *et al.*, 2004]. An impaired BBB and inflammatory state are common features of neurological diseases associated with the late onset of epilepsy. Proinflammatory cytokines are elevated in experimental animal brains after ischemia and in the CSF from patients after stroke and chronic epilepsy. Cytokine release causes subsequent up-regulation of endothelial and neutrophil adhesion molecules in human cerebrovascular endothelial cells during hypoxic injury [Zhang *et al.*, 2000], leading to transmigration of leukocytes across the endothelium and the BBB. Leukocyte recruitment triggers tight junction disorganization and BBB breakdown, a necessary component of epileptogenesis following brain injury.

BBB break down may not be a mere consequence, but rather a primary cause of seizures. Induction of BBB disruption by bile salt or serum albumin in animals [Ivens *et al.*, 2007] or by intra-arterial injection of mannitol in humans [Marchi *et al.*, 2007] increases seizure susceptibility and causes epileptiform discharges or focal seizures. Moreover, peripheral leukocytes appear to promote development of epilepsy by mediating the breakdown of the BBB [Kim *et al.*, 2009]. Suppression of adhesion between leukocytes and endothelial cells, either by genetically eliminating adhesion molecules or by blocking the interaction with neutralizing antibodies, abrogates the initiation of seizures and progression to epilepsy [Fabene *et al.*, 2008]. In a study of pediatric patients with chronic intractable focal epilepsy, an extensive perivascular space containing activated microglia, macrophages and T lymphocytes as well as splitting of the basal membrane were detected [Hildebrandt *et al.*, 2008]. This spongiform microangiopathy affecting arterioles and newly formed porous vascular elements is likely to compromise the BBB [Hildebrandt *et al.*, 2008; Marchi *et al.*, 2007].

10.2.2 *Adaptive immunity in epileptogenesis*

Our laboratory has pioneered the characterization of inflammatory cell infiltrates in surgically removed fresh brain samples from pediatric patients in search for novel therapeutic targets. Using an unbiased flow cytometric analysis of inflammatory leukocytes in resected brain tissues, we detected functionally activated lymphocytes within epileptogenic lesion of patients. Inflammatory myeloid cells and memory CD4+ and CD8+ T cells infiltrated the brains (Figure 10.1).

In the "two-hit" model of kainic acid (KA)-SE, we have detected significant increases in CNS-infiltrating peripheral inflammatory lymphocytes, macrophages and dendritic cells after KA-induced status ("second-hit") in the temporal lobes of mature animals with prior exposure to early-life seizures. Further work is needed to determine whether BBB breakdown is a pre-requisite for future development of epilepsy and to elucidate the potential for prophylactic treatment following an injury to prevent epilepsy.

10.2.3 *Autoimmune disease and epilepsy*

Pediatric infectious, inflammatory or autoimmune diseases are often accompanied by seizures during the course of illness thus implicating

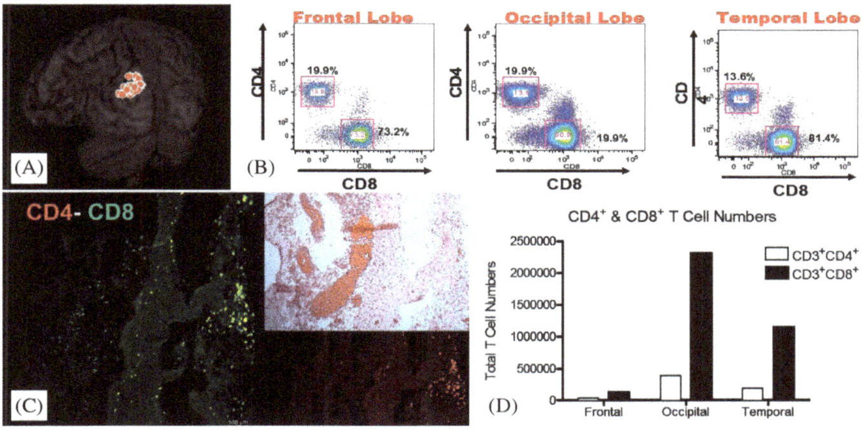

Figure 10.1. Influx of infiltrating leukocytes in the epileptogenic zone. (A) Magnetoencephalogram (MEG) localizes spike source to left occipital lobe behind the scar. (B&D) CNS mononuclear cells were isolated from the frontal, occipital and temporal lobes. Multi-color flow cytometry shows $CD8^+$ killer > $CD4^+$ helper T-cells in the occipital > temporal lobes. (C) $CD4^+$/$CD8^+$ cells are found near blood vessels.

brain inflammation as a common predisposing factor in epilepsy, particularly in childhood epilepsy.

10.2.3.1 *Rasmussen Encephalitis (RE)*

RE is the prototype inflammatory epilepsy. RE leads to progressive focal epilepsy, asymmetric cortical atrophy and deterioration of motor and cognitive function. The current histopathological criteria of RE include the presence of T-cell-dominated inflammation, microglial activation and formation of microglial nodules, neuronal loss, and astrocytic activation. Astrocytic apoptosis and subsequent loss have been demonstrated as a specific feature of RE [Bauer *et al.*, 2007]. A specific attack by cytotoxic T lymphocytes may be one possible mechanism responsible for astrocytic degeneration in RE [Bauer *et al.*, 2007].

The autoimmune nature of this condition was suspected after the discovery of autoantibodies against the glutamate AMPAR (α-3-hydroxy-5-methyl-4-isoxazole propionic acid receptor), GluR3.

Repeated plasma exchanges can reduce serum titers of GluR3 antibodies, decrease seizure frequency, and improve neurologic function [Rogers *et al.*, 1994]. Immunization of animals with GluR3 induces a disorder resembling the human disease [Rogers *et al.*, 1994]. Subsequently, antiGluR3 antibodies have been detected in two other epilepsy syndromes, early-onset noninflammatory focal epilepsy and catastrophic infantile epilepsy [Mantegazza *et al.*, 2002]. AntiGluR3 antibodies, therefore, appear to be a marker for intractable epilepsy not limited to RE. Long-term immunotherapy such as intravenous γ-globulin (IVIG) and corticosteroids may be beneficial for autoantibody-positive RE patients. A long term follow-up of 11 RE patients who received steroids showed that 45% of patients had significant improvement of motor function and reduction of seizure frequency with disappearance of epilepsia partialis continua, while 55% of patients had no benefit from steroid therapy and ultimately underwent hemispherotomy. Two initial responders to steroid treatment experienced progressive recurrence of seizures one to four years after the discontinuation of steroids and received a hemispherotomy [Bahi-Buisson *et al.*, 2007].

10.2.3.2 *Systemic Lupus Erythematosus (SLE)*

SLE is the most common rheumatic disease in children. The major organ systems involved in childhood SLE are similar to adult SLE, but the frequency of multiple organ involvement and severity of the disease are greater in children than adults. General clinical features include broad variations of rash, arthritis, constitutional symptoms, renal disease, and cardiovascular, pulmonary, and neuropsychiatric involvement. The prevalence of epilepsy in SLE patients is 10–20%, 8 times higher than in the general population. Notably, seizures can precede the diagnosis of SLE, and 5–10% of patients experience seizures several years before the clinical onset of SLE [Toubi *et al.*, 1995]. This finding suggests that long-term treatment with antiepileptic drugs may have precipitated SLE, or alternatively, that epilepsy and SLE are both manifestations of a genetically determined predisposition to altered immunity and inflammation. The presence of anti-phospholipid antibodies highly correlates with both epilepsy and abnormal brain MRI findings in SLE [Toubi *et al.*, 1995]. Patients with anti-phospholipid antibodies are at risk of thromboembolic manifestations, intrauterine fetal loss, and thrombocytopenia, a combination termed anti-phospholipid syndrome. In addition, anti-cardiolipin antibodies are found in 30–60% of SLE patients, and epilepsy is 3 times more frequent in patients with anti-cardiolipin antibodies than those without [Liou *et al.*, 1996]. These findings raise the possibility that autoantibodies may trigger seizures and contribute to epileptogenesis.

10.2.3.3 *Hashimoto thyroiditis*

Hashimoto thyroiditis is the most common thyroiditis in children and adults, affecting 1.2% of school-aged children. Hashimoto encephalopathy is a syndrome associated with high anti-thyroid antibody titer that can either begin abruptly, in the form of seizures or agitation, or develop gradually, in a relapsing-remitting manner manifested as cognitive deterioration and psychiatric illness. The occurrence of Hashimoto encephalopathy is unrelated to the patient's thyroid function, and most patients respond dramatically to corticosteroid therapy [Watemberg *et al.*, 2006]. The therapeutic efficacy of immunomodulation suggests a causative role of activated immunity and autoantibodies for the neurological symptoms in Hashimoto thyroiditis, including seizures and epilepsy.

10.2.3.4 *Behçet disease*

Behçet disease is a chronic systemic inflammatory disorder of unknown etiology defined by the classic triad of recurrent oral aphthous ulcers, genital ulcers, and inflammatory eye disease. The prevalence of CNS disease, often associated with significant morbidity, varies between 2.9% and 44%, with male predominance. In 22 patients with neuro-Behçet disease, 27% suffered either single or recurrent seizures [Joseph and Scolding, 2007]. CSF pleocytosis occurred in 50% of patients, and most showed improvement after immunosuppressant therapy.

10.2.3.5 *Autoimmune encephalitis*

Immune/inflammatory encephalitis falls under a broader category of autoimmune synaptopathies where autoantibodies target and disrupt the functional or structural integrity of CNS synapses [Crisp *et al.*, 2016]. Autoimmune epilepsies are immunologically mediated; recurrent seizures are prominent features. They include anti-N-methyl D-aspartate receptor (NMDAR) encephalitis, paraneoplastic (Hu, Ma2) or non-paraneoplastic (AMPAR) limbic encephalitis and limbic encephalitis with or without faciobrachial dystonic seizures (FBDS) associated with LGI1 autoantibodies. We are now able to test for an increasing number of antibodies that offer a definitive diagnosis for cases that would have been previously categorized as viral or idiopathic encephalitis [Armangue *et al.*, 2012; Flanagan *et al.*, 2010]. The California Encephalitis Project found that the frequency of autoimmune encephalitis was greater than any single viral etiology. Anti-NMDAR encephalitis was, in fact, the most frequent cause of immune mediated encephalitis in the pediatric population [Armangue *et al.*, 2012]. Any child who presents with such acute memory deficits, aphasia, seizures, movement disorder or behavioral changes of a subacute nature should have autoimmune encephalitis in the differential diagnosis. The initial presentation of these patients can vary depending on the receptor being targeted, but it is crucial to always consider immune-mediated encephalitis due to the potential for a successful outcome with prompt immunomodulatory therapy.

10.2.3.6 *Febrile Infection-Related Epilepsy Syndrome (FIRES)*

FIRES is a rare and devastating epileptic encephalopathy that typically affects school-aged children. It is clinically defined as a refractory, prolonged status epilepticus triggered by fever of unknown cause in the absence of a CNS infectious process that results in drug-resistant epilepsy and severe cognitive impairment [Nabbout *et al.*, 2010, 2011]. An inflammatory etiology is supported in FIRES [Nabbout *et al.*, 2011]. It remains poorly understood, however, how the fever generates such unrelenting repetitive seizures and how the refractory status epilepticus affects the developing brain [Nabbout *et al.*, 2010]. Although there have been good outcomes reported in some children diagnosed with FIRES, the majority of children develop significant neurological complications including refractory epilepsy with cognitive deficits, a vegetative state, or death [Kenney-Jung *et al.*, 2016; Nabbout *et al.*, 2011]. In addition to routinely used anticonvulsants and CNS depressants, anesthetic comas and ketogenic diets have been used to manage young children affected by FIRES [Nabbout *et al.*, 2010]. Effective treatments to adequately control seizures and its devastating consequences are lacking for patients with FIRES.

10.2.4 *Medically intractable childhood epilepsy improved by immunotherapy*

10.2.4.1 *Infantile Spasms (IS)*

IS is a unique age-specific epilepsy of early infancy. The electroencephalogram (EEG) characteristically shows hypsarrhythmia — disorganized, chaotic, high voltage polymorphic delta and theta rhythms with superimposed multifocal spikes and wave discharges. The onset of spasms is frequently associated with neurodevelopmental regression. The incidence varies from 0.25 to 0.60 per 1,000 live births [Cowan and Hudson, 1991], and the prevalence rate is 0.15 to 0.2 per 1,000 children age 10 or younger [Cowan *et al.*, 1989]. IS develop in infants with a variety of CNS pathologies, including structural abnormalities, prenatal and postnatal infection, stroke, trauma, chromosomal anomalies and genetic epilepsies [Berg *et al.*, 2017; Arzimanoglou *et al.*, 2004]. This disease entity of uniform semiology with diverse causes suggests that infantile spasms are an age-specific but cause-nonspecific final common response of the brain to insults [Baram, 1993; Riikonen, 1983].

Adrenocorticotrophic hormone (ACTH) and corticosteroids are well-known effective treatments for IS that not only result in seizure control, but also improve both behavior and EEG background. Meta-analysis reveals that ACTH is probably effective for short-term treatment of IS and leads to resolution of hypsarrhythmia [Mackay *et al.*, 2004]. Time to response is usually two weeks. Oral steroids can render as many as 60% of patients seizure-free. Further, early use of steroids is more effective; patients treated within one month of spasms onset had a better outcome than those treated after more than one month. A study of 18 children with Down syndrome and IS showed that spasms control was easier, subsequent seizures were less persistent, developmental quotients were higher, and there were fewer autistic features in children treated early [Eisermann *et al.*, 2003].

10.2.4.2 *Lennox-Gastaut Syndrome (LGS)*

LGS is diagnosed in children who have a minimum of two seizure types (usually atonic or astatic (drop) seizures, nocturnal tonic seizures, and atypical absence seizures), mental retardation, and bursts of generalized slow spike-waves on EEG. LGS is one of the epilepsy syndromes most resistant to the available antiepileptic medications. Corticosteroids and ACTH may be effective in treating children with LGS [Prasad *et al.*, 1996]. When 10 children with LGS and intractable seizures were treated with prednisolone for 12 weeks, 7 achieved seizure freedom and the other 3 experienced seizure reduction [Sinclair, 2003]. The patients' clinical improvement was generally reflected in improved EEGs. Another study of 45 children with LGS who received ACTH for 2 to 8 weeks found that while 51% of patients became seizure free for over 10 days, 78% of these children later relapsed [Yamatogi *et al.*, 1979].

10.2.4.3 *Landau-Kleffner Syndrome (LKS) and Epilepsy with continuous spike wave discharges (CSWS)*

Landau-Kleffner syndrome is an acquired epileptic aphasia presenting as progressive loss of speech in a previously well child with an abnormal and usually continuous epileptiform discharges on the EEG during slow wave sleep, with or without clinically apparent seizures. There are reports that corticosteroids improved both clinical features of the syndrome as well as the EEG, especially when instituted early [Sinclair and Snyder, 2005].

Continuous spike-waves during slow sleep syndrome (CSWSS) is a rare, sporadic childhood epilepsy characterized by the presence of spike waves during at least 85% of slow sleep and, clinically, by the existence of neuropsychological and behavioral disorders. LKS and CSWSS share some common features, including first appearance in childhood and mild epilepsy associated with severe neuropsychological disturbances. There are several case reports that CSWSS also responds to treatment with corticosteroids or ACTH, not only in terms of seizures and EEG, but also in language skills [Gallagher *et al.*, 2006; Veggiotti *et al.*, 2012].

10.2.4.4 *Myoclonic Atonic Epilepsy (MAE) and other refractory epilepsies*

MAE and myoclonic seizures have been treated with corticosteroids, possibly because of the frequent daily seizures, acute encephalopathic presentation, medical intractability, and tendency of the seizures to result in physical injury [Kelley and Kossoff, 2010]. In a study of myoclonic epilepsy, 34 children out of 64 were treated with prednisone and the remaining 30 children with ACTH. Seizures were effectively controlled in 73% of children treated with ACTH, but in none treated with prednisone [Snead *et al.*, 1983]. In another study of nine patients with myoclonic epilepsy treated with steroids, five became seizure free, two showed a reduction, and the remaining two exhibited no change [Sinclair, 2003]. In contrast, only a transient improvement was reported in 5 of 84 patients with myoclonic absence epilepsy treated with ACTH [Oguni *et al.*, 2001]. In a study of children with absence epilepsy, seven were treated with steroids. All improved and five became seizure free [Sinclair, 2003]. In 32 children with intractable epilepsy (IS excluded) treated with ACTH, 25% of patients became seizure-free and 47% showed significant reductions of seizures [Verhelst *et al.*, 2005].

10.3 Seizures cause acute and chronic brain inflammation — Evidence from experimental models

In many animal models of seizures and epilepsy, acute seizures cause glial activation and increased expression of transcription factors and cytokines that coordinate inflammatory responses [Plata-Salaman *et al.*, 2000]. After status epilepticus, members of the Toll-like receptor (TLR) family are significantly up-regulated in the microglia, leading to transcriptional activation of cytokines, chemokines, major histocompatibility complex (MHC) class I and II, and costimulatory molecules [Turrin and Rivest, 2004]. The activated glia and elevated cytokines, in turn, contribute to seizure-related pathology, such as neuronal death, neuronal birth, reactive gliosis, and mossy fiber sprouting [Jankowsky and Patterson, 2001; McNamara, 1994]. Accumulating experimental data also suggest that seizure-induced glial activation and up-regulation of pro-inflammatory cytokines can lead to neuronal excitability and neuronal injury either directly, by interacting with glutamatergic neurotransmission, or indirectly, by activating gene transcription.

10.3.1 *Microglial activation*

Microglia are myeloid lineage cells that comprise approximately 12% of the brain. Resting microglia with a ramified morphology are responsible for immune surveillance [Aloisi, 2001] and are activated at a very early stage in response to injury or immunological stimuli with transformation to an amoeboid shape [Kreutzberg, 1996]. Activated microglia up-regulate the expression of surface molecules, such as complement receptors and MHC molecules, and release a variety of pro-inflammatory and cytotoxic soluble factors [Block and Hong, 2005]. MHC class-I and class-II, IL-1, IL-2, IL-6, TGF-β1, the complement components and their receptors, M-CSF, and GM-CSF are all molecules considered to be signals in the activation process [Kreutzberg, 1996].

Widespread microglial activation accompanied by neuronal injury occurs after acute seizures [Rizzi *et al.*, 2003]. As a rapid response, activation of microglia may be responsible for neurodegeneration rather than a consequence of neurodegeneration. Within four hours after KA-induced status epilepticus, glial activation and cytokine expression are found in the hippocampus [Ravizza *et al.*, 2005]. Neuronal injury is detected 12–24 hours following status epilepticus, many hours after cytokines are induced in the glia [Ravizza *et al.*,

2005]. Status epilepticus, prolonged seizures over 30 minutes, can cause neuronal death through glutamate-mediated excitotoxicity, necrosis, and activation of apoptosis [Henshall, 2007]. One to three days after status epilepticus, both neuronal and astrocytic death are observed in the dentate hilus within the hippocampus [Kang *et al.*, 2006]. Injured neurons and glia and their fragmented DNA are rapidly cleared by activated microglia [Koh *et al.*, 1999]. The impaired neurogenesis in inflammation can be effectively restored by systemic administration of the tetracycline derivative minocycline, a specific inhibitor of microglia activation [Ekdahl *et al.*, 2003]. These findings suggest that microglial activation associated with inflammation induces neuronal injury and suppresses neurogenesis. The occurrence of spontaneous seizures has been correlated with the extent of glial activation, as well as astrocyte and neuron degeneration in the hippocampus, and blockade of neuronal death failed to prevent epileptogenesis [Borges *et al.*, 2003].

Cytokines released by microglia influence astrocytic function and proliferation. Increased levels of IFN-γ, IL-1, IL-2, IL-6, TNF-α, and M-CSF are associated with astrogliosis. IL-1Ra, an IL-1 receptor antagonist, is sufficient to prevent astroglial proliferation, suggesting a pivotal role of IL-1 in astrocyte activation [Hanisch, 2002]. In addition, these cytokines may modulate glutamate homeostasis by regulating glutamate receptors and transporters in astrocytes [Tilleux *et al.*, 2007]. Impaired handling of extracellular glutamate by gliotic astrocytes may lead to neuroexcitability and excitotoxic neuronal damage resulting from excessive glutamate levels [Seifert *et al.*, 2006]. These findings suggest that activation of microglia and the resultant increase in cytokines may influence epileptogenesis by altering glutamatergic transmission indirectly by modulating astrocytes.

To address the role of activated microglia in the pathogenesis of childhood epilepsy, we used minocycline to block seizure-induced inflammation and determine whether innate immunity plays a causal role in mediating the long-term epileptogenic effects of early-life seizure. First, status epilepticus was induced at postnatal day (P) 25 and a second status at P39. KA-SE at P25 caused nearly a two-fold increase in microglia activation within 24 h. Significant seizure-induced activation persisted for 7 days and returned to baseline by 14 days. P39 animals with prior exposure to KA-SE not only responded with greater microglial activation in response to "second hit" of KA, but had a shorter latency to seizure expression. Inhibition of seizure-induced inflammation by 7 day minocycline post-treatment abrogated both the exaggerated microglia activation and the increased susceptibility to the second seizure later in life. The priming effect of early-life seizures is accompanied by modified and rapidly reactivated microglia. Anti-inflammatory therapy after SE may be useful to block the epileptogenic process and mitigate the long-term damaging effects of early-life seizures [Abraham *et al.*, 2012].

10.3.2 *Astrogliosis*

For over 100 years, astroglial proliferation has been observed as a pathognomonic finding in surgically resected hippocampi in patients with intractable mesial temporal lobe epilepsy. Once regarded as an inert scar and consequence of the healing process after neuronal degeneration, recent studies suggest that reactive astrogliosis and modified astroglial function may have an important role in the generation and spread of seizure activity [Tian *et al.*, 2005].

Astrocytes are a critical component of the BBB and have many important roles in glutamate and potassium uptake and the production of growth factors, cytokines, and extracellular matrix proteins [Ekdahl *et al.*, 2003]. In response to immunologic challenges or brain injuries, astrocytes proliferate and become hypertrophic and fibrillary. Direct stimulation of astrocytes by photolysis of caged calcium and glutamate release in acute seizure models can induce a paroxysmal depolarization shift (PDS) abnormal prolonged depolarization observed during interictal activity [Tian *et al.*, 2005]. Cultured astrocytes isolated from the seizure focus of human epileptic tissue possess depolarized resting membrane potentials and are able to generate action potential-like responses upon injection of current [O'Connor *et al.*, 1998]. Astrocytes are initially activated by excessive neuronal activity, a potent trigger of astrocyte Ca^{2+} signaling. However, once activated, neuronal firing is no longer needed for continued astroglial activation. Activated astrocytes in the sclerotic hippocampus are not mere bystanders, but active players in epileptogenesis.

Within 24 to 48 hours after seizure induction, activation of GFAP-positive astrocytes is noted throughout the dentate gyrus and hippocampal subfields; this reactive astrogliosis persists chronically over three to four months [Somera-Molina *et al.*, 2007]. Newly generated astrocytes display distinct changes in glial membrane channels and receptors to promote neuronal hyperexcitability and seizure generation. These changes include GluR1 receptors with elevated flip-to-flop ratios [Seifert *et al.*, 2002], impaired uptake of potassium ion due to inwardly rectifying K^+ channels [Schroder *et al.*, 2000], over-expression of adenosine kinase [Fedele *et al.*, 2005], and down-regulation of glutamine synthase, glutamate dehydrogenase, and glial GABA transporter [Kang *et al.*, 2006].

10.3.3 *Pro-inflammatory cytokines and neuronal hyperexcitability*

Experimentally induced seizures in rodents trigger a prompt inflammatory response in brain areas recruited in the onset and propagation of epileptic activity [Jankowsky and Patterson, 2001]. Direct intra-cerebral injection of a cytokine worsens seizure activity, and cytokine receptor antibodies, such as IL-1-receptor antagonist, show powerful anticonvulsant activity [Vezzani *et al.*, 2000].

The mechanisms by which cytokines lead to neuronal excitability have been explored in several studies focusing on ictogenic and neurotoxic properties of IL-1β mediated by IL-1 receptor (IL-1RI) [Bernardino *et al.*, 2005; Vezzani *et al.*, 1999]. IL-1RI colocalizes with NMDA receptors on hippocampal pyramidal neurons, and IL-1RI-mediated modulation of glutamatergic transmission may contribute to excitotoxicity and spontaneous seizures [Ravizza *et al.*, 2008]. IL-1β binding to its receptor increases NMDA receptor-mediated Ca^{2+} influx and surface expression of AMPA receptors [Beattie *et al.*, 2002; Viviani *et al.*, 2003]. IL-1β acts on astrocytes to inhibit reuptake of glutamate [Ye and Sontheimer, 1996] and increase glutamate release via TNF-α production, both resulting in elevated extracellular glutamate levels and hyperexcitability. Furthermore, IL-1β can stimulate IL-6 release [Bezzi and Volterra, 2001]. Transgenic mice over-expressing astrocyte IL-6 show markedly increased astrogliosis and microgliosis, a loss of inhibitory interneurons, and are exquisitely and selectively sensitive to glutamatergic agonists [Samland *et al.*, 2003].

Cytokines are involved in the death of neurons. Direct intraventricular IL-1β injection concurrent with brain insult increases injury-induced cell death and brain edema [Patel *et al.*, 2003]. Inhibition of IL-1 signaling by IL-1 receptor antagonist injection just prior to chemoconvulsant administration significantly attenuates subsequent hippocampal cell loss, implicating endogenous IL-1 in seizure-associated cell death [Panegyres and Hughes, 1998]. Cytokines can influence the activation of astrocytes and microglia. Astrogliosis can be induced in healthy animals by the injection of cytokines such as IL-1, and injury-induced microglial activation is suppressed in TNF receptor knockout mice [Bruce *et al.*, 1996]. In turn, reactive microglia and astrocytes themselves provide a rich source of cytokines after injury or insult, especially IL-6, TGF-β, LIF and IL-1 [Ridet *et al.*, 1997].

10.4 Inflammatory reactions in chronic epilepsy — Evidence from human epilepsy

Increased expression of proinflammatory molecules has been demonstrated in brain tissue from patients who received surgery for drug resistant epilepsies. Brain inflammation may be a common factor contributing or predisposing to the occurrence of seizures and cell death in various forms of epilepsy of different etiologies.

10.4.1 *Blood and CSF from epilepsy patients*

Acute inflammatory reaction after seizures has long been suspected due to clinical observations. Mean peripheral blood and CSF-leukocyte counts as well as C-reactive protein, an acute phase reactant, are significantly elevated in patients who present with new onset generalized convulsions without any clinical evidence of CNS or systemic infection [Rider *et al.*, 1995]. Involvement of the "cytokine network" has also been implicated in febrile seizures. Significantly higher plasma IL-6 levels as well as a higher ratio of endogenous IL-1 receptor antagonist to IL-1β are found in children with febrile seizures compared to febrile children without seizures [Virta *et al.*, 2002] and in epilepsy patients with recent tonic-clonic convulsions [Peltola *et al.*, 2000].

Cytokine gene polymorphism has been linked to epilepsy susceptibility. The increased frequency of a biallelic polymorphism in the promoter region of IL-1β at the 511 position, which is suggested to have effects of higher IL-1β production, has been reported in patients with temporal lobe epilepsy with hippocampal sclerosis and prolonged febrile convulsions [Kanemoto *et al.*, 2003]. Sporadic simple febrile seizure patients exhibit significantly higher frequencies of IL1β -31C/-511T alleles and homozygotes than controls [Kira *et al.*, 2005]. These results suggest that genetic susceptibility to inflammation may contribute to epileptogenesis.

10.4.2 *Epileptogenic brains of children with epilepsy*

Active inflammation has been detected not only in prototypical inflammatory epilepsy such as Rasmussen encephalitis or limbic encephalitis, but also in pharmacoresistant epilepsy of diverse etiologies [Choi *et al.*, 2009]. Cortical tissue from 13 children who underwent epilepsy surgery were used to quantify cell death, astrocyte proliferation, microglial activation and cytokine release. Five autopsy patients with no history of seizures or neurological diseases were used as controls. We found marked glial activation and neuroinflammation in epileptogenic cortices. The majority of patients had intellectual disability. Numerous fibrillary astrocytes covered the entire cortex and converged onto blood vessels, neurons, and microglia. Large numbers of neurons and astrocytes displayed DNA fragmentation and the magnitude significantly correlated with seizure frequency. Panlaminar astrocytosis, diffuse microglial activation, and release of proinflammatory cytokines, especially IL-1β, IL-8, IL-12p70 and

MIP-1β, were present in the epileptogenic cortices, consistent with chronic neuroinflammatory responses. IL-6 and MCP-1 were significantly higher in patients with a family history of epilepsy, suggesting links between genetic susceptibility to inflammation and epilepsy. Our results suggest that active neuroinflammation may play a common pathogenic role in childhood epilepsies of diverse etiologies.

The role of peripherally derived CNS-infiltrating immune cells in pathogenesis of intractable pediatric epilepsy was highlighted recently [Xu *et al.*, 2018]. In surgically resected brain tissue from children with two leading causes of drug-resistant epilepsy, focal cortical dysplasia (n = 19) and encephalomalacia (n = 10), we found infiltration of activated memory CD4+helper and CD8+ cytotoxic T-lymphocytes as well as blood-borne antigen presenting cells (APCs). Moreover, proinflammatory IL-17-producing γδ T cells are concentrated in the epileptogenic zone and their numbers positively correlates with seizure frequency. In contrast, the number of brain infiltrating regulatory T cells (Treg) inversely correlate with seizure severity. Thus,

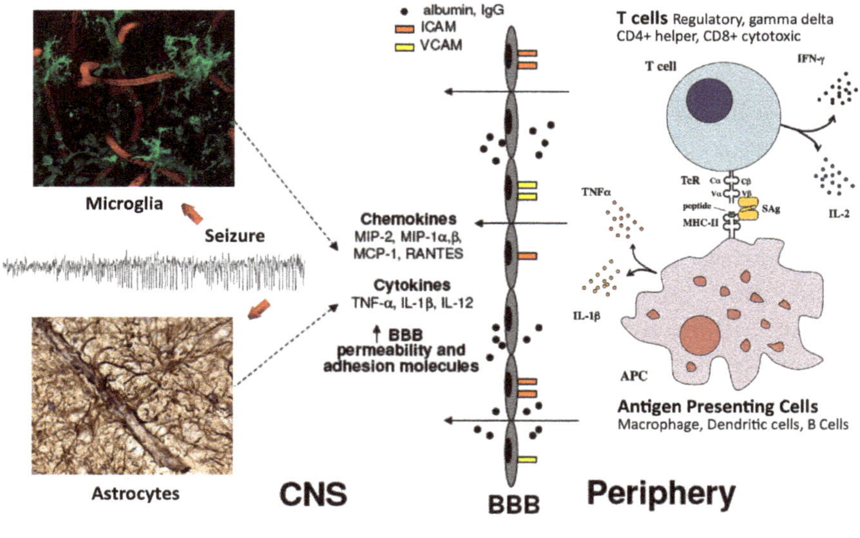

Figure 10.2. Amplifying feedback loop of innate and adaptive immunity triggered by seizures. Rapid microglia response and astrocyte activation → release of cytokines and chemokines, breakdown of blood brain barrier → infiltration of APCs and T-cells.

opposing roles of T cell subtypes, γδ T cells versus Treg are demonstrated in drug-resistant pediatric epilepsy. Immunomodulatory therapy targeting brain infiltration of peripheral immune cells has the potential to be a disease-modifying treatment [Xu *et al.*, 2018] (Figure 10.2).

10.5 Conclusion

Accumulating evidence indicates a critical role of immunity and neuroinflammation in the evolution of drug resistant childhood epilepsy. BBB breakdown and infiltration of peripheral immune cells are demonstrated both in humans and mice after recurrent seizures. Chronic brain inflammation may contribute both to intractability of seizures and comorbidity in children with epilepsy. No effective treatments currently exist to protect the brain from seizure-induced cell death and prevent future development of chronic epilepsy. Modulation of inflammatory reactions in the brain and targeting of inflammatory mediators may be effective therapeutic strategies to prevent or limit epileptogenesis in the vulnerable nervous system. Anti-inflammatory therapy may be particularly helpful when given shortly after the initial neurologic insult, but prior to the onset of epilepsy, before permanent changes can occur in neuronal aggregates that promote hyperexcitability and seizure spread.

Immune mechanisms in the evolution of drug-resistant pediatric epilepsy involve a non-linear, amplifying feedback loop of innate and adaptive immunity. Microglia in young brain react rapidly and robustly to recurrent seizures by releasing cytokines and chemokines, which then lead to infiltration of professional antigen presenting cells from the periphery and infiltration of T cells. Highlighted are the roles of proinflammatory T-cells in the pathogenesis of drug-resistant epilepsy. The ongoing, chronic neuroinflammation thus predisposes, precipitates, and perpetuates epileptogenesis in developing brain. The causative role of immunity in the pathogenesis of epilepsy and neurological sequelae of chronic intractable epilepsy needs to be proven and requires further investigation from both the clinic and basic science laboratory.

Acknowledgments

I thank Jieun Choi, MD, Douglas R. Nordli, Jr, MD, Dan Xu, PhD, Stephen D. Miller, PhD, Hyokwon Chung, MS, for their help, support and contributions to this chapter. Dr. Koh's research is supported by NIH/NINDS R01 NS073768.

References

Abraham, J., Fox, P.D., Condello, C., Bartolini, A., and Koh, S. (2012). Minocycline attenuates microglia activation and blocks the long-term epileptogenic effects of early-life seizures, *Neurobiol. Dis.*, 46, 425–430.

Aloisi, F. (2001). Immune function of microglia, *Glia*, 36, 165–179.

Armangue, T., Petit-Pedrol, M., and Dalmau, J. (2012). Autoimmune encephalitis in children, *J. Child. Neurol.*, 27, 1460–1469.

Arzimanoglou, A. Guerrini, R., and J. Aicardi, *Infantile spasms and related syndromes.* In: Aicardi's Epilepsy in Children, 3rd edition. ed. Arzimanoglou, A. Guerrini, R., and J. Aicardi. 2004, Philadelphia: Lippincott Williams & Wilkins. p. 14–37.

Bahi-Buisson, N., Villanueva, V., Bulteau, C., Delalande, O., Dulac, O., Chiron, C., and Nabbout, R. (2007). Long term response to steroid therapy in Rasmussen encephalitis, *Seizure*, 16, 485–492.

Ballabh, P., Braun, A., and Nedergaard, M. (2004). The blood-brain barrier: an overview: structure, regulation, and clinical implications, *Neurobiol. Dis.*, 16, 1–13.

Baram, T.Z. (1993). Pathophysiology of massive infantile spasms: perspective on the putative role of the brain adrenal axis, *Ann. Neurol.*, 33, 231–236.

Bauer, J., Elger, C.E., Hans, V.H., Schramm, J., Urbach, H., Lassmann, H., and Bien, C.G. (2007). Astrocytes are a specific immunological target in Rasmussen's encephalitis, *Ann. Neurol.*, 62, 67–80.

Beattie, E.C., Stellwagen, D., Morishita, W., Bresnahan, J.C., Ha, B.K., Von Zastrow, M., Beattie, M.S., and Malenka, R.C. (2002). Control of synaptic strength by glial TNF-alpha, *Science*, 295, 2282–2285.

Berg, A.T., Coryell, J., Saneto, R.P., Grinspan, Z.M., Alexander, J.J., Kekis, M., Sullivan, J.E., Wirrell, E.C., Shellhaas, R.A., Mytinger, J.R., Gaillard, W.D., Kossoff, E.H., Valencia, I., Knupp, K.G., Wusthoff, C., Keator, C., Dobyns, W.B., Ryan, N., Loddenkemper, T., Chu, C.J.,

Novotny, E.J., Jr., and Koh, S. (2017). Early-life epilepsies and the emerging role of genetic testing, *JAMA Pediatr.*, 171, 863–871.

Bernardino, L., Xapelli, S., Silva, A.P., Jakobsen, B., Poulsen, F.R., Oliveira, C.R., Vezzani, A., Malva, J.O., and Zimmer, J. (2005). Modulator effects of interleukin-1beta and tumor necrosis factor-alpha on AMPA-induced excitotoxicity in mouse organotypic hippocampal slice cultures, *J. Neurosci.*, 25, 6734–6744.

Bezzi, P. and Volterra, A. (2001). A neuron-glia signalling network in the active brain, *Curr. Opin. Neurobiol.*, 11, 387–394.

Block, M.L. and Hong, J.S. (2005). Microglia and inflammation-mediated neurodegeneration: multiple triggers with a common mechanism, *Prog. Neurobiol.*, 76, 77–98.

Borges, K., Gearing, M., McDermott, D.L., Smith, A.B., Almonte, A.G., Wainer, B.H., and Dingledine, R. (2003). Neuronal and glial pathological changes during epileptogenesis in the mouse pilocarpine model, *Exp. Neurol.*, 182, 21–34.

Bruce, A.J., Boling, W., Kindy, M.S., Peschon, J., Kraemer, P.J., Carpenter, M.K., Holtsberg, F.W., and Mattson, M.P. (1996). Altered neuronal and microglial responses to excitotoxic and ischemic brain injury in mice lacking TNF receptors, *Nat. Med.*, 2, 788–794.

Choi, J., Nordli, D.R., Jr., Alden, T.D., DiPatri, A., Jr., Laux, L., Kelley, K., Rosenow, J., Schuele, S.U., Rajaram, V., and Koh, S. (2009). Cellular injury and neuroinflammation in children with chronic intractable epilepsy, *J. Neuroinflammation*, 6, 38.

Cowan, L.D., Bodensteiner, J.B., Leviton, A., and Doherty, L. (1989). Prevalence of the epilepsies in children and adolescents, *Epilepsia*, 30, 94–106.

Cowan, L.D. and Hudson, L.S. (1991). The epidemiology and natural history of infantile spasms, *J. Child Neurol.*, 6, 355–364.

Crespel, A., Coubes, P., Rousset, M.C., Brana, C., Rougier, A., Rondouin, G., Bockaert, J., Baldy-Moulinier, M., and Lerner-Natoli, M. (2002). Inflammatory reactions in human medial temporal lobe epilepsy with hippocampal sclerosis, *Brain Res.*, 952, 159–169.

Crisp, S.J., Kullmann, D.M., and Vincent, A. (2016). Autoimmune synaptopathies, *Nat. Rev. Neurosci.*, 17, 103–117.

Eisermann, M.M., DeLaRaillere, A., Dellatolas, G., Tozzi, E., Nabbout, R., Dulac, O., and Chiron, C. (2003). Infantile spasms in Down syndrome — effects of delayed anticonvulsive treatment, *Epilepsy Res.*, 55, 21–27.

Ekdahl, C.T., Claasen, J.H., Bonde, S., Kokaia, Z., and Lindvall, O. (2003). Inflammation is detrimental for neurogenesis in adult brain, *Proc. Natl. Acad. Sci. U. S. A.*, 100, 13632–13637.

Fabene, P.F., Navarro Mora, G., Martinello, M., Rossi, B., Merigo, F., Ottoboni, L., Bach, S., Angiari, S., Benati, D., Chakir, A., Zanetti, L., Schio, F., Osculati, A., Marzola, P., Nicolato, E., Homeister, J.W., Xia, L., Lowe, J.B., McEver, R.P., Osculati, F., Sbarbati, A., Butcher, E.C., and Constantin, G. (2008). A role for leukocyte-endothelial adhesion mechanisms in epilepsy, *Nat. Med.*, 14, 1377–1383.

Fedele, D.E., Gouder, N., Guttinger, M., Gabernet, L., Scheurer, L., Rulicke, T., Crestani, F., and Boison, D. (2005). Astrogliosis in epilepsy leads to overexpression of adenosine kinase, resulting in seizure aggravation, *Brain*, 128, 2383–2395.

Flanagan, E.P., McKeon, A., Lennon, V.A., Boeve, B.F., Trenerry, M.R., Tan, K.M., Drubach, D.A., Josephs, K.A., Britton, J.W., Mandrekar, J.N., Lowe, V., Parisi, J.E., and Pittock, S.J. (2010). Autoimmune dementia: clinical course and predictors of immunotherapy response, *Mayo Clin. Proc.*, 85, 881–897.

Gallagher, S., Weiss, S., Oram Cardy, J., Humphries, T., Harman, K.E., and Menascu, S. (2006). Efficacy of very high dose steroid treatment in a case of Landau-Kleffner syndrome, *Dev. Med. Child Neurol.*, 48, 766–769.

Hanisch, U.K. (2002). Microglia as a source and target of cytokines, *Glia*, 40, 140–155.

Henshall, D.C. (2007). Apoptosis signalling pathways in seizure-induced neuronal death and epilepsy, *Biochem. Soc. Trans.*, 35, 421–423.

Hildebrandt, M., Amann, K., Schroder, R., Pieper, T., Kolodziejczyk, D., Holthausen, H., Buchfelder, M., Stefan, H., and Blumcke, I. (2008). White matter angiopathy is common in pediatric patients with intractable focal epilepsies, *Epilepsia*, 49, 804–815.

Ivens, S., Kaufer, D., Flores, L.P., Bechmann, I., Zumsteg, D., Tomkins, O., Seiffert, E., Heinemann, U., and Friedman, A. (2007). TGF-beta receptor-mediated albumin uptake into astrocytes is involved in neocortical epileptogenesis, *Brain*, 130, 535–547.

Jankowsky, J.L. and Patterson, P.H. (2001). The role of cytokines and growth factors in seizures and their sequelae, *Prog. Neurobiol.*, 63, 125–149.

Joseph, F.G. and Scolding, N.J. (2007). Neuro-Behcet's disease in Caucasians: a study of 22 patients, *Eur. J. Neurol.*, 14, 174–180.

Kanemoto, K., Kawasaki, J., Yuasa, S., Kumaki, T., Tomohiro, O., Kaji, R., and Nishimura, M. (2003). Increased frequency of interleukin-1beta-511T allele in patients with temporal lobe epilepsy, hippocampal sclerosis, and prolonged febrile convulsion, *Epilepsia*, 44, 796–799.

Kang, T.C., Kim, D.S., Kwak, S.E., Kim, J.E., Won, M.H., Kim, D.W., Choi, S.Y., and Kwon, O.S. (2006). Epileptogenic roles of astroglial death and regeneration in the dentate gyrus of experimental temporal lobe epilepsy, *Glia*, 54, 258–271.

Kelley, S.A. and Kossoff, E.H. (2010). Doose syndrome (myoclonic-astatic epilepsy): 40 years of progress, *Dev. Med. Child Neurol.*, 52, 988–993.

Kenney-Jung, D.L., Vezzani, A., Kahoud, R.J., LaFrance-Corey, R.G., Ho, M.L., Muskardin, T.W., Wirrell, E.C., Howe, C.L., and Payne, E.T. (2016). Febrile infection-related epilepsy syndrome treated with anakinra, *Ann. Neurol.*, 80, 939–945.

Khalili, K., White, M.K., Lublin, F., Ferrante, P., and Berger, J.R. (2007). Reactivation of JC virus and development of PML in patients with multiple sclerosis, *Neurology*, 68, 985–990.

Kim, J.V., Kang, S.S., Dustin, M.L., and McGavern, D.B. (2009). Myelomonocytic cell recruitment causes fatal CNS vascular injury during acute viral meningitis, *Nature*, 457, 191–195.

Kira, R., Torisu, H., Takemoto, M., Nomura, A., Sakai, Y., Sanefuji, M., Sakamoto, K., Matsumoto, S., Gondo, K., and Hara, T. (2005). Genetic susceptibility to simple febrile seizures: interleukin-1beta promoter polymorphisms are associated with sporadic cases, *Neurosci. Lett.*, 384, 239–244.

Koh, S., Storey, T.W., Santos, T.C., Mian, A.Y., and Cole, A.J. (1999). Early-life seizures in rats increase susceptibility to seizure-induced brain injury in adulthood, *Neurology*, 53, 915–921.

Kreutzberg, G.W. (1996). Microglia: a sensor for pathological events in the CNS, *Trends Neurosci.*, 19, 312–318.

Liou, H.H., Wang, C.R., Chen, C.J., Chen, R.C., Chuang, C.Y., Chiang, I.P., and Tsai, M.C. (1996). Elevated levels of anticardiolipin antibodies and epilepsy in lupus patients, *Lupus*, 5, 307–312.

Mackay, M.T., Weiss, S.K., Adams-Webber, T., Ashwal, S., Stephens, D., Ballaban-Gill, K., Baram, T.Z., Duchowny, M., Hirtz, D., Pellock, J.M., Shields, W.D., Shinnar, S., Wyllie, E., Snead, O.C., 3rd, American Academy of, N., and Child Neurology, S. (2004). Practice parameter: medical treatment of infantile spasms: report of the American Academy of Neurology and the Child Neurology Society, *Neurology*, 62, 1668–1681.

Mantegazza, R., Bernasconi, P., Baggi, F., Spreafico, R., Ragona, F., Antozzi, C., Bernardi, G., and Granata, T. (2002). Antibodies against GluR3 peptides are not specific for Rasmussen's encephalitis but are also present in epilepsy patients with severe, early onset disease and intractable seizures, *J. Neuroimmunol.*, 131, 179–185.

Marchi, N., Angelov, L., Masaryk, T., Fazio, V., Granata, T., Hernandez, N., Hallene, K., Diglaw, T., Franic, L., Najm, I., and Janigro, D. (2007). Seizure-promoting effect of blood-brain barrier disruption, *Epilepsia*, 48, 732–742.

McNamara, J.O. (1994). Cellular and molecular basis of epilepsy, *J. Neurosci.*, 14, 3413–3425.

Nabbout, R., Mazzuca, M., Hubert, P., Peudennier, S., Allaire, C., Flurin, V., Aberastury, M., Silva, W., and Dulac, O. (2010). Efficacy of ketogenic diet in severe refractory status epilepticus initiating fever induced refractory epileptic encephalopathy in school age children (FIRES), *Epilepsia*, 51, 2033–2037.

Nabbout, R., Vezzani, A., Dulac, O., and Chiron, C. (2011). Acute encephalopathy with inflammation-mediated status epilepticus, *Lancet Neurol.*, 10, 99–108.

O'Connor, E.R., Sontheimer, H., Spencer, D.D., and de Lanerolle, N.C. (1998). Astrocytes from human hippocampal epileptogenic foci exhibit action potential-like responses, *Epilepsia*, 39, 347–354.

Oguni, H., Hayashi, K., Awaya, Y., Fukuyama, Y., and Osawa, M. (2001). Severe myoclonic epilepsy in infants — a review based on the Tokyo Women's Medical University series of 84 cases, *Brain Dev.*, 23, 736–748.

Panegyres, P.K. and Hughes, J. (1998). The neuroprotective effects of the recombinant interleukin-1 receptor antagonist rhIL-1ra after excitotoxic stimulation with kainic acid and its relationship to the amyloid precursor protein gene, *J. Neurol. Sci.*, 154, 123–132.

Patel, H.C., Boutin, H., and Allan, S.M. (2003). Interleukin-1 in the brain: mechanisms of action in acute neurodegeneration, *Ann. N. Y. Acad. Sci.*, 992, 39–47.

Peltola, J., Palmio, J., Korhonen, L., Suhonen, J., Miettinen, A., Hurme, M., Lindholm, D., and Keranen, T. (2000). Interleukin-6 and interleukin-1 receptor antagonist in cerebrospinal fluid from patients with recent tonic-clonic seizures, *Epilepsy Res.*, 41, 205–211.

Plata-Salaman, C.R., Ilyin, S.E., Turrin, N.P., Gayle, D., Flynn, M.C., Romanovitch, A.E., Kelly, M.E., Bureau, Y., Anisman, H., and McIntyre, D.C. (2000). Kindling modulates the IL-1beta system, TNF-alpha, TGF-beta1, and neuropeptide mRNAs in specific brain regions, *Brain Res. Mol. Brain Res.*, 75, 248–258.

Prasad, A.N., Stafstrom, C.F., and Holmes, G.L. (1996). Alternative epilepsy therapies: the ketogenic diet, immunoglobulins, and steroids, *Epilepsia*, 37 Suppl 1, S81–95.

Ravizza, T., Gagliardi, B., Noe, F., Boer, K., Aronica, E., and Vezzani, A. (2008). Innate and adaptive immunity during epileptogenesis and spontaneous seizures: evidence from experimental models and human temporal lobe epilepsy, *Neurobiol. Dis.*, 29, 142–160.

Ravizza, T., Rizzi, M., Perego, C., Richichi, C., Velíšková, J., Moshé, S.L., De Simoni, M.G., and Vezzani, A. (2005). Inflammatory response and glia activation in developing rat hippocampus after status epilepticus, *Epilepsia*, 46 Suppl 5, 113–117.

Rider, L.G., Thapa, P.B., Del Beccaro, M.A., Gale, J.L., Foy, H.M., Farwell, J.R., and Mendelman, P.M. (1995). Cerebrospinal fluid analysis in children with seizures, *Pediatr. Emerg. Care*, 11, 226–229.

Ridet, J.L., Malhotra, S.K., Privat, A., and Gage, F.H. (1997). Reactive astrocytes: cellular and molecular cues to biological function, *Trends Neurosci.*, 20, 570–577.

Riikonen, R. (1983). Infantile spasms: some new theoretical aspects, *Epilepsia*, 24, 159–168.

Rizzi, M., Perego, C., Aliprandi, M., Richichi, C., Ravizza, T., Colella, D., Velíšková, J., Moshé, S.L., De Simoni, M.G., and Vezzani, A. (2003). Glia activation and cytokine increase in rat hippocampus by kainic acid-induced status epilepticus during postnatal development, *Neurobiol. Dis.*, 14, 494–503.

Rogers, S.W., Andrews, P.I., Gahring, L.C., Whisenand, T., Cauley, K., Crain, B., Hughes, T.E., Heinemann, S.F., and McNamara, J.O. (1994). Autoantibodies to glutamate receptor GluR3 in Rasmussen's encephalitis, *Science*, 265, 648–651.

Samland, H., Huitron-Resendiz, S., Masliah, E., Criado, J., Henriksen, S.J., and Campbell, I.L. (2003). Profound increase in sensitivity to glutamatergic- but not cholinergic agonist-induced seizures in transgenic mice with astrocyte production of IL-6, *J. Neurosci. Res.*, 73, 176–187.

Schroder, W., Hinterkeuser, S., Seifert, G., Schramm, J., Jabs, R., Wilkin, G.P., and Steinhauser, C. (2000). Functional and molecular properties of human astrocytes in acute hippocampal slices obtained from patients with temporal lobe epilepsy, *Epilepsia*, 41 Suppl 6, S181–184.

Seifert, G., Schilling, K., and Steinhauser, C. (2006). Astrocyte dysfunction in neurological disorders: a molecular perspective, *Nat. Rev. Neurosci.*, 7, 194–206.

Seifert, G., Schroder, W., Hinterkeuser, S., Schumacher, T., Schramm, J., and Steinhauser, C. (2002). Changes in flip/flop splicing of astroglial AMPA receptors in human temporal lobe epilepsy, *Epilepsia*, 43 Suppl 5, 162–167.

Sinclair, D.B. (2003). Prednisone therapy in pediatric epilepsy, *Pediatr. Neurol.*, 28, 194–198.

Sinclair, D.B. and Snyder, T.J. (2005). Corticosteroids for the treatment of Landau-kleffner syndrome and continuous spike-wave discharge during sleep, *Pediatr. Neurol.*, 32, 300–306.

Snead, O.C., 3rd, Benton, J.W., and Myers, G.J. (1983). ACTH and prednisone in childhood seizure disorders, *Neurology*, 33, 966–970.

Somera-Molina, K.C., Robin, B., Somera, C.A., Anderson, C., Stine, C., Koh, S., Behanna, H.A., Van Eldik, L.J., Watterson, D.M., and Wainwright, M.S. (2007). Glial activation links early-life seizures and long-term neurologic dysfunction: evidence using a small molecule inhibitor of proinflammatory cytokine upregulation, *Epilepsia*, 48, 1785–1800.

Tian, G.F., Azmi, H., Takano, T., Xu, Q., Peng, W., Lin, J., Oberheim, N., Lou, N., Wang, X., Zielke, H.R., Kang, J., and Nedergaard, M. (2005). An astrocytic basis of epilepsy, *Nat. Med.*, 11, 973–981.

Tilleux, S., Berger, J., and Hermans, E. (2007). Induction of astrogliosis by activated microglia is associated with a down-regulation of metabotropic glutamate receptor 5, *J. Neuroimmunol.*, 189, 23–30.

Toubi, E., Khamashta, M.A., Panarra, A., and Hughes, G.R. (1995). Association of antiphospholipid antibodies with central nervous system disease in systemic lupus erythematosus, *Am. J. Med.*, 99, 397–401.

Turrin, N.P. and Rivest, S. (2004). Innate immune reaction in response to seizures: implications for the neuropathology associated with epilepsy, *Neurobiol. Dis.*, 16, 321–334.

Veggiotti, P., Pera, M.C., Teutonico, F., Brazzo, D., Balottin, U., and Tassinari, C.A. (2012). Therapy of encephalopathy with status epilepticus during sleep (ESES/CSWS syndrome): an update, *Epileptic Disord.*, 14, 1–11.

Verhelst, H., Boon, P., Buyse, G., Ceulemans, B., D'Hooghe, M., Meirleir, L.D., Hasaerts, D., Jansen, A., Lagae, L., Meurs, A., Coster, R.V., and Vonck, K. (2005). Steroids in intractable childhood epilepsy: clinical experience and review of the literature, *Seizure*, 14, 412–421.

Vezzani, A., Aronica, E., Mazarati, A., and Pittman, Q.J. (2013). Epilepsy and brain inflammation, *Exp. Neurol.*, 244, 11–21.

Vezzani, A., Conti, M., De Luigi, A., Ravizza, T., Moneta, D., Marchesi, F., and De Simoni, M.G. (1999). Interleukin-1beta immunoreactivity and microglia are enhanced in the rat hippocampus by focal kainate application: functional evidence for enhancement of electrographic seizures, *J. Neurosci.*, 19, 5054–5065.

Vezzani, A., Moneta, D., Conti, M., Richichi, C., Ravizza, T., De Luigi, A., De Simoni, M.G., Sperk, G., Andell-Jonsson, S., Lundkvist, J., Iverfeldt, K., and Bartfai, T. (2000). Powerful anticonvulsant action of IL-1 receptor antagonist on intracerebral injection and astrocytic overexpression in mice, *Proc. Natl. Acad. Sci. U. S. A.*, 97, 11534–11539.

Virta, M., Hurme, M., and Helminen, M. (2002). Increased frequency of interleukin-1beta (-511) allele 2 in febrile seizures, *Pediatr. Neurol.*, 26, 192–195.

Viviani, B., Bartesaghi, S., Gardoni, F., Vezzani, A., Behrens, M.M., Bartfai, T., Binaglia, M., Corsini, E., Di Luca, M., Galli, C.L., and Marinovich, M. (2003). Interleukin-1beta enhances NMDA receptor-mediated intracellular calcium increase through activation of the Src family of kinases, *J. Neurosci.*, 23, 8692–8700.

Watemberg, N., Greenstein, D., and Levine, A. (2006). Encephalopathy associated with Hashimoto thyroiditis: pediatric perspective, *J. Child. Neurol.*, 21, 1–5.

Xu, D., Robinson, A.P., Ishii, T., Duncan, D.S., Alden, T.D., Goings, G.E., Ifergan, I., Podojil, J.R., Penaloza-MacMaster, P., Kearney, J.A., Swanson, G.T., Miller, S.D., and Koh, S. (2018). Peripherally derived T regulatory and gammadelta T cells have opposing roles in the pathogenesis of intractable pediatric epilepsy, *J. Exp. Med.*, 218, 1169–1186.

Yamatogi, Y., Ohtsuka, Y., Ishida, T., Ichiba, N., Ishida, S., Miyake, S., Oka, E., and Ohtahara, S. (1979). Treatment of the Lennox syndrome with ACTH: a clinical and electroencephalographic study, *Brain Dev.*, 1, 267–276.

Ye, Z.C. and Sontheimer, H. (1996). Cytokine modulation of glial glutamate uptake: a possible involvement of nitric oxide, *Neuroreport*, 7, 2181–2185.

Zhang, W., Smith, C., Howlett, C., and Stanimirovic, D. (2000). Inflammatory activation of human brain endothelial cells by hypoxic astrocytes in vitro is mediated by IL-1beta, *J. Cereb. Blood Flow Metab.*, 20, 967–978.

Chapter 11
Developmental Dysplasias and Epilepsy

Jeffrey Goodman, PhD

Department of Developmental Neurobiology, Institute for Basic Research, Staten Island, New York and Department of Physiology and Pharmacology, SUNY Downstate Medical Center, Brooklyn, New York, USA

11.1 Introduction

It has become increasingly apparent from anatomical and radiological evidence that a significant cause of intractable seizures in children and adults is an underlying malformation of cortical development (MCD) [Fauser *et al.*, 2006; Vinters *et al.*, 2008; Blumcke *et al.*, 2011; Barkovich *et al.*, 2012, 2015]. Vinters and colleagues [Vinters *et al.*, 2008] examined surgically-resected tissue from over 500 children diagnosed with intractable seizures. They estimate that in those children under the age of three, over 80% had a cortical malformation. As the resolution of magnetic resonance imaging (MRI) increases, smaller defects are being identified in children and adults that are related to clinical epilepsy [Bastos *et al.*, 1999; Li *et al.*, 1995; Leventer *et al.*, 1999].

MCDs are diverse in their size, location, the amount of brain tissue involved, the degree of altered cortical architecture and types and number of abnormal cells. Often the patient will exhibit a combination of different types of malformation [Li *et al.*, 1995; Mathew *et al.*,

2010] and multiple malformations can be present in more than one lobe. While most malformations occur due to a genetic defect, they can also result from an intrauterine or perinatal insult or infection [Reutens *et al.*, 1993; Raymond *et al.*, 1995; Chen *et al.*, 2012].

The formation of MCD results from a disruption in one of three phases of cortical development: neuronal proliferation, migration and differentiation [Kuzniecky and Barkovich, 2001; Bast *et al.*, 2006]. The earlier in development the lesion first appears the more tissue likely to be involved and the type of epilepsy associated with the malformation often correlates with the timing of when the lesion occurred during development [Jellinger, 1987]. Seizures originating from a malformation can exacerbate the condition by further interfering with subsequent developmental processes [Ben-Ari and Holmes, 2006]. Most malformations associated with epilepsy are believed to originate from disruption of cortical development after 6 weeks gestation [Vintners *et al.*, 2008].

Initially, MCD were classified by size and cellular morphology identified after surgical resection and histological analysis [Taylor *et al.*, 1971]. However, with the development of high-resolution MRI, smaller, previously unidentified lesions have been shown to be the cause of seizures [Li *et al.*, 1995; Bastos *et al.*, 1999; Veersema *et al.*, 2017]. MCD can range in size from a small population of abnormal cells, microdysgenesis [Meencke and Janz, 1985], to involve an entire hemisphere, hemimegalencephalopathy [Gupta *et al.*, 2004]. Broad categories of malformation that are often associated with epilepsy include: lissencephaly, heterotopias, polymicrogyria and cortical dysplasia [Porter *et al.*, 2002].

This chapter focuses on the different types of focal cortical dysplasias (FCD), a subtype of MCD and one of the most frequent causes of drug resistant epilepsy in children [Serino *et al.*, 2015]. The morphological characteristics of the different types of FCD and the resulting epilepsies are described. When possible, the genetic abnormality underlying the malformation is identified. The difficulties associated with localization and surgical removal are addressed. Finally, some novel therapies (other than surgery) currently being investigated to treat seizures in this patient population are presented (see Chapter 1 for additional details).

11.2 Prevalence

MCD have been estimated to cause between 25–40% of intractable seizures in children [Kuzniecky, 1994; Leventer *et al.*, 2008] and it has been predicted that 75–80% of patients with MCD will develop epilepsy [Leventer *et al.*, 1999]. Often these seizures are refractory to antiepileptic drug (AED) therapy [Serino *et al.*, 2015]. FCD have been estimated to be responsible for the cause of seizures in 10–15% of patients diagnosed with epilepsy [Bast *et al.*, 2006]. Given the sensitivity of current methods of detection and diagnosis, these numbers likely underestimate the number of patients whose epilepsy is caused by an FCD. A recent retrospective study by Maynard *et al.* [2017] examined the prevalence of epilepsy and drug-resistant epilepsy in 97 pediatric patients up to the age of 18 who were diagnosed with FCD by MRI. They found that 71% of the patients were diagnosed with epilepsy and 33% were drug resistant. Unexpectedly, 29% had not developed epilepsy. However, it is reasonable to speculate that many of these patients will develop epilepsy later in adulthood. The results from this study likely underestimate the prevalence of FCD and epilepsy since only patients who were suspected of having an FCD were evaluated by MRI. Not all subtypes of FCD are equally identified by MRI with FCD Type II more readily identified by MRI than FCD Type I [Lerner *et al.*, 2009; Leach *et al.*, 2014].

11.3 Classification of FCD

Over a number of years, a series of studies have attempted to classify MCD by their size and cellular morphology. An initial characterization was developed by Taylor *et al.* [1971] who performed a microscopic examination of resected tissue from ten patients with epilepsy. In each case the resected area had been identified electrographically as the likely site of the seizure focus. Some of the abnormal features identified in these isolated lesions were: the blurring of the gray/white matter junction, localized disruption of cortical lamination and the presence of large aberrant neurons defined as balloon cells, randomly distributed throughout the deeper cortical layers and underlying white matter. These histopathological features were similar to those that had been observed in patients with tuberous sclerosis (TSC) but the MCD patients did not exhibit any of the other features associated with TSC. This type of MCD became known as FCD of the Taylor type [Foldvary *et al.*, 2004].

Barkovich *et al.* [1996, 2005, 2012] developed and modified a classification system of different types of MCDs based on the first step in the developmental process that was disturbed: cell proliferation, neuronal migration, or cortical organization. Palmini *et al.* [2004] provided the first comprehensive system that correlated clinical observations with the different histopathological features observed in different types of FCD. Most recently the Task Force of the ILAE Diagnostic Methods Commission [Blümcke *et al.*, 2011] developed a series of definitions to specify the structural and cellular abnormalities observed in different types of FCD and used these characteristics to develop a three-tiered classification system: FCD Type I through Type III. An increase in number correlates with an increase in complexity of the malformation.

11.3.1 *Terminology of the ILAE Taskforce [Blümcke et al., 2011]*

The following terms have been used in a number of studies that have attempted to characterize the histopathology observed in different types of FCD. The Taskforce developed the following definitions to provide a consistent, uniform meaning for each of the terms.

(1) **Dysmorphic neurons** — Abnormally large soma and nucleus accompanied by an abnormal accumulation of Nissl substance and neurofilaments.
(2) **Hypertrophic neurons** — Similar to layer 5 pyramidal cells but found in layers 1–4. Dendritic orientation and arborization can be altered. No evidence of intracellular pathology.
(3) **Immature neurons** — Develop from neuroblasts and have a small size. No accumulation of non-phosphorylated neurofilaments. Oriented vertically in minicolumns.

(4) **Dysplastic neurons** — Neuronal component of glio-neuronal tumors.
(5) **Balloon cells** — Large cell body with opaque eosinophilic cytoplasm. Lack Nissl substance. May contain multiple nuclei.
(6) **Heterotopia** — Misplaced tissue or cells within their normal organ of origin.
(7) **Dyslamination** — Compromised cortical architecture due to altered radial or tangential organization.
(8) **Double pathology** — Two independent lesions affecting one or multiple lobes that are believed to have developed independent of each other.

11.3.2 *ILAE Taskforce classification of the different types of FCD [Blümcke et al., 2011]. The Taskforce used the above definitions to characterize the different types of FCD*

11.3.2.1 **FCD Type I** — *Presents with abnormal cortical layering due to compromised radial or tangential migration. The mechanism underlying the development of FCD Type I is unknown and the malformation can be present in more than one lobe within the same patient*

FCD Type Ia is characterized by microcolumns of more than 8 neurons oriented vertically. Cellular abnormalities in this malformation include immature small diameter neurons as well as hypertrophic pyramidal neurons outside of layer 5.

FCD Type Ib is characterized by a failure to form a layered cortex. This lack of layering can be present throughout the entire cortex or can be limited to layers 2 or 4 or both. There is often a blurring of the transition between different cortical layers with some layers missing entirely. FCD Type Ib can include the cellular abnormalities observed in FCD Type Ia.

FCD Type Ic is characterized by isolated lesions that contain both compromised radial and tangential migration.

11.3.2.2 FCD Type II — *Disrupted lamination with specific cytologic abnormalities. This malformation is more frequently found extra temporally*

FCD Type IIa — This FCD is characterized by dysmorphic neurons with an enlarged soma and nucleus with an altered orientation. There is an abnormal distribution of Nissl substance and an accumulation of neurofilaments in the cytoplasm. There are no identifiable cortical layers except layer 1 and dysmorphic neurons can be present in the white matter. There can also be a blurring of the gray/white matter junction with heterotopic neurons in the white matter. Most importantly, there are no balloon cells in this FCD.

FCD Type IIb — All of the histopathologies present in FCD Type IIa are present in FCD Type IIb with the presence of balloon cells in addition to dysmorphic neurons. The dysmorphic neurons can include principal neurons as well as interneurons. An abnormal cell type that exhibits glial and neuronal features, defined as an Intermediate cell, can also be present. In addition, the myelin content of the subcortical white matter may be reduced.

11.3.2.3 FCD Type III — *These malformations are characterized by cortical dyslamination combined with another lesion in the same lobe. Some of these FCD may develop secondary to the presence of the primary lesion*

FCD Type IIIa — Specific to the temporal lobe, this FCD presents with cortical dyslamination or abnormal hypertrophic cells outside of layer 5 combined with hippocampal sclerosis. This type of FCD can have a number of different combinations of features such as hippocampal sclerosis plus temporal lobe sclerosis, hippocampal sclerosis combined with lentiform-shaped heterotopias or heterotopic neurons in the white matter, or hippocampal sclerosis combined with any other type of principal lesion in the temporal lobe.

FCD Type IIIb — Characterized by altered cortical architecture combined with the presence of an adjacent tumor.

FCD Type IIIc — Characterized by altered cortical architecture adjacent to a vascular malformation. The altered cortical architecture could have developed as a consequence of the primary lesion.

FCD Type IIId — A cortical dysplasia associated with any other lesion acquired early in life. This FCD is characterized by cortical dyslamination of the cytoarchitecture adjacent to a lesion acquired early in life. The primary lesion can include a traumatic brain injury, ischemic injury or infection.

11.4 Neocortical development and types of mutations leading to MCD

11.4.1 *Normal neocortical development*

11.4.1.1 *Radial glial migration*

Radial glial migration is the process by which cells destined to become glutaminergic principal neurons proliferate and migrate into the developing neocortex [Noctor *et al.*, 2001]. During corticogenesis, neuroepithelial cells and radial glial cells that line the lateral ventricle create the ventricular zone (VZ) [Noctor *et al.*, 2001]. Cells in the VZ undergo a number of mitotic divisions forming the preplate. A second proliferative zone called the subventricular zone (SVZ) develops between the VZ and the preplate. Future neurons generated in the proliferative zones migrate first into the preplate, splitting it into the more superficial marginal zone and a deeper subplate [Kriegstein and Noctor, 2004]. The cells that split the preplate form the cortical plate which will eventually become the neocortex as newly generated cells continue to migrate into the cortical plate [Kriegstein *et al.*, 2006].

Radial glial cells in the VZ extend a process from the VZ to the pial surface forming a guide for subsequent migration of newly-born principal neurons into what will become the neocortex [Rakic, 1978]. These cells undergo an asymmetric division renewing the proliferative radial glial cell but also generating an intermediate progenitor cell that migrates into the cortical plate and becomes a cortical projection neuron [Miyata *et al.*, 2001]. This process is referred to as the "direct pathway" of cortical neurogenesis [Hevner, 2006] and is responsible for the generation of the majority of cortical projection neurons [Anthony *et al.*, 2004]. Some neurons proliferate via an "indirect pathway" of neurogenesis. In the indirect pathway, intermediate progenitor cells migrate into the SVZ where they undergo symmetric division generating 2 progenitors that will eventually also migrate into the cortical plate such that the SVZ becomes a second proliferative zone [Noctor *et al.*, 2004]. Expansion of the cortical plate into the 6 layered cortex follows an inside-out pattern with neurons destined for the more superficial layers being born later in development and migrating past neurons born earlier to get to their appropriate location [Kriegstein *et al.*, 2006] (see Chapter 1 for more details).

11.4.1.2 *Tangential migration*

Cells destined to become GABAergic inhibitory neurons in the developing neocortex originate in the medial ganglionic eminence and migrate into the cortical plate by a process called tangential migration [de Carlos *et al.*, 1996; Tan *et al.*, 1998; Jimenez *et al.*, 2002; Marin and Rubenstein, 2001]. Cortical interneurons exhibit the same inside-out pattern of cortical layering observed with principal neurons [Cavanagh and Parnavelas, 1989; Andersen *et al.*, 2002].

11.4.2 *Germline and somatic mutations*

Genetic mutations are likely responsible for the majority of MCD associated with epilepsy. Abnormalities in over 30 genes have been identified as contributing to the formation of cortical malformations [Aronica *et al.*, 2012]. These mutations can be inherited through the germ cells from either parent or they can develop *de novo* in the form of a somatic mutation that occurs during development [Poduri *et al.*, 2013]. The ultimate impact of these mutations depends on the timing of their occurrence during development and for a somatic mutation, the type of cells involved. Mutations that occur in the germ cell of the parent before conception will be present in all of the cells of the offspring. A somatic mutation will have a more limited impact but still has the potential to be present in multiple cell types throughout the body. A somatic mutation that occurs in progenitor cells of brain development will result in a malformation limited to the brain [Poduri *et al.*, 2013].

Somatic mutations occuring during cortical development can result in a mosaic pattern with some cells expressing the mutation while others do not [Poduri *et al.*, 2013]. The pattern of mosaicism is also dependent on the timing of when the mutation occurred and the type of cell in which it occurred [Guerrini, 2005]. This situation can be further complicated because mutations in the same gene can result in dramatically different malformations depending on the timing of mutation during brain development [D'Gama *et al.*, 2017]. In some malformations, the abnormal cells will be highly localized while in others the abnormal cells are widely distributed [Franco and Muller, 2013; Poduri *et al.*, 2013] and in women, mutations in the X chromosome can lead to a variety of mosaics due to X inactivation. In some instances, a two-hit hypothesis has been proposed when a germ cell mutation combines with a somatic mutation or two separate somatic mutations combine to form an FCD [Poduri *et al.*, 2013; Baulac *et al.*, 2015].

11.4.3 *Timing of disruption of cortical development and types of MCD*

As stated above, the timing of when a mutation occurs during cortical development can affect the location, size and the types of cells present in the malformation. Excellent reviews by Guerrini [Guerrini *et al.*, 2003; Guerrini, 2005] identified the phase of neocortical development that is disrupted for a number of the different types of MCD. The following is a modification of a list from Guerrini *et al.* [2003] that identified the phase of cortical development that is altered for different types of cortical malformations. Briefly, malformations caused by alterations in neuronal and glial proliferation include tuberous sclerosis complex, FCD, and hemimegaencephaly. Malformations that occur because of abnormal neuronal migration include lissencephaly, cobblestone complex, and heterotopias. Malformations that occur due to alterations in cortical organization include polymicrogyria, schizencephaly, cortical dysplasias without balloon cells and microdysgenesis [Shrot *et al.*, 2018].

11.4.4 *Tuberous Sclerosis Complex (TSC) and FCD — mTORopathies*

The observation by Taylor *et al.* [1971] that many of the abnormal histopathological features observed in the FCD are similar to those that have been observed in patients with tuberous sclerosis (TSC) provided a clue to some of the genes responsible for the formation of FCD [Crino, 2015]. TSC is an autosomal dominant, multisystem disorder that results from a mutation in one of two genes, *TSC1* or *TSC2* which regulate the function of the mTOR signaling pathway [Chu-Shore *et al.*, 2010] (see also Chapter 12). Some of the many functions regulated by the mTOR pathway during normal development include cell proliferation, differentiation and axonal and dendritic growth [Lee, 2015; Lim *et al.*, 2017]. The loss of function of one of these two genes leads to hyperactivation of the mTOR pathway, which is likely responsible for the formation of the cortical tubers observed in TSC and malformations in patients with FCD Type IIb [Wong, 2013; D'Gama *et al.*, 2015]. While a germline mutation in *TSC1* or *TSC2* is responsible for TSC, FCD can develop from a somatic mutation in the *TSC1* or *TSC2* gene as well as genes that regulate mTOR activity [D'Gama *et al.*, 2015, 2017; Lim and Lee, 2016; Lim *et al.*, 2017; Marsan and Baulac, 2018]. Enhanced mTOR signaling has been observed in cells located within FCD Type IIb malformations [Baybis *et al.*, 2004; Miyata *et al.*, 2004]. It has been estimated that somatic mutations that result in mTOR hyperactivation account for 15–25% of patients with FCD Type II [Lim *et al.*, 2015, 2017; Nakashima *et al.*, 2015]. In addition to mutations in *TSC1* and *TSC2*, mutations in several genes that regulate mTOR activity have also been identified that underlie the formation of FCD. These include somatic mutations in *PIK3CA* and *AKT3* and germline mutations in *DEPDC5*, *NPRL2*, and *NPRL3*

[Poduri *et al.*, 2013; Poduri, 2014; Scheffer *et al.*, 2014, D'Gama *et al.*, 2015, 2017; Moller *et al.*, 2016; Sim *et al.*, 2016]. Somatic mutations that result in the hyperactivation of the mTOR pathway are the most frequent mutations found in resected FCD tissue [Marsan and Baulac, 2018].

11.5 Epilepsy and mechanisms of epileptogenicity associated with FCD

11.5.1 *Clinical seizure semiology*

Palmini *et al.* [1995] used intraoperative electrocorticography (ECoG) to identify the following three patterns of epileptic discharges from dysplastic cortex in 67% of the patients examined: 1) repetitive electrographic seizures, 2) repetitive burst discharges and 3) continuous rhythmic spiking. They concluded that cortical dysplastic lesions are highly epileptogenic and that removal of all of the tissue exhibiting epileptogenic discharges is necessary for a favorable outcome. The inherent epileptogenicity of dysplastic tissue was confirmed by Avoli's group who used *in vitro* slice electrophysiology to record epileptiform activity in neocortical slices from patients with FCD [Mattia *et al.*, 1995; Avoli *et al.*, 2003]. They observed that slices containing dysplastic tissue had an intrinsic ability to generate ictal- like epileptiform activity when treated with the convulsant 4-aminopyridine (4-AP). This was not observed in neocortical slices that did not contain a lesion. The 4-AP-induced epileptiform activity was shown to be mediated through blockade of voltage-activated potassium channels.

Several retrospective studies evaluated the combination of electrographic localization, neuroimaging and histological analysis of resected tissue to confirm that FCD is a frequent cause of focal epilepsy [Tassi *et al.*, 2002, 2012; Lortie *et al.*, 2002; Fauser *et al.*, 2006; Bast *et al.*, 2006; Maynard *et al.*, 2017]. Epilepsy in patients with FCD usually begins in the first year of life [Bast *et al.*, 2006] with the majority of the patients becoming refractory to AED therapy [Serino *et al.*, 2015].

A variety of types of epilepsy have been observed in this diverse patient population including infantile spasms, focal seizures and generalized-tonic clonic seizures, status epilepticus and febrile seizures [Porter *et al.*, 2002; Fauser *et al.*, 2006]. In some patients, the seizure semiology changes over time [Fauser *et al.*, 2006]. In one study, the initial seizure in a majority of patients was focal but these focal seizures could secondarily generalize or be accompanied by infantile spasms [Lortie *et al.*, 2002].

The ictal manifestations of focal seizures depend on the location of the malformation. Serino *et al.* [2015] correlated seizure type with FCD location in patients with seizure onset in the first year. In a sample of 41 patients, 21 had focal seizures, 11 had infantile spasms and 9 had focal seizures followed by infantile spasms. In those patients with only infantile spasms, 90.9% had a FCD localized to the frontal lobe.

11.5.2 *Mechanisms of epileptogenicity*

11.5.2.1 *Assessment of human dysplastic tissue*

The tissue within the FCD is inherently epileptogenic and when all of the dysplastic tissue is successfully removed, seizure freedom can be obtained [Palmini *et al.*, 1995; Avoli *et al.*, 2003; Chassoux *et al.*, 2012]. However, the mechanisms underlying the epileptogenicity of the malformation are less clear. A number of studies have examined alterations in the expression of glutamate and GABA receptors on neurons in tissue surgically resected from patients with FCD [Najm *et al.*, 2000]. Alterations in the expression of NMDAR2 and AMPA GluR2/3 have been reported to be present on human dysplastic neurons which could underlie the inherent epileptogenicity present in the malformation [Ying *et al.*, 1998]. Immunohistochemical analysis of microdissected dysplastic neurons from human cortical dysplasia specimens also revealed an abnormal expression of mRNA for glutamate and GABA receptor subunits that could contribute to epileptogenesis [Crino *et al.*, 2001; White *et al.*, 2001]. An earlier study reported a decrease in the number of parvalbumin and calbindin D28k expressing inhibitory interneurons in dysplastic human tissue which is also consistent with a hyperexcitable network [Ferrer *et al.*, 1994].

Specific cell types within the malformation may be the seizure generators. Whole-cell patch clamping combined with biocytin labeling revealed the presence of excitatory and inhibitory cytomegalic neurons within FCD Type IIb dysplasias, with both cell types hyperexcitable [Cepeda *et al.*, 2005; Andre *et al.*, 2007]. The presence of an abundance of immature neurons within the dysplasia led Cepeda *et al.* [2006] to propose the Dysmature Cerebral Development hypothesis. They proposed that the cytomegalic neurons within the dysplasia resemble human subplate neurons and that balloon cells have similar features to radial glial cells. The presence of these immature neurons within the dysplasia would result from a failure of prenatal cell death in the later stages of cortical development [Andres *et al.*, 2005]. Further evidence that the cells within the dysplasia resembled immature cortex was the unexpected observations that: 1) NMDA receptors on these cells had a reduced sensitivity to Mg^{2+} and 2) GABA was depolarizing [Cepeda *et al.*, 2007, 2012; Abdijadid *et al.*, 2015]. Both of these changes would be proconvulsive.

A possible explanation for why patients with a FCD are resistant to AED therapy is the increased expression of multidrug-resistant proteins in FCD tissue [Sisodiya *et al.*, 2001, 2002; Aronica *et al.*, 2003; Ak *et al.*, 2007]. Functionally, multidrug transporters act as outwardly directed pumps, transferring therapeutic agents from the brain back into the capillaries [Loscher and Potschka, 2002]. The overexpression of multidrug resistance gene-1 p-glycoprotein (*MDR1*) and multidrug resistance-associated protein-1 (*MRP1*) has been detected in endothelial cells and glia of epileptogenic tissue [Tishler *et al.*, 1995; Sisodiya *et al.*, 2001, 2002]. More recently, Ak *et al.* [2007] observed the overexpression of *MDR1* and *MRP1* in neurons and reactive astrocytes in epileptogenic tissue surgically-resected from patients with FCD. The overexpression of these transporters in dysplasic tissue may lead to inadequate levels of AED at the epileptogenic zone [Loscher and Potschka, 2002; Aronica *et al.*, 2003].

11.5.2.2 *Experimental models*

There are a limited number of experimental models specific for FCD that result in a lesion that is accompanied by spontaneous seizure activity [Wong, 2009]. In many of the models that result in a brain malformation, the seizure activity can only be detected *in vitro* although some have reduced seizure threshold to other experimental methods of seizure induction. Fetal insults that induce an FCD include prenatal exposure to methylazoxymethanol acetate (MAM), which induces a hippocampal heterotopia [Baraban *et al.*, 2000] and the in utero irradiation rat model which induces a cortical dysplasia and a hippocampal heterotopia [Roper *et al.*, 1998, Kellinghaus *et al.*, 2004; Marin-Padilla *et al.*, 2013]. The incidence of spontaneous seizure activity in both of these models is less than 20% [Wong, 2009]. Recently, in utero electroporation of a plasmid encoding the constitutively active form of RheB, the activator of mTORC1, has been used to create a mouse model of FCB Type II [Hsieh *et al.*, 2016]. The resulting increase in mTOR activity generated cortical dysplasia in layer 2/3 of the medial prefrontal cortex that was accompanied by spontaneous behavioral and electrographic seizures. Importantly, postnatal treatment with rapamycin starting on postnatal day one prevented generation of the FCD and seizure activity.

The neonatal freeze lesion model results in a lesion similar to polymicrogyria in which epileptiform activity can be evoked in vitro. The seizure activity appears to arise from tissue adjacent to the malformation, not from the malformation itself [Jacobs *et al.*, 1999; Najm *et al.*, 2007].

11.6 Treatment options

11.6.1 *Localization and surgical resection*

Seizures in patients with FCD are difficult to treat. Many patients with FCD are refractory to AED therapy and even when the epileptogenic zone can be identified with improved imaging and neurophysiologic detection, the location of the FCD may be surgically inaccessible [Guerrini *et al.*, 2015]. However, for most patients diagnosed with FCD, surgical resection is the primary treatment and the one with the greatest chance of success, especially when all of the epileptic tissue is removed which requires accurate localization of the epileptogenic zone [Thornton *et al.*, 2011]. When surgical removal is successful, a remission rate as high as 90% has been reported (Engel class 1) [Chassoux *et al.*, 2012]. However, typical surgical success rates are lower, dependent on location and the type of malformation [Guerrini *et al.*, 2003, 2015; Leach *et al.*, 2014; Fauser *et al.*, 2015]. In most cases, surgical outcome is better in patients with FCD Type II than FCD Type I [Tassi *et al.*, 2002], probably because for many cases of FCD Type I, interictal and ictal EEG are not reliable determinants of the epileptogenic zone [Krsek *et al.*, 2009]. Also, the diagnostic sensitivity of the MRI increases with the severity of pathology in the FCD such that FCD Type II is easier to detect than FCD Type I [Krsek *et al.*, 2009; Kim *et al.*, 2012; Lee and Kim, 2013]. In addition, imaging may fail to detect the presence of an FCD [Krsek *et al.*, 2009; Lerner *et al.*, 2009; Veersema *et al.*, 2017]. Lerner *et al.* [2009] reported that the MRI failed to detect 37% of FCD Type I and 15% of FCD Type II malformations in patients who underwent epilepsy surgery. The accuracy of FCD detection improves as the field strength of the MRI increases [Veersema *et al.*, 2017].

11.6.1.1 *Methods of enhanced localization*

Several different approaches are currently being examined to better target the epileptogenic zone in patients with FCD with the goal of improving surgical outcome. One approach is to combine EEG with fMRI [Grouiller *et al.*, 2011; Thornton *et al.*, 2011; Pittau *et al.*, 2012; Guerrini *et al.*, 2015]. Thornton *et al.* [2011] reported improved detection of the seizure onset zone when the blood oxygen level dependent (BOLD) signal correlated with interictal electrographic activity. Surgical success was improved if the resected tissue included maximal BOLD activity.

High-frequency oscillations (HFOs) have also been used to localize the epileptogenic zone in patients with FCD but the presence of HFOs could not be used to identify the specific type of lesion underlying the epileptiform activity [Jacobs *et al.*, 2009; Ferrari-Marinho *et al.*, 2015; Guerrini *et al.*, 2015; Sato *et al.*, 2015].

Combining MRI with fluorodeoxyglucose positron emission tomography (FDG-PET) has become an effective means of identifying the epileptogenic zone [Moeller *et al.*, 2009] and also identifying MRI-negative FCD malformations [Kim *et al.*, 2000]. FDG-PET has also been combined with MRI and DTI to improve detection of cortical tubers associated TSC [Chandra *et al.*, 2006]. This combination should also be useful in the identification of FCD. Other methods used to improve the location and borders of the epileptogenic zone of FCD include magnetoencephalography (MEG) [Ishii *et al.*, 2008; Colombo *et al.*, 2009; Heers *et al.*, 2014], stereoencephalogaphy (SEEG) [Varotto *et al.*, 2010, 2012], and ictal single-photon emission computed tomography (SPECT) [Widdess-Walsh *et al.*, 2006; Lee and Kim, 2013; Delev *et al.*, 2018].

11.6.2 *Nonsurgical treatment options*

A number of nonsurgical treatments are being investigated as antiepileptic therapies for FCD. These include the ketogenic diet, mTOR inhibitors, and vagus nerve stimulation (VNS) [Guerrini *et al.*, 2015]. Perhaps the most promising is the ketogenic diet. A retrospective study by Jung *et al.* [2008] evaluated 47 patients with a FCD identified by MRI who were treated with the ketogenic diet prior to becoming candidates for surgery. The group included patients diagnosed with infantile spasms, Lennox-Gastaut and focal seizures. Three months after starting the diet, 61.7% of the patients had a reduction in seizure frequency greater than 50%, with 45% becoming seizure-free. Ten of the patients remained seizure-free up to 3 years after going off the diet with 22 eventually undergoing epilepsy surgery.

There is great enthusiasm for the potential of mTOR inhibitors to stop or prevent seizures in patients with FCD given the neuropathological similarities between the cortical tubers present in TSC and FCD Type II and the observation that hyperactivated mTOR has been linked to many forms of epilepsy [Citraro *et al.*, 2016]. (Involvement of the mTOR pathway in developmental epilepsy is further detailed in Chapter 12.) Most of the supporting evidence has come from experimental models [Galanopoulou *et al.*, 2012; Wong, 2013] but there is clinical evidence that mTOR inhibitors have antiepileptic efficacy in TSC patients. Everolimus, a rapamycin analog approved for patients with TSC and epilepsy has clinical efficacy in patients with TSC [Krueger *et al.*, 2010, 2016].

There is also evidence that VNS can be efficacious in some patients with MCD. A retrospective study that examined the efficacy of VNS in 46 children with pharmacoresistant epilepsy included patients with TSC, lissencephaly, polymicrogyria, and subependymal nodules. While not all of these patients responded, one patient became seizure-free and several had a decrease in seizure frequency greater than 50% [Alexopoulos *et al.*, 2006].

11.7 Conclusions

MCD are a frequent cause of pediatric and adult epilepsy with the resultant seizures often refractory to currently available antiepileptic drug therapy. Increases in the resolution of MR imaging combined with neuropathological examination of resected tissue have led to a recognition that subtle defects in cortical development are likely responsible for many cases of epilepsy whose etiology was previously undetermined. While an intrauterine or a perinatal insult can contribute to the development of a cortical malformation, the most likely cause is a genetic defect. Mutations in over 30 genes have been shown to lead to the development of a MCD. These mutations can occur in the germ cells or occur as *de novo* somatic mutations. The timing of mutation occurrence during development can determine the size and location of the malformation with some malformations limited to a small number of cells while others involve an entire hemisphere. Germline and somatic mutations that result in enhanced activation of the mTOR pathway have been implicated in the formation of some types of FCD.

Surgical resection remains the primary treatment if the location of the FCD can be identified and is accessible. However, the effectiveness of surgery is greater for FCD Type II than FCD Type I. Combining EEG with fMRI, PET, MEG and the detection of HFOs can improve localization of the epileptogenic zone, epileptic network, and boundaries of the FCD which can lead to a more accurate resection and better surgical outcome. Alternative therapies, including the ketogenic diet, mTOR inhibitors, and neurostimulation can be effective in patients who are not candidates for surgery or in whom surgery has failed.

References

Abdijadid, S., Mathern, G.W., Levine, M.S., and Cepeda, C. (2015). Basic mechanisms of epileptogenesis in pediatric cortical dysplasia, *CNS Neurosci. Ther.*, 21, 92–103.

Ak, H., Ay, B., Tanriverdi, T., Sanus, G.Z., Is, M., Sar, M., Oz, B., Ozkara, C., Ozyurt, E., and Uzan, M. (2007). Expression and cellular distribution of multidrug resistance-related proteins in patients with focal cortical dysplasia, *Seizure*, 16, 493–503.

Alexopoulos, A.V., Kotagal, P., Loddenkemper, T., Hammel, J., and Bingaman, W.E. (2006). Long-term results with vagus nerve stimulation in children with pharmacoresistant epilepsy, *Seizure*, 15, 491–503.

Anderson, S.A., Kaznowski, C.E., Horn, C., Rubenstein, J.L.R., and McConnell, S.K. (2002). Distinct origins of neocortical projection neurons and interneurons in vivo, *Cereb. Cortex*, 12, 702–709.

André, V.M., Wu, N., Yamazaki, I., Nguyen, S.T., Fisher, R.S., Vinters, H.V., Mathern, G.W., Levine, M.S., and Cepeda, C. (2007). Cytomegalic interneurons: a new abnormal cell type in severe pediatric cortical dysplasia, *J. Neuropathol. Exp. Neurol.*, 66, 491–504.

Andres, M., Andre, V.M., Nguyen, S., Salamon, N., Cepeda, C., Levine, M.S., Leite, J.P., Neder, L., Vinters, H.V., and Mathern, G.W. (2005). Human cortical dysplasia and epilepsy: an ontogenetic hypothesis based on volumetric MRI and NeuN neuronal density and size measurements, *Cereb. Cortex*, 15, 194–210.

Anthony, T.E., Klein, C., Fishell, G., and Heintz, N. (2004). Radial glia serve as neuronal progenitors in all regions of the central nervous system, *Neuron*, 41, 881–890.

Aronica, E., Becker, A.J., and Spreafico, R. (2012). Malformations of cortical development, *Brain Pathol.*, 22, 380–401.

Aronica, E., Gorter, J.A., Jansen, G.H. van Veelen, C.W., van Jien, P.C. Leenstra, S., Ramkema, M., Sceffer, G.L., Scheper, R.J., Troost, D. (2003). Expression and cellular distribution of multidrug transporter proteins in two major causes of medically intractable epilepsy: foacl cortical dysplasia and glioneuronal tumors, *Neuroscience*, 118, 417–429.

Avoli, M., Louvel, J., Mattia, D., Olivier, A., Esposito, V., Pumain, R., and D'Antuono, M. (2003). Epileptiform synchronization in the human dysplastic cortex, *Epileptic Disord.*, 5 Suppl 2, S45–50.

Baraban, S.C., Wenzel, H.J., Hochman, D.W., and Schwartzkroin, P.A. (2000). Characterization of heterotopic cell clusters in the hippocampus of rats exposed to methylazoxymethanol in utero, *Epilepsy Res.*, 39, 87–102.

Barkovich, A.J., Kuzniecky, R.I., Dobyns, W.B., Jackson, G.D., Becker, L.E., and Evrard, P. (1996). A classification scheme for malformations of cortical development, *Neuropediatrics*, 27, 59–63.

Barkovich, A.J., Guerrini, R., Kuzniecky, R.I., Jackson, G.D., and Dobyns, W.B. (2012). A developmental and genetic classification for malformations of cortical development: update 2012, *Brain*, 135, 1348–1369.

Barkovich, A.J., Dobyns, W.B., and Guerrini, R. (2015). Malformations of cortical development and epilepsy, *Cold Spring Harb. Perspect. Med.*, 5, a022392.

Bast, T., Ramantani, G., Seitz, A., and Rating, D. (2006). Focal cortical dysplasia: prevalence, clinical presentation and epilepsy in children and adults, *Acta Neurol. Scand.*, 113, 72–81.

Bastos, A.C., Comeau, R.M., Andermann, F., Melanson, D., Cendes, F., Dubeau, F., Fontaine, S., Tampieri, D., and Olivier, A. (1999). Diagnosis of subtle focal dysplastic lesions: curvilinear reformatting from three-dimensional magnetic resonance imaging, *Ann. Neurol.*, 46, 88–94.

Baulac, S., Ishida, S., Marsan, E., Miquel, C., Biraben, A., Nguyen, D.K., Nordli, D., Cossette, P., Nguyen, S., Lambrecq, V., *et al.* (2015). Familial focal epilepsy with focal cortical dysplasia due to DEPDC5 mutations, *Ann. Neurol.*, 77, 675–683.

Baybis, M., Yu, J., Lee, A., Golden, J.A., Weiner, H., McKhann, G., Aronica, E., and Crino, P.B. (2004). mTOR cascade activation distinguishes tubers from focal cortical dysplasia, *Ann. Neurol.*, 56, 478–487.

Ben-Ari, Y. and Holmes, G.L. (2006). Effects of seizures on developmental processes in the immature brain, *Lancet Neurol.*, 5, 1055–1063.

Blümcke, I., Thom, M., Aronica, E., Armstrong, D.D., Vinters, H.V., Palmini, A., Jacques, T.S., Avanzini, G., Barkovich, A.J., Battaglia, G., *et al.* (2011). The clinicopathologic spectrum of focal cortical dysplasias: a consensus classification proposed by an ad hoc Task Force of the ILAE Diagnostic Methods Commission, *Epilepsia*, 52, 158–174.

de Carlos, J.A., López-Mascaraque, L., and Valverde, F. (1996). Dynamics of cell migration from the lateral ganglionic eminence in the rat, *J. Neurosci.*, 16, 6146–6156.

Cavanagh, M.E. and Parnavelas, J.G. (1989). Development of vasoactive-intestinal-polypeptide-immunoreactive neurons in the rat occipital cortex: a combined immunohistochemical-autoradiographic study, *J. Comp. Neurol.*, 284, 637–645.

Cepeda, C., André, V.M., Vinters, H.V., Levine, M.S., and Mathern, G.W. (2005). Are cytomegalic neurons and balloon cells generators of epileptic activity in pediatric cortical dysplasia?, *Epilepsia*, 46, 82–88.

Cepeda, C., André, V.M., Levine, M.S., Salamon, N., Miyata, H., Vinters, H.V., and Mathern, G.W. (2006). Epileptogenesis in pediatric cortical dysplasia: the dysmature cerebral developmental hypothesis, *Epilepsy Behav.*, 9, 219–235.

Cepeda, C., André, V.M., Wu, N., Yamazaki, I., Uzgil, B., Vinters, H.V., Levine, M.S., and Mathern, G.W. (2007). Immature neurons and GABA networks may contribute to epileptogenesis in pediatric cortical dysplasia, *Epilepsia*, 48 Suppl 5, 79–85.

Cepeda, C., André, V.M., Hauptman, J.S., Yamazaki, I., Huynh, M.N., Chang, J.W., Chen, J.Y., Fisher, R.S., Vinters, H.V., Levine, M.S., *et al.* (2012). Enhanced GABAergic network and receptor function in pediatric cortical dysplasia Type IIB compared with Tuberous Sclerosis Complex, *Neurobiol. Dis.*, 45, 310–321.

Chandra, P.S., Salamon, N., Huang, J., Wu, J.Y., Koh, S., Vinters, H.V., and Mathern, G.W. (2006). FDG-PET/MRI coregistration and diffusion-tensor imaging distinguish epileptogenic tubers and cortex in patients with tuberous sclerosis complex: a preliminary report, *Epilepsia*, 47, 1543–1549.

Chassoux, F., Landré, E., Mellerio, C., Turak, B., Mann, M.W., Daumas-Duport, C., Chiron, C., and Devaux, B. (2012). Type II focal cortical dysplasia: electroclinical phenotype and surgical outcome related to imaging, *Epilepsia*, 53, 349–358.

Chen, J., Tsai, V., Parker, W.E., Aronica, E., Baybis, M., and Crino, P.B. (2012). Detection of human papillomavirus in human focal cortical dysplasia type IIB, *Ann. Neurol.*, 72, 881–892.

Chu-Shore, C.J., Major, P., Camposano, S., Muzykewicz, D., and Thiele, E.A. (2010). The natural history of epilepsy in tuberous sclerosis complex, *Epilepsia*, 51, 1236–1241.

Citraro, R., Leo, A., Constanti, A., Russo, E., and De Sarro, G. (2016). mTOR pathway inhibition as a new therapeutic strategy in epilepsy and epileptogenesis, *Pharmacol. Res.*, 107, 333–343.

Colombo, N., Salamon, N., Raybaud, C., Ozkara, C., and Barkovich, A.J. (2009). Imaging of malformations of cortical development, *Epileptic Disord.*, 11, 194–205.

Crino, P.B. (2015). mTOR signaling in epilepsy: insights from malformations of cortical development, *Cold Spring Harb. Perspect. Med.*, 5, pii: a022442. doi: 10.1101/cshperspect.a022442.

Crino, P.B., Duhaime, A.C., Baltuch, G., and White, R. (2001). Differential expression of glutamate and GABA-A receptor subunit mRNA in cortical dysplasia, *Neurology*, 56, 906–913.

Delev, D., Quesada, C.M., Grote, A., Boström, J.P., Elger, C., Vatter, H., and Surges, R. (2018). A multimodal concept for invasive diagnostics and surgery based on neuronavigated voxel-based morphometric MRI postprocessing data in previously nonlesional epilepsy, *J. Neurosurg.*, 128, 1178–1186.

D'Gama, A.M., Geng, Y., Couto, J.A., Martin, B., Boyle, E.A., LaCoursiere, C.M., Hossain, A., Hatem, N.E., Barry, B., Kwiatkowski, D.J., *et al.* (2015). mTOR pathway mutations cause hemimegalencephaly and focal cortical dysplasia, *Ann. Neurol.*, 77, 720–725.

D'Gama, A.M., Woodworth, M.B., Hossain, A.A., Bizzotto, S., Hatem, N.E., LaCoursiere, C.M., Najm, I., Ying, Z., Yang, E., Barkovich, A.J., *et al.* (2017). Somatic mutations activating the mTOR pathway in dorsal telencephalic progenitors cause a continuum of cortical dysplasias, *Cell Rep.*, 21, 3754–3766.

Fauser, S., Huppertz, H.-J., Bast, T., Strobl, K., Pantazis, G., Altenmueller, D.-M., Feil, B., Rona, S., Kurth, C., Rating, D., *et al.* (2006). Clinical characteristics in focal cortical dysplasia: a retrospective evaluation in a series of 120 patients, *Brain*, 129, 1907–1916.

Fauser, S., Essang, C., Altenmüller, D.-M., Staack, A.M., Steinhoff, B.J., Strobl, K., Bast, T., Schubert-Bast, S., Stephani, U., Wiegand, G., *et al.* (2015). Long-term seizure outcome in 211 patients with focal cortical dysplasia, *Epilepsia*, 56, 66–76.

Ferrari-Marinho, T., Perucca, P., Mok, K., Olivier, A., Hall, J., Dubeau, F., and Gotman, J. (2015). Pathologic substrates of focal epilepsy influence the generation of high-frequency oscillations, *Epilepsia*, 56, 592–598.

Ferrer, I., Oliver, B., Russi, A., Casas, R., and Rivera, R. (1994). Parvalbumin and calbindin-D28k immunocytochemistry in human neocortical epileptic foci, *J. Neurol. Sci.*, 123, 18–25.

Foldvary-Schaefer, N., Bautista, J., Andermann, F., Cascino, G., and Spencer, S. (2004). Focal malformations of cortical development, *Neurology*, 62, S14–19.

Franco, S.J. and Müller, U. (2013). Shaping our minds: stem and progenitor cell diversity in the mammalian neocortex, *Neuron*, 77, 19–34.

Galanopoulou, A.S., Gorter, J.A., and Cepeda, C. (2012). Finding a better drug for epilepsy: the mTOR pathway as an antiepileptogenic target, *Epilepsia*, 53, 1119–1130.

Grouiller, F., Thornton, R.C., Groening, K., Spinelli, L., Duncan, J.S., Schaller, K., Siniatchkin, M., Lemieux, L., Seeck, M., Michel, C.M., *et al.* (2011). With or without spikes: localization of focal epileptic activity by simultaneous electroencephalography and functional magnetic resonance imaging, *Brain*, 134, 2867–2886.

Guerrini, R. (2005). Genetic malformations of the cerebral cortex and epilepsy, *Epilepsia*, 46 Suppl 1, 32–37.

Guerrini, R., Sicca, F., and Parmeggiani, L. (2003). Epilepsy and malformations of the cerebral cortex, *Epileptic Disord.*, 5 Suppl 2, S9–26.

Guerrini, R., Duchowny, M., Jayakar, P., Krsek, P., Kahane, P., Tassi, L., Melani, F., Polster, T., Andre, V.M., Cepeda, C., *et al.* (2015). Diagnostic methods and treatment options for focal cortical dysplasia, *Epilepsia*, 56, 1669–1686.

Gupta, A., Carreño, M., Wyllie, E., and Bingaman, W.E. (2004). Hemispheric malformations of cortical development, *Neurology*, 62, S20–26.

Heers, M., Hirschmann, J., Jacobs, J., Dümpelmann, M., Butz, M., von Lehe, M., Elger, C.E., Schnitzler, A., and Wellmer, J. (2014). Frequency domain beamforming of magnetoencephalographic beta band activity in epilepsy patients with focal cortical dysplasia, *Epilepsy Res.*, 108, 1195–1203.

Hevner, R.F. (2006). From radial glia to pyramidal-projection neuron: transcription factor cascades in cerebral cortex development, *Mol. Neurobiol.*, 33, 33–50.

Hsieh, L.S., Wen, J.H., Claycomb, K., Huang, Y., Harrsch, F.A., Naegele, J.R., Hyder, F., Buchanan, G.F., and Bordey, A. (2016). Convulsive seizures from experimental focal cortical dysplasia occur independently of cell misplacement, *Nat. Commun.*, 7, 11753.

Ishii, R., Canuet, L., Ochi, A., Xiang, J., Imai, K., Chan, D., Iwase, M., Takeda, M., Snead, O.C., and Otsubo, H. (2008). Spatially filtered magnetoencephalography compared with electrocorticography to identify intrinsically epileptogenic focal cortical dysplasia, *Epilepsy Res.*, 81, 228–232.

Jacobs, J., Levan, P., Châtillon, C.-E., Olivier, A., Dubeau, F., and Gotman, J. (2009). High frequency oscillations in intracranial EEGs mark epileptogenicity rather than lesion type, *Brain.*, 132, 1022–1037.

Jacobs, K.M., Hwang, B.J., and Prince, D.A. (1999). Focal epileptogenesis in a rat model of polymicrogyria, *J. Neurophysiol.*, 81, 159–173.

Jellinger, K. (1987). Neuropathological aspects of infantile spasms, *Brain Dev.*, 9, 349–357.

Jiménez, D., López-Mascaraque, L.M., Valverde, F., and De Carlos, J.A. (2002). Tangential migration in neocortical development, *Dev. Biol.*, 244, 155–169.

Jung, D.E., Kang, H.C., and Kim, H.D. (2008). Long-term outcome of the ketogenic diet for intractable childhood epilepsy with focal malformation of cortical development, *Pediatrics*, 122, e330–333.

Kellinghaus, C., Kunieda, T., Ying, Z., Pan, A., Lüders, H.O., and Najm, I.M. (2004). Severity of histopathologic abnormalities and in vivo epileptogenicity in the in utero radiation model of rats is dose dependent, *Epilepsia*, 45, 583–591.

Kim, D.W., Kim, S., Park, S.-H., Chung, C.-K., and Lee, S.K. (2012). Comparison of MRI features and surgical outcome among the subtypes of focal cortical dysplasia, *Seizure*, 21, 789–794.

Kim, S.K., Na, D.G., Byun, H.S., Kim, S.E., Suh, Y.L., Choi, J.Y., Yoon, H.K., and Han, B.K. (2000). Focal cortical dysplasia: comparison of MRI and FDG-PET, *J. Comput. Assist. Tomogr.*, 24, 296–302.

Kriegstein, A.R. and Noctor, S.C. (2004). Patterns of neuronal migration in the embryonic cortex, *Trends Neurosci.*, 27, 392–399.

Kriegstein, A., Noctor, S., and Martínez-Cerdeño, V. (2006). Patterns of neural stem and progenitor cell division may underlie evolutionary cortical expansion, *Nat. Rev. Neurosci.*, 7, 883–890.

Krsek, P., Pieper, T., Karlmeier, A., Hildebrandt, M., Kolodziejczyk, D., Winkler, P., Pauli, E., Blümcke, I., and Holthausen, H. (2009). Different presurgical characteristics and seizure outcomes in children with focal cortical dysplasia type I or II, *Epilepsia*, 50, 125–137.

Krueger, D.A., Care, M.M., Holland, K., Agricola, K., Tudor, C., Mangeshkar, P., Wilson, K.A., Byars, A., Sahmoud, T., and Franz, D.N. (2010). Everolimus for subependymal giant-cell astrocytomas in tuberous sclerosis, *N. Engl. J. Med.*, 363, 1801–1811.

Krueger, D.A., Wilfong, A.A., Mays, M., Talley, C.M., Agricola, K., Tudor, C., Capal, J., Holland-Bouley, K., and Franz, D.N. (2016). Long-term treatment of epilepsy with everolimus in tuberous sclerosis, *Neurology*, 87, 2408–2415.

Kuzniecky, R.I. (1994). Magnetic resonance imaging in developmental disorders of the cerebral cortex, *Epilepsia*, 35 Suppl 6, S44–56.

Kuzniecky, R.I. and Barkovich, A.J. (2001). Malformations of cortical development and epilepsy. *Brain Dev.*, 23, 2–11.

Leach, J.L., Miles, L., Henkel, D.M., Greiner, H.M., Kukreja, M.K., Holland, K.D., Rose, D.F., Zhang, B., and Mangano, F.T. (2014). Magnetic resonance imaging abnormalities in the resection region correlate with histopathological type, gliosis extent, and postoperative outcome in pediatric cortical dysplasia, *J. Neurosurg. Pediatr.*, 14, 68–80.

Lee, D.Y. (2015). Roles of mTOR Signaling in brain development, *Exp. Neurobiol.*, 24, 177–185.

Lee, S.K. and Kim, D.-W. (2013). Focal cortical dysplasia and epilepsy surgery, *J. Epilepsy Res.*, 3, 43–47.

Lerner, J.T., Salamon, N., Hauptman, J.S., Velasco, T.R., Hemb, M., Wu, J.Y., Sankar, R., Donald Shields, W., Engel, J., Fried, I., *et al.* (2009). Assessment and surgical outcomes for mild type I and severe type II cortical dysplasia: a critical review and the UCLA experience, *Epilepsia*, 50, 1310–1335.

Leventer, R.J., Phelan, E.M., Coleman, L.T., Kean, M.J., Jackson, G.D., and Harvey, A.S. (1999). Clinical and imaging features of cortical malformations in childhood, *Neurology*, 53, 715–722.

Leventer, R.J., Guerrini, R., and Dobyns, W.B. (2008). Malformations of cortical development and epilepsy, *Dialogues Clin. Neurosci.*, 10, 47–62.

Li, L.M., Fish, D.R., Sisodiya, S.M., Shorvon, S.D., Alsanjari, N., and Stevens, J.M. (1995). High resolution magnetic resonance imaging in adults with partial or secondary generalised epilepsy attending a tertiary referral unit, *J. Neurol. Neurosurg. Psychiatry*, 59, 384–387.

Lim, J.S., and Lee, J.H. (2016). Brain somatic mutations in MTOR leading to focal cortical dysplasia, *BMB Rep.*, 49, 71–72.

Lim, J.S., Kim, W., Kang, H.-C., Kim, S.H., Park, A.H., Park, E.K., Cho, Y.-W., Kim, S., Kim, H.M., Kim, J.A., *et al.* (2015). Brain somatic mutations in MTOR cause focal cortical dysplasia type II leading to intractable epilepsy, *Nat. Med.*, 21, 395–400.

Lim, J.S., Gopalappa, R., Kim, S.H., Ramakrishna, S., Lee, M., Kim, W.-I., Kim, J., Park, S.M., Lee, J., Oh, J.-H., *et al.* (2017). Somatic mutations in TSC1 and TSC2 cause focal cortical dysplasia, *Am. J. Hum. Genet.*, 100, 454–472.

Lortie, A., Plouin, P., Chiron, C., Delalande, O., and Dulac, O. (2002). Characteristics of epilepsy in focal cortical dysplasia in infancy, *Epilepsy Res.*, 51, 133–145.

Loscher, W. and Potschka, H. (2002). Role of multidrug transporters in pharmacoresistance to antiepileptic drugs, *J. Pharmacol. Exp. Ther.*, 301, 7–14.

Marín, O. and Rubenstein, J.L. (2001). A long, remarkable journey: tangential migration in the telencephalon, *Nat. Rev. Neurosci.*, 2, 780–790.

Marín-Padilla, M., Tsai, R.J., King, M.A., and Roper, S.N. (2003). Altered corticogenesis and neuronal morphology in irradiation-induced cortical dysplasia: a Golgi-Cox study, *J. Neuropathol. Exp. Neurol.*, 62, 1129–1143.

Marsan, E. and Baulac, S. (2018). Review: Mechanistic target of rapamycin (mTOR) pathway, focal cortical dysplasia and epilepsy, *Neuropathol. Appl. Neurobiol.*, 44, 6–17.

Mathew, T., Srikanth, S.G., and Satishchandra, P. (2010). Malformations of cortical development (MCDs) and epilepsy: experience from a tertiary care center in south India, *Seizure*, 19, 147–152.

Mattia, D., Olivier, A., and Avoli, M. (1995). Seizure-like discharges recorded in human dysplastic neocortex maintained in vitro, *Neurology*, 45, 1391–1395.

Maynard, L.M., Leach, J.L., Horn, P.S., Spaeth, C.G., Mangano, F.T., Holland, K.D., Miles, L., Faist, R., and Greiner, H.M. (2017). Epilepsy prevalence and severity predictors in MRI-identified focal cortical dysplasia, *Epilepsy Res.*, 132, 41–49.

Meencke, H.J. and Janz, D. (1985). The significance of microdysgenesia in primary generalized epilepsy: an answer to the considerations of Lyon and Gastaut, *Epilepsia*, 26, 368–371.

Miyata, H., Chiang, A.C.Y., and Vinters, H.V. (2004). Insulin signaling pathways in cortical dysplasia and TSC-tubers: tissue microarray analysis, *Ann. Neurol.*, 56, 510–519.

Miyata, T., Kawaguchi, A., Okano, H., and Ogawa, M. (2001). Asymmetric inheritance of radial glial fibers by cortical neurons, *Neuron*, 31, 727–741.

Moeller, F., Tyvaert, L., Nguyen, D.K., LeVan, P., Bouthillier, A., Kobayashi, E., Tampieri, D., Dubeau, F., and Gotman, J. (2009). EEG-fMRI: adding to standard evaluations of patients with nonlesional frontal lobe epilepsy, *Neurology*, 73, 2023–2030.

Møller, R.S., Weckhuysen, S., Chipaux, M., Marsan, E., Taly, V., Bebin, E.M., Hiatt, S.M., Prokop, J.W., Bowling, K.M., Mei, D., *et al.* (2016). Germline and somatic mutations in the MTORgene in focal cortical dysplasia and epilepsy, *Neurol. Genet.*, 2, e118.

Najm, I.M., Ying, Z., Babb, T., Mohamed, A., Hadam, J., LaPresto, E., Wyllie, E., Kotagal, P., Bingaman, W., Foldvary, N., *et al.* (2000). Epileptogenicity correlated with increased N-methyl-D-aspartate receptor subunit NR2A/B in human focal cortical dysplasia, *Epilepsia*, 41, 971–976.

Najm, I.M., Tilelli, C.Q., and Oghlakian, R. (2007). Pathophysiological mechanisms of focal cortical dysplasia: a critical review of human tissue studies and animal models, *Epilepsia*, 48 Suppl 2, 21–32.

Nakashima, M., Saitsu, H., Takei, N., Tohyama, J., Kato, M., Kitaura, H., Shiina, M., Shirozu, H., Masuda, H., Watanabe, K., *et al.* (2015). Somatic Mutations in the MTOR gene cause focal cortical dysplasia type IIb, *Ann. Neurol.*, 78, 375–386.

Noctor, S.C., Flint, A.C., Weissman, T.A., Dammerman, R.S., and Kriegstein, A.R. (2001). Neurons derived from radial glial cells establish radial units in neocortex, *Nature*, 409, 714–720.

Noctor, S.C., Martínez-Cerdeño, V., Ivic, L., and Kriegstein, A.R. (2004). Cortical neurons arise in symmetric and asymmetric division zones and migrate through specific phases, *Nat. Neurosci.*, 7, 136–144.

Palmini, A., Gambardella, A., Andermann, F., Dubeau, F., da Costa, J.C., Olivier, A., Tampieri, D., Gloor, P., Quesney, F., and Andermann, E. (1995). Intrinsic epileptogenicity of human dysplastic cortex as suggested by corticography and surgical results, *Ann. Neurol.*, 37, 476–487.

Palmini, A., Najm, I., Avanzini, G., Babb, T., Guerrini, R., Foldvary-Schaefer, N., Jackson, G., Lüders, H.O., Prayson, R., Spreafico, R., *et al.* (2004). Terminology and classification of the cortical dysplasias, *Neurology*, 62, S2–8.

Pittau, F., Dubeau, F., and Gotman, J. (2012). Contribution of EEG/fMRI to the definition of the epileptic focus, *Neurology*, 78, 1479–1487.

Poduri, A. (2014). DEPDC5 does it all: shared genetics for diverse epilepsy syndromes, *Ann. Neurol.*, 75, 631–633.

Poduri, A., Evrony, G.D., Cai, X., and Walsh, C.A. (2013). Somatic mutation, genomic variation, and neurological disease, *Science*, 341, 1237758.

Porter, B.E., Brooks-Kayal, A., and Golden, J.A. (2002). Disorders of cortical development and epilepsy, *Arch. Neurol.*, 59, 361–365.

Rakic, P. (1978). Neuronal migration and contact guidance in the primate telencephalon, *Postgrad. Med. J.*, 54 Suppl 1, 25–40.

Raymond, A.A., Fish, D.R., Sisodiya, S.M., Alsanjari, N., Stevens, J.M., and Shorvon, S.D. (1995). Abnormalities of gyration, heterotopias, tuberous sclerosis, focal cortical dysplasia, microdysgenesis, dysembryoplastic neuroepithelial tumour and dysgenesis of the archicortex in epilepsy. Clinical, EEG and neuroimaging features in 100 adult patients, *Brain*, 118, 629–660.

Reutens, D.C., Berkovic, S.F., Kalnins, R.M., McKelvie, P., Saling, M.M., and Fabinyi, G.C. (1993). Localised neuronal migration disorder and intractable epilepsy: a prenatal vascular aetiology, *J. Neurol. Neurosurg. Psychiatry*, 56, 314–316.

Roper, S.N. (1998). In utero irradiation of rats as a model of human cerebrocortical dysgenesis: a review, *Epilepsy Res.*, 32, 63–74.

Sato, Y., Doesburg, S.M., Wong, S.M., Ochi, A., and Otsubo, H. (2015). Dynamic preictal relations in FCD type II: potential for early seizure detection in focal epilepsy, *Epilepsy Res.*, 110, 26–31.

Scheffer, I.E., Heron, S.E., Regan, B.M., Mandelstam, S., Crompton, D.E., Hodgson, B.L., Licchetta, L., Provini, F., Bisulli, F., Vadlamudi, L., *et al.* (2014). Mutations in mammalian target of rapamycin regulator DEPDC5 cause focal epilepsy with brain malformations, *Ann. Neurol.*, 75, 782–787.

Serino, D., Freri, E., Ragona, F., D'Incerti, L., Bernardi, B., Di Ciommo, V., Granata, T., Vigevano, F., and Fusco, L. (2015). Focal seizures versus epileptic spasms in children with focal cortical dysplasia and epilepsy onset in the first year, *Epilepsy Res.*, 109, 203–209.

Shrot S, Hwang M, Stafstrom CE, Huisman TAGM, Soares BP. (2018). Dysplasia and overgrowth: magnetic resonance imaging of pediatric brain abnormalities secondary to alterations in the mechanistic target of rapamycin pathway, *Neuroradiology*, 60, 137–150.

Sim, J.C., Scerri, T., Fanjul-Fernández, M., Riseley, J.R., Gillies, G., Pope, K., van Roozendaal, H., Heng, J.I., Mandelstam, S.A., McGillivray, G., *et al.* (2016). Familial cortical dysplasia caused by mutation in the mammalian target of rapamycin regulator NPRL3, *Ann. Neurol.*, 79, 132–137.

Sisodiya, S.M., Lin, W.R., Harding, B.N., Squier, M.V., Thom, M. (2002). Drug resistance in epilepsy: expression of drug resistance proteins in common causes of refractory epilepsy, *Brain*, 125, 22–31.

Sisodiya, S.M., Lin, W.R., Squier, M.V., Thom, M. (2001). Multidrug-resistance protein-1 in focal cortical dysplasia, *Lancet*, 357, 42–43.

Tan, S.S., Kalloniatis, M., Sturm, K., Tam, P.P., Reese, B.E., and Faulkner-Jones, B. (1998). Separate progenitors for radial and tangential cell dispersion during development of the cerebral neocortex, *Neuron*, 21, 295–304.

Tassi, L., Colombo, N., Garbelli, R., Francione, S., Lo Russo, G., Mai, R., Cardinale, F., Cossu, M., Ferrario, A., Galli, C., *et al.* (2002). Focal cortical dysplasia: neuropathological subtypes, EEG, neuroimaging and surgical outcome, *Brain*, 125, 1719–1732.

Tassi, L., Garbelli, R., Colombo, N., Bramerio, M., Russo, G.L., Mai, R., Deleo, F., Francione, S., Nobili, L., and Spreafico, R. (2012). Electroclinical, MRI and surgical outcomes in 100 epileptic patients with type II FCD, *Epileptic Disord.*, 14, 257–266.

Taylor, D.C., Falconer, M.A., Bruton, C.J., and Corsellis, J.A.N. (1971). Focal dysplasia of the cerebral cortex in epilepsy, *J. Neurol. Neurosurg. Psychiatry*, 34, 369–387.

Thornton, R., Vulliemoz, S., Rodionov, R., Carmichael, D.W., Chaudhary, U.J., Diehl, B., Laufs, H., Vollmar, C., McEvoy, A.W., Walker, M.C., *et al.* (2011). Epileptic networks in focal cortical dysplasia revealed using electroencephalography-functional magnetic resonance imaging, *Ann. Neurol.*, 70, 822–837.

Tishler, D.M., Weinberg, K.I., Hinton, D.R., Barbaro, N., Annett, G.M., and Raffel, C. (1995). MDR1 gene expression in brain of patients with medically intractable epilepsy, *Epilepsia*, 36, 1–6.

Varotto, G., Franceschetti, S., Spreafico, R., Tassi, L., and Panzica, F. (2010). Partial directed coherence estimated on stereo-EEG signals in patients with Taylor's type focal cortical dysplasia, *Conf. Proc. IEEE Eng. Med. Biol. Soc.*, 2010, 4646–4649.

Varotto, G., Tassi, L., Franceschetti, S., Spreafico, R., and Panzica, F. (2012). Epileptogenic networks of type II focal cortical dysplasia: a stereo-EEG study, *NeuroImage*, 61, 591–598.

Veersema, T.J., Ferrier, C.H., van Eijsden, P., Gosselaar, P.H., Aronica, E., Visser, F., Zwanenburg, J.M., de Kort, G.A.P., Hendrikse, J., Luijten, P.R., *et al.* (2017). Seven tesla MRI improves detection of focal cortical dysplasia in patients with refractory focal epilepsy, *Epilepsia Open*, 2, 162–171.

Vinters, H., Salamon, S., Miyata, H., Khanlou, N., and Mathern, G. W. (2008). Neuropathology of developmental disorders associated with epilepsy. In Epilepsy: A Comprehensive Textbook, (Philadelphia, USA: Lippincott, Willianms & Wilkins), pp. 137–160.

White, R., Hua, Y., Scheithauer, B., Lynch, D.R., Henske, E.P., and Crino, P.B. (2001). Selective alterations in glutamate and GABA receptor subunit mRNA expression in dysplastic neurons and giant cells of cortical tubers, *Ann. Neurol.*, 49, 67–78.

Widdess-Walsh, P., Diehl, B., and Najm, I. (2006). Neuroimaging of focal cortical dysplasia, *J. Neuroimaging*, 16, 185–196.

Wong, M. (2009). Animal models of focal cortical dysplasia and tuberous sclerosis complex: recent progress toward clinical applications, *Epilepsia*, 50 Suppl 9, 34–44.

Wong, M. (2013). Mammalian target of rapamycin (mTOR) activation in focal cortical dysplasia and related focal cortical malformations, *Exp. Neurol.*, 244, 22–26.

Ying, Z., Babb, T.L., Comair, Y.G., Bingaman, W., Bushey, M., and Touhalisky, K. (1998). Induced expression of NMDAR2 proteins and differential expression of NMDAR1 splice variants in dysplastic neurons of human epileptic neocortex, *J. Neuropathol. Exp. Neurol.*, 57, 47–62.

Chapter 12
mTORopathies as Signaling Pathway Disorders in Developmental Epilepsies

Michael Wong, MD, PhD

Department of Neurology and the Hope Center for Neurological Disorders, Washington University School of Medicine, St. Louis, Missouri, USA

12.1 Introduction

Normal brain development requires a complex, tightly-regulated interplay of physiological processes on multiple levels from gross anatomical structure, circuit and cellular components, and biochemical and molecular machinery (see Chapter 1). On the molecular level, cell signaling pathways have the capacity to be the master coordinators of the overall developmental blueprint, serving as the central upstream switch or gateway to otherwise divergent and independent downstream biological mechanisms. Conversely, defects in cell signaling at critical developmental time periods have the potential to cause widespread, severe abnormalities in brain development, again on multiple biological levels. The developing brain is particularly susceptible to seizures given the finely balanced and rapidly evolving physiological maturation between excitatory and inhibitory mechanisms. As a result, disruption of cell signaling pathways predispose to epilepsy by leading to aberrant molecular, cellular, and anatomical properties in the developing brain. In particular, the mechanistic target of rapamycin pathway (mTOR) pathway has received increasing attention as a central signaling mechanism that is critical for normal brain development and is implicated in causing a spectrum of developmental epilepsies. In this chapter, the role of the mTOR pathway in normal brain development and developmental epilepsies is reviewed.

12.2 mTOR pathway during normal brain development

mTOR is a relatively ubiquitous serine-threonine protein kinase found in a wide range of cell types [Saxton and Sabatini, 2017; Weber and Gutmann, 2012]. TOR was originally identified in yeast as the molecular target of the drug rapamycin and was subsequently found to be highly conserved across species, including invertebrates (such as Drosophila), and mammals (originally labeled mammalian target of rapamycin, but now generally referred to as mechanistic target of rapamycin). mTOR typically exists in one of two complexes, mTOR complex 1 (mTORC1) and mTOR complex 2 (mTORC2). In addition to the catalytic subunit of mTOR itself, mTORC1 consists of a primary regulatory subunit, raptor, which controls complex assembly and dictates downstream effector mechanisms, as well as a series of other accessory subunits. In contrast, the primary regulatory component of mTORC2 is rictor. mTORC1 is involved in an extensive variety of cellular physiological functions, including cell growth, proliferation, metabolism, and autophagy, primarily by regulating protein translation, although transcriptional and posttranslational mechanisms have also been implicated. The functions of mTORC2 are not as well-delineated, but include cell survival and cytoskeletal organization. A key pharmacological difference between mTORC1 and mTORC2 is that mTORC1 is strongly inhibited by rapamycin, whereas mTORC2 is relatively insensitive to rapamycin, at least acutely, although mTORC2 has also been reported to also be inhibited by rapamycin with chronic, long-term administration [Sarbassov *et al.*, 2006].

The mTOR pathway consists of a larger network of signaling molecules, with mTORC1 and to a lesser degree mTORC2 as central components, but involving a number of upstream regulators and downstream mediators, as well as complex feedback regulation among the different components and potential cross-talk between mTORC1 and mTORC2 [Saxton and Sabatini, 2017; Weber and Gutmann, 2012] (Figure 12.1). On the upstream side, a couple of major regulatory mechanisms include the insulin-Akt-PI3K pathway, which responds to nutrient and energy signals to stimulate mTOR and

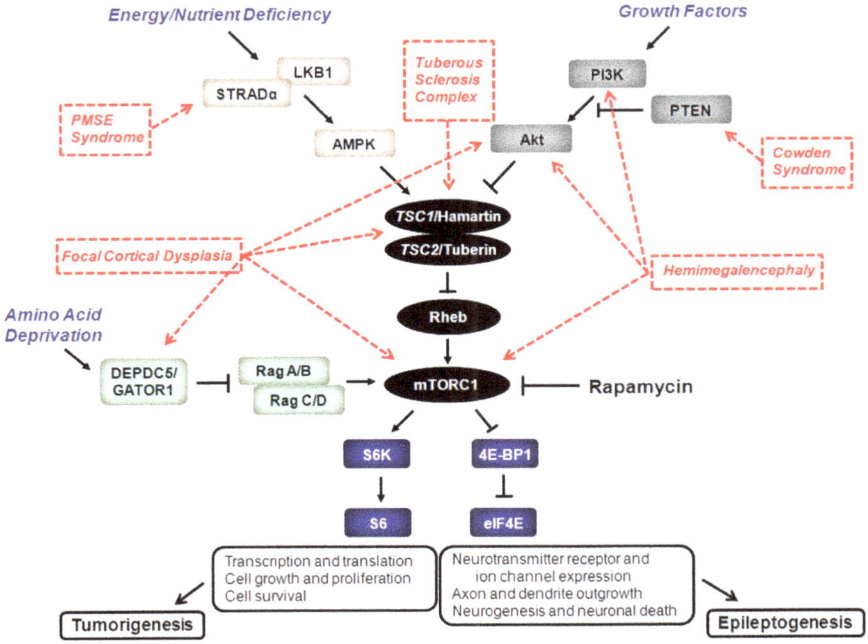

Figure 12.1 mTORopathies in Developmental Epilepsy. The mTOR pathway involves a number of upstream and downstream signaling mechanisms, with the central components being the rapamycin-sensitive, mTORC1, and the relatively rapamycin-insensitive, mTORC2 (not shown, as its role in developmental epilepsy is not clear). mTORC1 is regulated by upstream regulators (PI3K/Akt/Pten and LKB1/AMPK/STADα via TSC1/TSC2/Rheb; and DEPDC5/GATOR1 complex via Rag GTPases) in response to various physiological and pathological stimuli involved in energy, nutrient, and growth regulation. In turn, mTORC1 stimulates multiple downstream signaling mechanisms, primarily involved in ribosomal biogenesis (S6K, S6) and protein translation (4E-BP1, eIF4E), which affect a variety of cellular and molecular processes that may promote tumorigenesis and epileptogenesis. Genetic mutations in different components of the mTOR pathway have been identified that cause hyperactivation of mTORC1 and may lead to different malformations of cortical development (shown in red) and epilepsy.

promote cellular growth, and the LKB1/AMPK pathway, which inhibits mTOR in response to hypoxia or metabolic stress. *Tuberous sclerosis complex (TSC) 1* and *2* genes integrate converging upstream inputs and inhibit mTOR via Rheb GTPase. On the downstream side, mTORC1 in particular primarily regulates protein synthesis by phosphorylating S6 kinase and ribosomal S6, involved in ribosomal biosynthesis, and 4EBP1/eIF4E, translation initiating factors (Figure 12.1).

Given the large variety of cellular and physiological functions of mTOR, particularly involving cell growth and differentiation, the mTOR pathway has been strongly implicated in normal brain development [Lee, 2015; Takei and Nawa, 2014]. First of all, mTOR is clearly established in a range of developmental processes in neurons. Synapse formation is a fundamental aspect of brain development, including both dendritic and axonal components. mTOR regulates dendritic growth, arborization and spine formation [Jaworski *et al.*, 2005; Kumar *et al.*, 2005]. mTOR is also involved in axonal elongation [Sherman *et al.*, 2012]. On the molecular level, mTOR may regulate the expression of various ion channels and neurotransmitter receptors that demonstrate developmental changes, such as potassium channels and glutamate receptors [Raab-Graham *et al.*, 2006; Wang *et al.*, 2006]. Furthermore, mTOR may influence neuronal differentiation and neuronal migration [Tee *et al.*, 2016]. In addition to neurons, mTOR may be involved in astrocyte and microglial function during normal brain development [Dello Russo *et al.*, 2009], which also influences synapse formation and pruning. Finally, both neurogenesis and gliogenesis may be dependent on mTOR [Cloetta *et al.*, 2013; Tee *et al.*, 2016]. Experimentally, transgenic mice with deletion of mTOR exhibit severe microcephaly or other developmental malformations [Cloetta *et al.*, 2013], whereas mice with hyperactivation of mTOR leads to progressive macrocephaly [Zeng *et al.*, 2008], establishing the importance of mTOR in normal brain development.

12.3 mTORopathy as a general cause of developmental epilepsies

Given mTOR's important role in normal brain development, dysfunction of the mTOR signaling pathway has been strongly linked to certain types of developmental epilepsies, which have been aptly labeled "mTORopathies". This is most evident in genetic epilepsies, involving mutations in various aspects of the mTOR pathway and leading to malformations of cortical development [Crino, 2007], with the prototypical mTORopathy causing epilepsy being tuberous sclerosis complex (TSC). Given advances in neuroimaging, non-syndromic cortical malformations, ranging from subtle focal cortical dysplasia to extensive hemimegalencephaly, have been increasingly recognized as causes of developmental epilepsies and, in some cases, have been associated with mTOR pathway mutations, particularly mTORC1 (Figure 12.1). In addition, there is some evidence, at least in animal models, that mTOR could be involved in other types of developmental epilepsy syndromes due to acquired brain injury, such as neonatal seizures or infantile spasms. Overall, mTOR could be viewed as a potential common mechanistic pathway linking a variety of genetic and acquired epilepsies during early brain development. The practical and translational application of this general concept is that rapamycin or other mTOR inhibitors could represent novel rational treatments for this group of epilepsies due to mTOR-opathies, including potential disease-modifying or antiepileptogenic therapies.

In theory, either decreased or increased mTOR signaling could affect brain development and predispose to developmental epilepsies. However, the majority of documented examples, including both human cases and animal models, involve hyperactivation of mTOR. In these examples, the proximal cause of mTOR hyperactivation is either a genetic mutation (gain-of-function mutation in mTOR itself or an upstream activator of mTOR, or disinhibition of mTOR due to loss-of-function mutation of an upstream inhibitor of mTOR) or an environmental/acquired increase in upstream activation of mTOR. Less is known about the mechanisms downstream from mTOR that lead to epileptogenesis, but given the wide range of normal biological functions of mTOR, a variety of anatomical, cellular, and molecular mechanisms have been implicated. Perhaps the most obvious examples involve the formation of epilepsy-associated focal cortical malformations, which are at least partially due to abnormal mTOR-driven cellular growth, proliferation, differentiation, and migration within the brain. In addition to or independent of focal structural lesions, mTOR may stimulate a number of other downstream mechanisms on the cellular or molecular level that may also promote epileptogenesis, such as synaptic reorganization, metabolic disturbances, or abnormal expression of ion channels and neurotransmitter receptors.

In the following sections, the clinical and pathophysiological features of different mTORpathies associated with developmental epilepsies are discussed in turn. TSC will first be presented as the model mTORopathy causing epilepsy, as the role of mTOR in the pathophysiology of TSC is most firmly established and clinical trials now support the use of mTOR inhibitors for TSC-related epilepsy. Second, the list of related malformations of cortical development linked to mTOR pathway mutations continues to grow. Finally, the evidence will be analyzed, primarily from animal models, that mTOR could also be involved in epileptogenesis in acquired developmental epilepsies due to brain injury.

12.4 Tuberous sclerosis complex as the model mTORopathy causing developmental epilepsy

TSC is an autosomal dominant genetic disorder caused by mutation in either the *TSC1* or *TSC2* gene and is associated with tumor or hamartoma formation in multiple organs throughout the body [DiMario *et al.*, 2015; Islam and Roach, 2015; Orlova and Crino, 2010]. In the brain, TSC patients commonly develop one or more typical neuropathological lesions of cortical tubers, subependymal nodules, and subependymal giant cell astrocytomas (SEGAs). Cortical tubers are focal malformations of cortical development, which are pathologically indistinguishable from focal cortical dysplasia type IIB, whereas SEGAs are true, benign brain tumors that may grow progressively. In terms of neurological symptoms, TSC is highly associated with epilepsy, intellectual disability or other developmental delays, and autism. The causative relationship between the neurological symptoms and the different brain lesions of TSC is not always clear or precise, but epilepsy is most closely linked to cortical tubers.

Epilepsy is particularly common in TSC, occurring in up to 80–90% of patients, and often features multiple seizure types, including focal and generalized seizures, as well as infantile spasms [Chu-Shore *et al.*, 2010]. Epilepsy in TSC is often intractable to treatment, with about two-thirds of TSC patients with epilepsy meeting the definition of drug-resistant epilepsy (as opposed to about one-third in the overall epilepsy population) [Sparagana *et al.*, 2003]. Furthermore, while some TSC patients can be helped by epilepsy surgery [Madhavan *et al.*, 2007], particularly tuberectomy, many TSC patients are not good surgical candidates due to the poor localization or multifocal nature of seizures. Finally, epilepsy in TSC definitely qualifies as a developmental epilepsy. While TSC patients occasionally present with their first seizure in adulthood, in one large study 63% developed epilepsy in the first year of life and 80% within three years of age [Chu-Shore *et al.*, 2010]. Furthermore, about 40% of TSC patients with epilepsy have a history of infantile spasms, and approximately 20% have Lennox-Gastaut syndrome [Chu-Shore *et al.*, 2010].

The role of mTOR in the pathogenesis of tumors in TSC is well-established. *TSC1* and *TSC2* gene products bind together to form a complex that normally inhibits the mTORC1 pathway. In TSC, mutation of either *TSC1* or *TSC2* leads to a disinhibition, or hyperactivation, of mTORC1, which may have a number of downstream effects, but definitely may promote increased cell growth and proliferation. The classic giant cell, a large undifferentiated cell with immature markers of both neurons and glia, represents the hallmark pathological finding of TSC brains and can be directly attributed to increased mTOR activity causing cytomegaly. Furthermore, increased mTOR-driven cellular growth and proliferation logically account for tumor formation in TSC and would represent a rational mechanistic basis for utilizing mTOR inhibitors for treating tumors in this disease. In fact, controlled clinical trials support efficacy of mTOR inhibitors, everolimus (Afinitor) or sirolimus (rapamycin), for different tumors in TSC patients, including SEGAs, renal angiomyolipomas, and pulmonary lymphangioleiomyomatosis [Bissler *et al.*, 2013; Krueger *et al.*, 2010; McCormack *et al.*, 2011], leading to FDA approval for these indications.

While mTOR clearly represents a rational, effective target for treating tumors in TSC, the link of mTOR to epilepsy is likely more complex. Epilepsy in TSC is generally not directly caused by tumor growth per se, but in many cases is more related to the relatively static, developmental malformations, the cortical tubers. However, mTOR may activate a number of abnormalities on the network, cellular, and molecular levels that promote epileptogenesis, either within tubers or in the perituberal region surrounding tubers, such as synaptic reorganization, cytomegaly of neurons, astrogliosis, and altered expression or function of ion channels and neurotransmitter receptors. A number of mouse models of TSC have been created, involving inactivation of *Tsc1* or *Tsc2* in different cell types in the brain, and most of these TSC knockout mice exhibit seizures [Carson *et al.*, 2012; Goto *et al.*, 2011; Meikle *et al.*, 2007; Uhlmann *et al.*, 2002; Way *et al.*, 2009]. The role of mTOR in epileptogenesis in these mouse models is strongly supported by the effectiveness of rapamycin in suppressing or even preventing epilepsy in these mice [Anderl *et al.*, 2011; Meikle *et al.*, 2008; Way *et al.*, 2012; Zeng *et al.*, 2008]. The downstream mechanisms mediating epileptogenesis are not as clearly established and may vary depending on the model, but a variety of mechanisms have been implicated involving both neurons and glia, such as megalencephaly, neuronal cytomegaly, hypomyelination, impaired astrocyte glutamate transport, upregulated glutamate receptors, microglia activation, and inflammatory mechanisms, to name just a few [Lozovaya *et al.*, 2014; Meikle *et al.*, 2007; Uhlmann *et al.*, 2002; Wong *et al.*, 2003; Zhang *et al.*, 2015].

From a therapeutic standpoint, the potential utility and translational applications of mTOR inhibitors for epilepsy in TSC are tremendous. First of all, recent placebo-controlled trials have demonstrated efficacy of the mTOR inhibitor, everolimus, against drug-resistant focal seizures in TSC patients [French *et al.*, 2016; Krueger *et al.*, 2013]. These studies have led to official approval of everolimus for this indication by the FDA in the United States. The establishment of an mTOR inhibitor as an approved treatment for epilepsy, albeit specifically for TSC patients with epilepsy, represents a significant advance from a mechanistic standpoint in targeting a cell signaling pathway, as most existing medications for epilepsy modulate ion channels or neurotransmitter systems as the primary mechanism of action. In addition, based on mechanism of action, mTOR inhibitors may have even greater potential as preventative or anti-epileptogenic treatments for epilepsy in TSC [Wong, 2013]. Current medications for epilepsy are viewed primarily as symptomatic treatments that suppress seizures, but do not appear to have disease-modifying or anti-epileptogenic properties to prevent the development or progression of epilepsy. In contrast, the TSC animal models suggest that rapamycin has true anti-epileptogenic actions in not only preventing epilepsy, but also preventing the underlying pathological and molecular abnormalities that cause epileptogenesis in these models [Zeng *et al.*, 2008]. Furthermore, some patients are diagnosed with TSC during infancy due to non-neurological findings (i.e., prior to onset of seizures); these patients are at high risk for epilepsy in the future, suggesting that it is rational and feasible to target these patients with anti-epileptogenic therapy to prevent epilepsy. As preventative drug trials are practically more difficult to conduct than standard clinical trials in patients with drug-resistant epilepsy, a preventative clinical trial with mTOR inhibitors in TSC has not yet been undertaken. However, plans for such a trial are under discussion and could be modeled after novel preventative trials of vigabatrin in TSC patients [Jozwiak *et al.*, 2011].

12.5 mTORopathies in developmental epilepsies due to other malformations of cortical development

The etiologies of developmental epilepsies are diverse, but, given advances in neuroimaging, a major, increasingly recognized cause of developmental epilepsies is the spectrum of malformations of cortical development. While TSC can be viewed as a model mTORopathy causing epilepsy associated with cortical malformations (tubers), there is accumulating evidence that other related malformations of cortical development are also due to genetic defects affecting different components of the mTOR pathway (Figure 12.1). In comparison to the multifocal tubers typical of TSC, isolated, non-syndromic focal cortical dysplasia is a common cause of drug-resistant epilepsy in the pediatric age group that is often amenable to epilepsy surgery [Madhavan *et al.*, 2007]. Cases of focal cortical dysplasia type IIB, which again has striking pathological similarities to tubers of TSC, have recently been reported to be due to somatic mutations in *TSC1* or *TSC2* [Lim *et al.*, 2017]. In addition, mutations in mTOR itself or other upstream aspects of the mTOR pathway, particularly *AKT* and *DEPDC5*, are associated with other types of focal cortical dysplasia [Baulac *et al.*, 2015; D'Gama *et al.*, 2015; Jansen *et al.*, 2015; Mirzaa *et al.*, 2016; Nakashima *et al.*, 2015]. Similarly, hemimegalencephaly, which invariably presents in infancy with intractable seizures [Di Rocco *et al.*, 2006], has been associated with somatic mutations in *mTOR*, *AKT*, and *PI3K* [D'Gama *et al.*, 2015; Lee *et al.*, 2012; Poduri *et al.*, 2012]. On the cellular level, these focal malformations of cortical development share features with TSC, particularly cytomegaly in the form of balloon cells, which are similar to the giant cells of TSC and are likely a result of mTOR hyperactivation in these cases.

In addition to isolated, non-syndromic cortical malformations, there are other genetic syndromes which, like TSC, feature cortical malformation, epilepsy, and other associated systemic manifestations, such as tumor growth in other organs. PMSE syndrome (polyhydramnios, megalencephaly, and symptomatic epilepsy; also known as Pretzel syndrome) is a severe neurodevelopmental disorder found in the Old Order Mennonite population and characterized by developmental delay and drug-resistant epilepsy presenting in early childhood with diffuse megalencephaly of the brain. PMSE has been linked to homozygous mutations in the STE20-related kinase alpha (*STRADA*) gene, which encodes a pseudokinase that binds to and enhances the catalytic activity of *LKB1*, an upstream regulator of mTOR signaling [Parker *et al.*, 2013]. Thus, mutation of *STRADA* results in dysregulated mTOR signaling due a decrease in the inhibitory upstream LKB1/AMPK pathway. Conversely, mutations in the *PTEN* gene, which normally inhibit PI3K, result in increased mTOR signaling due to elevated AKT/PI3K activity. *PTEN* mutations are associated with

Cowden syndrome, which features multiple hamartomas, as well as isolated focal cortical dysplasia [Cheung *et al.*, 2014].

The downstream mechanisms mediating epileptogenesis in these other cortical malformation-associated mTORopathies are not known, but likely share some cellular and molecular features with TSC. Similar to TSC mouse models, *Pten* knockout mice exhibit megalencephaly and cytomegaly and rapamycin can decrease seizures in these mice, establishing the importance of mTOR [Kwon *et al.*, 2003; Ljungberg *et al.*, 2009; Sunnen *et al.*, 2011]. While it may be rational to consider treating patients with these other mTORopathies with rapamycin, there is minimal clinical data on the efficacy of mTOR inhibitors in these other mTORopathies besides TSC. In particular, the effect of mTOR inhibitors has not been reported in other isolated cortical malformations, such as focal cortical dysplasia and hemimegalencephaly. However, in an uncontrolled small trial, rapamycin has been reported to decrease seizures and improve cognitive function in a series of patients with PMSE syndrome [Parker *et al.*, 2013].

12.6 mTORopathies in developmental epilepsies due to acquired brain injury

While genetic mTORpathies causing malformations of cortical development and epilepsy are now well-established, an interesting and important question is whether mTOR may also be relevant to non-genetic types of epilepsy due to acquired brain injury at certain developmental stages. As the mTOR pathway responds to various environmental cues and stimuli, particularly nutrient and energy status, it is rational to hypothesize that acquired brain injuries with associated metabolic or energetic stress may regulate mTOR activity, which could also influence epileptogenesis. Most of the data supporting a possible role of mTOR in acquired epilepsy due to brain injuries derive from animal models.

In terms of acquired developmental epilepsies, neonatal hypoxia is a major risk factor for future neurological problems, including epilepsy [Fatemi *et al.*, 2009]. In a rat model of neonatal hypoxic seizures, mTOR activity is transiently elevated following acute hypoxia

[Talos *et al.*, 2012]. This is associated with subsequent elevation of AMPA-type glutamate receptor function and development of chronic epilepsy. Treatment with rapamycin can prevent this mTOR activation and increased glutamate receptor function and correspondingly decrease the later development of epilepsy. This study provides proof-of-principle that mTOR may be involved in a developmental epilepsy related to hypoxic brain injury in the neonatal period and that mTOR inhibitors could be considered as potential preventative therapy for the long-term neurological consequences of neonatal hypoxia and perinatal brain injury.

Another common, often devastating, developmental epilepsy syndrome is infantile spasms. Although infantile spasms has a variety of causes, including genetic disorders such as TSC, various acquired brain injuries during this critical developmental period often result in the final common outcome of infantile spasms and associated comorbidities. A "multiple hit" rat model of symptomatic infantile spasms has been developed using a combination of neurotoxic drugs during the neonatal period [Scantlebury *et al.*, 2010]. Markers of elevated mTOR activity were detected around the age of onset of spasms in rat pups. Rapamycin treatment could block this increased mTOR activity and suppress the infantile spasms in this model [Raffo *et al.*, 2011]. This suggests that mTOR could also be involved in the pathophysiology of infantile spasms due to brain injury. However, another rodent model of infantile spasms related to prenatal stress showed no response to rapamycin [Chachua *et al.*, 2011], so mTOR may not be universally involved in all conditions or models.

A final consideration regarding the potential role of mTOR in epileptic encephalopathies and potential progressive epilepsies in early life is the direct effect of seizures on mTOR activity. Independent of an underlying etiology, seizures themselves induce increased mTOR activity. In normal rodents, acute induction of seizures by chemoconvulsants causes transient elevation of mTOR activity independent of preexisting or subsequent brain injury [Zhang and Wong, 2012]. This implies that seizures may contribute to a process of progressive epileptogenesis involving mTOR, where seizures induce mTOR activity, which in turn may activate downstream mechanisms that promote additional seizures. Although seizure-induced mTOR activation has also been observed in a variety of seizure models in adult rodents, this positive feedback cycle may be particularly relevant during critical developmental periods when epileptic encephalopathies emerge.

12.7 Conclusions/future directions

The mTOR pathway represents a common, shared signaling mechanism that may be involved in epileptogenesis in a variety of genetic and acquired developmental epilepsies. The role of mTOR in epileptogenesis is most clearly established in the genetic disorder, TSC. However, recent genetic studies demonstrate that TSC is part of a larger family of genetic mTORopathies involving various malformations of cortical development and intractable epilepsy, including isolated focal cortical dysplasia, hemimegalencephaly, and other developmental epilepsy syndromes. Based primarily on animal models, mTOR may also be involved in acquired epilepsy due to brain injury during critical developmental periods, such as related to neonatal hypoxia and infantile spasms. Finally, seizures themselves may contribute to progressive epileptogenesis in epileptic encephalopathies via seizure-induced mTOR activation.

Given that mTOR is the target of the clinically-available drug, rapamycin, as well as other mTOR inhibitors, the potential therapeutic applications of exploiting the mTOR mechanism are direct and immediate. Multiple TSC animal models support the efficacy of rapamycin in inhibiting established seizures and also preventing the development of epilepsy in the first place. These consistent preclinical data have already been translated to TSC patients, as a recent Phase 3, placebo-controlled trial confirmed efficacy of the mTOR inhibitor, everolimus, in decreasing seizures in TSC patients with drug-resistant epilepsy [French *et al.*, 2016]. There are minimal clinical data testing effect of mTOR inhibitors on other genetic mTORpathies and cortical malformations besides TSC, although there is some anecdotal data of rapamycin effectiveness in the PMSE syndrome.

There are a number of obvious future directions in this field related to both basic science mechanisms and clinical applications of mTORopathies related to developmental epilepsies. While mTOR may be centrally involved in epileptogenesis in these disorders, the critical downstream mechanisms involved are not well-established. mTOR may regulate a wide variety of biological processes on multiple levels from gross anatomical structure and circuit organization to cellular and molecular mechanisms, thus implicating a large number of potential downstream mediators of epileptogenesis. In reality, there are likely multiple downstream mechanisms that contribute at least partially to epileptogenesis and seizure generation. If one or a small subset of such mechanisms can be identified as the most influential, these mechanisms can potentially be selectively targeted with treatments that may improve efficacy or decrease side effects compared with inhibiting mTOR, which has widespread downstream effects.

Future therapeutic applications of mTOR inhibitors can also be further refined and expanded. In TSC, the mTOR inhibitor, everolimus, is already approved in Europe and the United States for treating drug-resistant epilepsy in TSC patients. However, efficacy of everolimus against drug-resistant epilepsy in TSC is quantitatively similar to other standard anti-seizure medications already approved for epilepsy, with everolimus causing a significant reduction in seizure frequency in some patients, but very few patients actually become seizure-free, which is the ultimate goal in treating drug-resistant epilepsy. In this regard, timing may be critical and, based on mechanism of action, mTOR inhibitors may have much greater potential as early preventative or antiepileptogenic treatments in TSC. As preventative epilepsy trials in treating infants newly diagnosed with TSC due to non-neurological reasons are feasible and have a recent precedent in early treatment with vigabatrin, the next major step would be a clinical trial of an mTOR inhibitor as preventative therapy against epilepsy for TSC infants.

Beyond TSC, future clinical trials should test efficacy of mTOR inhibitors against other genetic mTORopathies causing other cortical malformations and epilepsy, particularly focal cortical dysplasia and hemimegalencephaly. However, similar limitations to treatment will likely be encountered for drug-resistant epilepsy related to these other disorders. Again, timing may be critical and earlier preventative treatment is key. However, unlike some cases of TSC, isolated, non-syndromic cortical malformations usually present with seizures, so there may not be a window of opportunity to diagnose and treat preventatively before onset of epilepsy.

Finally, more clinical data are needed as to whether the mTOR pathway is dysregulated in patients with acquired epilepsy due to brain injury. While animal models support a potential role of mTOR in acquired epileptogenesis, there is a paucity of human pathological studies investigating mTOR markers in acquired developmental epilepsies. If such evidence can be obtained, this would add support to considering treatment with mTOR inhibitors for acquired epilepsy following brain injury.

References

Anderl, S., Freeland, M., Kwiatkowski, D.J., and Goto, J. (2011). Therapeutic value of prenatal rapamycin treatment in a mouse brain model of tuberous sclerosis complex, *Hum. Mol. Genet.*, 20, 4597–4604.

Baulac, S., Ishida, S., Marsan, E., Miquel, C., Biraben, A., Nguyen, D.K., Nordli, D., Cossette, P., Nguyen, S., Lambrecq, V., Vlaicu, M., Daniau, M., Bielle, F., Andermann, E., Andermann, F., Leguern, E., Chassoux, F., and Picard, F. (2015). Familial focal epilepsy with focal cortical dysplasia due to DEPDC5 mutations, *Ann. Neurol.*, 77, 675–683.

Bissler, J.J., Kingswood, J.C., Radzikowska, E., Zonnenberg, B.A., Frost, M., Belousova, E., Sauter, M., Nonomura, N., Brakemeier, S., de Vries, P.J., Whittemore, V.H., Chen, D., Sahmoud, T., Shah, G., Lincy, J., Lebwohl, D., and Budde, K. (2013). Everolimus for angiomyolipoma associated with tuberous sclerosis complex or sporadic lymphangioleiomyomatosis (EXIST-2): a multicentre, randomised, double-blind, placebo-controlled trial, *Lancet*, 381, 817–824.

Carson, R.P., Van Nielen, D.L., Winzenburger, P.A., and Ess, K.C. (2012). Neuronal and glia abnormalities in Tsc1-deficient forebrain and partial rescue by rapamycin, *Neurobiol. Dis.*, 45, 369–380.

Chachua, T., Yum, M.S., Velíšková, J., and Velíšek, L. (2011). Validation of the rat model of cryptogenic infantile spasms, *Epilepsia*, 52, 1666–1677.

Cheung, K.M., Lam, C.W., Chan, Y.K., Siu, W.K., and Yong, L. (2014). Atypical focal cortical dysplasia in a patient with Cowden syndrome, *Hong Kong Med. J.*, 20, 165–167.

Chu-Shore, C.J., Major, P., Camposano, S., Muzykewicz, D., and Thiele, E.A. (2010). The natural history of epilepsy in tuberous sclerosis complex, *Epilepsia*, 51, 1236–1241.

Cloetta, D., Thomanetz, V., Baranek, C., Lustenberger, R.M., Lin, S., Oliveri, F., Atanasoski, S., and Ruegg, M.A. (2013). Inactivation of mTORC1 in the developing brain causes microcephaly and affects gliogenesis, *J. Neurosci.*, 33, 7799–7810.

Crino, P.B. (2007). Focal brain malformations: a spectrum of disorders along the mTOR cascade, *Novartis Found. Symp.*, 288, 260–272; discussion 272–281.

D'Gama, A.M., Geng, Y., Couto, J.A., Martin, B., Boyle, E.A., LaCoursiere, C.M., Hossain, A., Hatem, N.E., Barry, B.J., Kwiatkowski, D.J., Vinters, H.V., Barkovich, A.J., Shendure, J., Mathern, G.W., Walsh, C.A., and Poduri, A. (2015). Mammalian target of rapamycin pathway mutations cause hemimegalencephaly and focal cortical dysplasia, *Ann. Neurol.*, 77, 720–725.

Dello Russo, C., Lisi, L., Tringali, G., and Navarra, P. (2009). Involvement of mTOR kinase in cytokine-dependent microglial activation and cell proliferation, *Biochem. Pharmacol.*, 78, 1242–1251.

Di Rocco, C., Battaglia, D., Pietrini, D., Piastra, M., and Massimi, L. (2006). Hemimegalencephaly: clinical implications and surgical treatment, *Childs Nerv. Sys.*, 22, 852–866.

DiMario, F.J., Jr., Sahin, M., and Ebrahimi-Fakhari, D. (2015). Tuberous sclerosis complex, *Pediatr. Clin. North Am.*, 62, 633–648.

Fatemi, A., Wilson, M.A., and Johnston, M.V. (2009). Hypoxic-ischemic encephalopathy in the term infant, *Clin. Perinatol.*, 36, 835–858, vii.

French, J.A., Lawson, J.A., Yapici, Z., Ikeda, H., Polster, T., Nabbout, R., Curatolo, P., de Vries, P.J., Dlugos, D.J., Berkowitz, N., Voi, M., Peyrard, S., Pelov, D., and Franz, D.N. (2016). Adjunctive everolimus therapy for treatment-resistant focal-onset seizures associated with tuberous sclerosis (EXIST-3): a phase 3, randomised, double-blind, placebo-controlled study, *Lancet*, 388, 2153–2163.

Goto, J., Talos, D.M., Klein, P., Qin, W., Chekaluk, Y.I., Anderl, S., Malinowska, I.A., Di Nardo, A., Bronson, R.T., Chan, J.A., Vinters, H.V., Kernie, S.G., Jensen, F.E., Sahin, M., and Kwiatkowski, D.J. (2011). Regulable neural progenitor-specific Tsc1 loss yields giant cells with organellar dysfunction in a model of tuberous sclerosis complex, *Proc. Natl. Acad. Sci. U.S.A.*, 108, E1070–1079.

Islam, M.P. and Roach, E.S. (2015). Tuberous sclerosis complex, *Handb. Clin. Neurol.* 132, 97–109.

Jansen, L.A., Mirzaa, G.M., Ishak, G.E., O'Roak, B.J., Hiatt, J.B., Roden, W.H., Gunter, S.A., Christian, S.L., Collins, S., Adams, C., Riviere, J.B., St-Onge, J., Ojemann, J.G., Shendure, J., Hevner, R.F., and Dobyns, W.B. (2015). PI3K/AKT pathway mutations cause a spectrum of brain malformations from megalencephaly to focal cortical dysplasia, *Brain*, 138, 1613–1628.

Jaworski, J., Spangler, S., Seeburg, D.P., Hoogenraad, C.C., and Sheng, M. (2005). Control of dendritic arborization by the phosphoinositide-3'-kinase-Akt-mammalian target of rapamycin pathway, *J. Neurosci.*, 25, 11300–11312.

Jozwiak, S., Kotulska, K., Domanska-Pakiela, D., Lojszczyk, B., Syczewska, M., Chmielewski, D., Dunin-Wasowicz, D., Kmiec, T., Szymkiewicz-Dangel, J., Kornacka, M., Kawalec, W., Kuczynski, D., Borkowska, J., Tomaszek, K., Jurkiewicz, E., and Respondek-Liberska, M. (2011). Antiepileptic treatment before the onset of seizures reduces epilepsy severity and risk of mental retardation in infants with tuberous sclerosis complex, *Eur. J. Paediatr. Neurol.*, 15, 424–431.

Krueger, D.A., Care, M.M., Holland, K., Agricola, K., Tudor, C., Mangeshkar, P., Wilson, K.A., Byars, A., Sahmoud, T., and Franz, D.N. (2010). Everolimus for subependymal giant-cell astrocytomas in tuberous sclerosis, *NEJM*, 363, 1801–1811.

Krueger, D.A., Wilfong, A.A., Holland-Bouley, K., Anderson, A.E., Agricola, K., Tudor, C., Mays, M., Lopez, C.M., Kim, M.O., and Franz, D.N. (2013). Everolimus treatment of refractory epilepsy in tuberous sclerosis complex, *Ann. Neurol.*, 74, 679–687.

Kumar, V., Zhang, M.X., Swank, M.W., Kunz, J., and Wu, G.Y. (2005). Regulation of dendritic morphogenesis by Ras-PI3K-Akt-mTOR and Ras-MAPK signaling pathways, *J. Neurosci.*, 25, 11288–11299.

Kwon, C.H., Zhu, X., Zhang, J., and Baker, S.J. (2003). mTor is required for hypertrophy of Pten-deficient neuronal soma in vivo, *Proc. Natl. Acad. Sci. U.S.A.*, 100, 12923–12928.

Lee, D.Y. (2015). Roles of mTOR signaling in brain development, *Exp. Neurobiol.*, 24, 177–185.

Lee, J.H., Huynh, M., Silhavy, J.L., Kim, S., Dixon-Salazar, T., Heiberg, A., Scott, E., Bafna, V., Hill, K.J., Collazo, A., Funari, V., Russ, C., Gabriel, S.B., Mathern, G.W., and Gleeson, J.G. (2012). De novo somatic mutations in components of the PI3K-AKT3-mTOR pathway cause hemimegalencephaly, *Nat. Gen.*, 44, 941–945.

Lim, J.S., Gopalappa, R., Kim, S.H., Ramakrishna, S., Lee, M., Kim, W.I., Kim, J., Park, S.M., Lee, J., Oh, J.H., Kim, H.D., Park, C.H., Lee, J.S., Kim, S., Kim, D.S., Han, J.M., Kang, H.C., Kim, H.H., and Lee, J.H. (2017). Somatic mutations in TSC1 and TSC2 cause focal cortical dysplasia, *Am. J. Hum. Genet.*, 100, 454–472.

Ljungberg, M.C., Sunnen, C.N., Lugo, J.N., Anderson, A.E., and D'Arcangelo, G. (2009). Rapamycin suppresses seizures and neuronal hypertrophy in a mouse model of cortical dysplasia, *Dis. Model Mech.*, 2, 389–398.

Lozovaya, N., Gataullina, S., Tsintsadze, T., Tsintsadze, V., Pallesi-Pocachard, E., Minlebaev, M., Goriounova, N.A., Buhler, E., Watrin, F., Shityakov, S., Becker, A.J., Bordey, A., Milh, M., Scavarda, D., Bulteau, C., Dorfmuller, G., Delalande, O., Represa, A., Cardoso, C., Dulac, O., Ben-Ari, Y., and Burnashev, N. (2014). Selective suppression of excessive GluN2C expression rescues early epilepsy in a tuberous sclerosis murine model, *Nat. Commun.*, 5, 4563.

Madhavan, D., Schaffer, S., Yankovsky, A., Arzimanoglou, A., Renaldo, F., Zaroff, C.M., LaJoie, J., Weiner, H.L., Andermann, E., Franz, D.N., Leonard, J., Connolly, M., Cascino, G.D., and Devinsky, O. (2007). Surgical outcome in tuberous sclerosis complex: a multicenter survey, *Epilepsia*, 48, 1625–1628.

McCormack, F.X., Inoue, Y., Moss, J., Singer, L.G., Strange, C., Nakata, K., Barker, A.F., Chapman, J.T., Brantly, M.L., Stocks, J.M., Brown, K.K., Lynch, J.P., 3rd, Goldberg, H.J., Young, L.R., Kinder, B.W., Downey, G.P., Sullivan, E.J., Colby, T.V., McKay, R.T., Cohen, M.M., Korbee, L., Taveira-DaSilva, A.M., Lee, H.S., Krischer, J.P., and Trapnell, B.C. (2011). Efficacy and safety of sirolimus in lymphangioleiomyomatosis, *N. Engl. J. Med.*, 364, 1595–1606.

Meikle, L., Pollizzi, K., Egnor, A., Kramvis, I., Lane, H., Sahin, M., and Kwiatkowski, D.J. (2008). Response of a neuronal model of tuberous sclerosis to mammalian target of rapamycin (mTOR) inhibitors: effects on mTORC1 and Akt signaling lead to improved survival and function, *J. Neurosci.*, 28, 5422–5432.

Meikle, L., Talos, D.M., Onda, H., Pollizzi, K., Rotenberg, A., Sahin, M., Jensen, F.E., and Kwiatkowski, D.J. (2007). A mouse model of tuberous sclerosis: neuronal loss of Tsc1 causes dysplastic and ectopic neurons, reduced myelination, seizure activity, and limited survival, *J. Neurosci.*, 27, 5546–5558.

Mirzaa, G.M., Campbell, C.D., Solovieff, N., Goold, C., Jansen, L.A., Menon, S., Timms, A.E., Conti, V., Biag, J.D., Adams, C., Boyle, E.A., Collins, S., Ishak, G., Poliachik, S., Girisha, K.M., Yeung, K.S., Chung, B.H.Y., Rahikkala, E., Gunter, S.A., McDaniel, S.S., Macmurdo, C.F., Bernstein, J.A., Martin, B., Leary, R., Mahan, S., Liu, S., Weaver, M., Doerschner, M., Jhangiani, S., Muzny, D.M., Boerwinkle, E., Gibbs, R.A., Lupski, J.R., Shendure, J., Saneto, R.P., Novotny, E.J., Wilson, C.J., Sellers, W.R., Morrissey, M., Hevner, R.F., Ojemann, J.G., Guerrini, R., Murphy, L.O., Winckler, W., and Dobyns, W.B. (2016). Association of mTOR mutations with developmental brain disorders, including megalencephaly, focal cortical dysplasia, and pigmentary mosaicism, *JAMA Neurol.*, 73, 836–845.

Nakashima, M., Saitsu, H., Takei, N., Tohyama, J., Kato, M., Kitaura, H., Shiina, M., Shirozu, H., Masuda, H., Watanabe, K., Ohba, C., Tsurusaki, Y., Miyake, N., Zheng, Y., Sato, T., Takebayashi, H., Ogata, K., Kameyama, S., Kakita, A., and Matsumoto, N. (2015). Somatic Mutations in the MTOR gene cause focal cortical dysplasia type IIb, *Ann. Neurol.*, 78, 375–386.

Orlova, K.A. and Crino, P.B. (2010). The tuberous sclerosis complex, *Ann. N.Y. Acad. Sci.*, 1184, 87–105.

Parker, W.E., Orlova, K.A., Parker, W.H., Birnbaum, J.F., Krymskaya, V.P., Goncharov, D.A., Baybis, M., Helfferich, J., Okochi, K., Strauss, K.A., and Crino, P.B. (2013). Rapamycin prevents seizures after depletion of STRADA in a rare neurodevelopmental disorder, *Sci. Transl. Med.*, 5, 182ra153.

Poduri, A., Evrony, G.D., Cai, X., Elhosary, P.C., Beroukhim, R., Lehtinen, M.K., Hills, L.B., Heinzen, E.L., Hill, A., Hill, R.S., Barry, B.J., Bourgeois, B.F., Riviello, J.J., Barkovich, A.J., Black, P.M., Ligon, K.L., and Walsh, C.A. (2012). Somatic activation of AKT3 causes hemispheric developmental brain malformations, *Neuron*, 74, 41–48.

Raab-Graham, K.F., Haddick, P.C., Jan, Y.N., and Jan, L.Y. (2006). Activity- and mTOR-dependent suppression of Kv1.1 channel mRNA translation in dendrites, *Science*, 314, 144–148.

Raffo, E., Coppola, A., Ono, T., Briggs, S.W., and Galanopoulou, A.S. (2011). A pulse rapamycin therapy for infantile spasms and associated cognitive decline, *Neurobiol. Dis.*, 43, 322–329.

Sarbassov, D.D., Ali, S.M., Sengupta, S., Sheen, J.H., Hsu, P.P., Bagley, A.F., Markhard, A.L., and Sabatini, D.M. (2006). Prolonged rapamycin treatment inhibits mTORC2 assembly and Akt/PKB, *Mol. Cell*, 22, 159–168.

Saxton, R.A. and Sabatini, D.M. (2017). mTOR signaling in growth, metabolism, and disease, *Cell*, 168, 960–976.

Scantlebury, M.H., Galanopoulou, A.S., Chudomelova, L., Raffo, E., Betancourth, D., and Moshe, S.L. (2010). A model of symptomatic infantile spasms syndrome, *Neurobiol. Dis.*, 37, 604–612.

Sherman, D.L., Krols, M., Wu, L.M., Grove, M., Nave, K.A., Gangloff, Y.G., and Brophy, P.J. (2012). Arrest of myelination and reduced axon growth when Schwann cells lack mTOR, *J. Neurosci.*, 32, 1817–1825.

Sparagana, S.P., Delgado, M.R., Batchelor, L.L., and Roach, E.S. (2003). Seizure remission and antiepileptic drug discontinuation in children with tuberous sclerosis complex, *Arch. Neurol.*, 60, 1286–1289.

Sunnen, C.N., Brewster, A.L., Lugo, J.N., Vanegas, F., Turcios, E., Mukhi, S., Parghi, D., D'Arcangelo, G., and Anderson, A.E. (2011). Inhibition of the mammalian target of rapamycin blocks epilepsy progression in NS-Pten conditional knockout mice, *Epilepsia*, 52, 2065–2075.

Takei, N. and Nawa, H. (2014). mTOR signaling and its roles in normal and abnormal brain development, *Front. Mol. Neurosci.*, 7, 28.

Talos, D.M., Sun, H., Zhou, X., Fitzgerald, E.C., Jackson, M.C., Klein, P.M., Lan, V.J., Joseph, A., and Jensen, F.E. (2012). The interaction between early life epilepsy and autistic-like behavioral consequences: a role for the mammalian target of rapamycin (mTOR) pathway, *PloS One*, 7, e35885.

Tee, A.R., Sampson, J.R., Pal, D.K., and Bateman, J.M. (2016). The role of mTOR signalling in neurogenesis, insights from tuberous sclerosis complex, *Semin. Cell. Dev. Biol.*, 52, 12–20.

Uhlmann, E.J., Wong, M., Baldwin, R.L., Bajenaru, M.L., Onda, H., Kwiatkowski, D.J., Yamada, K., and Gutmann, D.H. (2002). Astrocyte-specific TSC1 conditional knockout mice exhibit abnormal neuronal organization and seizures, *Ann. Neurol.*, 52, 285–296.

Wang, Y., Barbaro, M.F., and Baraban, S.C. (2006). A role for the mTOR pathway in surface expression of AMPA receptors, *Neurosci. Lett.*, 401, 35–39.

Way, S.W., McKenna, J., 3rd, Mietzsch, U., Reith, R.M., Wu, H.C., and Gambello, M.J. (2009). Loss of Tsc2 in radial glia models the brain pathology of tuberous sclerosis complex in the mouse, *Hum. Mol. Genet.*, 18, 1252–1265.

Way, S.W., Rozas, N.S., Wu, H.C., McKenna, J., 3rd, Reith, R.M., Hashmi, S.S., Dash, P.K., and Gambello, M.J. (2012). The differential effects of prenatal and/or postnatal rapamycin on neurodevelopmental defects and cognition in a neuroglial mouse model of tuberous sclerosis complex, *Hum. Mol. Genet.*, 21, 3226–3236.

Weber, J.D. and Gutmann, D.H. (2012). Deconvoluting mTOR biology, *Cell Cycle*, 11, 236–248.

Wong, M. (2013). A critical review of mTOR inhibitors and epilepsy: from basic science to clinical trials, *Expert Rev. Neurother.*, 13, 657–669.

Wong, M., Ess, K.C., Uhlmann, E.J., Jansen, L.A., Li, W., Crino, P.B., Mennerick, S., Yamada, K.A., and Gutmann, D.H. (2003). Impaired glial glutamate transport in a mouse tuberous sclerosis epilepsy model, *Ann. Neurol.*, 54, 251–256.

Zeng, L.H., Xu, L., Gutmann, D.H., and Wong, M. (2008). Rapamycin prevents epilepsy in a mouse model of tuberous sclerosis complex, *Ann. Neurol.*, 63, 444–453.

Zhang, B. and Wong, M. (2012). Pentylenetetrazole-induced seizures cause acute, but not chronic, mTOR pathway activation in rat, *Epilepsia*, 53, 506–511.

Zhang, B., Zou, J., Rensing, N.R., Yang, M., and Wong, M. (2015). Inflammatory mechanisms contribute to the neurological manifestations of tuberous sclerosis complex, *Neurobiol. Dis.*, 80, 70–79.

Chapter 13
Neurobiology of Cognitive Impairment in Developmental Epilepsy: Seeing the Forest Through the Trees

Jeremy M. Barry, PhD
Gregory L. Holmes, MD

*Department of Neurological Sciences,
University of Vermont Larner College of Medicine,
Burlington, Vermont, USA*

13.1 Introduction

Although seizures are the most striking clinical manifestation of the epilepsies, children with epilepsy are at risk for a myriad of other co-morbid health problems that occur at a higher rate in individuals with epilepsy than would be expected by chance [Committee on the Public Health Dimensions of the Epilepsies, 2012]. Among the co-morbidities associated with epilepsy in children, cognitive abnormalities are among the most common and troublesome [Holmes, 2014; Holmes, 2015]. The distribution of IQ scores of children with epilepsy is skewed toward lower values [Farwell *et al.*, 1985; Neyens *et al.*, 1999] and the number of children with epilepsy experiencing difficulties in school because of learning disabilities is greater than children without epilepsy [Bailet and Turk, 2000; Buelow *et al.*, 2012; Prasad *et al.*,

2014a; Prasad *et al.*, 2014b; Sillanpaa *et al.*, 1998; Wakamoto *et al.*, 2000; Williams *et al.*, 1998].

While most children with epilepsy maintain stable IQ scores, there is now compelling evidence that some children with epilepsy slow, or even regress, in their mental development [Bourgeois *et al.*, 1983; Hermann *et al.*, 2002; Neyens *et al.*, 1999]. In one large community-based cohort study of children who developed epilepsy before age 8 years, an 11 point drop in mean IQ was seen in those children with medically refractory epilepsy [Berg *et al.*, 2012]. Children with status epilepticus (SE), including febrile SE, are also at risk for cognitive impairment [Chang *et al.*, 2001; Martinos *et al.*, 2012; Martinos *et al.*, 2013; van Esch *et al.*, 1996; Weiss *et al.*, 2016].

When considering the pathophysiological mechanisms of the cognitive and behavioral consequences of epilepsy, it is helpful to distinguish between impairments caused by the etiology of the epilepsy and those due to the epilepsy itself. Epilepsy can result from a large variety of brain insults including acquired disorders such as hypoxic-ischemic insults, trauma, and infectious and genetic disorders, such as Dravet syndrome, Rett syndrome, and tuberous sclerosis complex. In addition to causing seizures, these etiologies may result in cognitive and behavioral disturbances, independent of the seizures. While the cognitive and behavioral issues associated with these brain insults may evolve over time due to maturational changes in the brain, they are relatively fixed and remain attributable to the underlying brain disorder. Independent of etiology, there is also evidence that seizures and interictal epileptiform discharges on the EEG, also termed spikes, can result in both transitory and long-term cognitive impairment. This chapter discusses the pathophysiological mechanisms by which seizures and interictal spikes result in cognitive impairment. Whereas cognitive deficits caused by the etiology of the epilepsy are difficult to treat, preventing or reducing the length and severity of seizures and interictal spikes have the potential of reducing the cognitive deficits [Barry and Holmes, 2016; Holmes, 2014; Holmes and Lenck-Santini, 2006].

Children with epilepsy have varying age of onset, etiology, antiepileptic drug exposure, and seizure frequencies, severity, and type.

Attempting to tease out the pathophysiological mechanisms leading to cognitive impairment from heterogeneous populations of children has been challenging. For that reason, much of the information available regarding the neurobiology of cognitive deficits in children comes from animal models. With animal models, variables such as age and seizure duration and frequency can be controlled and invasive electrophysiological techniques used to understand the physiological consequences of both seizures and interictal epileptiform discharges. Another advantage of using rodent animal models is that the field has made advances in understanding the relationship between physiology and neural coding mechanisms that underpin cognition in normal animals [Wilson *et al.*, 2015]. Translational science has therefore profited greatly from these advances, allowing for direct comparisons between animals that have experienced early-life seizures as a function of physiological changes at the level of genes to networks, both as a function of development and changes in cognitive demand. In particular, we focus on the meso-scale interactions of single cell activity with regard to local field potentials and how these are dynamically coordinated both within and between neuronal circuits that underpin cognition [Barry *et al.*, 2015; Barry *et al.*, 2016a; Barry and Holmes, 2016; Patterson *et al.*, 2017].

To conceptualize the focus on these meso-scale interactions, first imagine a long series of dominos. The falling of the first domino represents the occurrence of a seizure at an early stage of development. The event that initiated the seizure may have had genetic predeterminants such as those that alter key ion channels, or a complex mixture of genetic pre-determinants and environmental factors such as high fever. Despite the precedent, our falling domino will cause a further cascade of falling dominos that over time will branch out in complex patterns while gaining momentum toward an unknown trajectory. Such is the challenge to translational systems neuroscience. Recognizing that the developing brain is dynamic and complex — and that predicting cognitive function from the physiological and morphological changes of individual ensembles of cells is difficult — there has been a movement towards adapting a systems biology approach to quantitatively measure the behavior of groups of interacting components, using both single cell and network oscillations, in relation to performance on complex cognitive tasks.

13.2 Animal models and cognitive impairment

While there are numerous models of early-life seizures (ELS), this chapter concentrates on two: 1) Recurrent flurothyl seizures (RFS) that mimic frequent brief generalized tonic-clonic seizures in children; and 2) Experimental febrile status epilepticus (eFSE), which uses hyperthermia induction of seizures to model prolonged seizures that result from fever. In the RFS model, rat pups are subjected to multiple brief tonic-clonic seizures through inhalation of flurothyl, a convulsant that blocks γ-aminobutyric acid (GABA)-type A receptors. The seizures are brief, lasting <5 minutes and have a low mortality rate. In the eFSE model, hyperthermia induces a generalized tonic seizure, which is typically maintained until the rat has a 30–40 minute seizure. Both of these models result in cognitive impairment when the animals are tested as adolescents or adults [Barry *et al.*, 2015; Barry *et al.*, 2016a; de Rogalski Landrot *et al.*, 2001; Dube *et al.*, 2009; Gatt *et al.*, 1993; Hoffmann *et al.*, 2004; Holmes, 1991; Holmes *et al.*, 1998; Huang *et al.*, 1999; Karnam *et al.*, 2009a; Karnam *et al.*, 2009b; Kleen *et al.*, 2011a; Neill *et al.*, 1996; Sogawa *et al.*, 2001; Zhou *et al.*, 2007b]. What is the nature of these cognitive impairments and what physiological alterations lay at their root? Can the precedents of these changes be measured to improve predictions for those most susceptible and, more importantly, can these changes be prevented or repaired?

The primary form of cognition that we shall focus on is spatial cognition. If we break down the components of spatial cognition, it may include the encoding, retrieval (learning and memory), and long-term maintenance of spatial information as well as the ability to pay attention to relevant cues and ignore irrelevant ones. ELS-induced deficits of spatial cognition have predominantly been found on that workhorse of behavioral neuroscience, the Morris water maze [Morris, 1984], as well as the radial-arm water maze [Huang *et al.*, 1999; Karnam *et al.*, 2009b; Lucas *et al.*, 2011] which involve remembering the static location of an unseen, submerged platform that allows for escape from a pool of opaque water. Similarly, performance deficits have been shown in ELS animals on the active avoidance task [Barry *et al.*, 2015; Barry *et al.*, 2016a; Barry *et al.*, 2016b; Patterson *et al.*, 2017]. In this task, animals learn to associate an unmarked region of space with a mild shock on a constantly rotating arena. The rats must attend to their ever-changing position in the room frame lest they be rotated into a pre-determined shock zone where they receive a mildly painful electrical shock. Specifically, a subset of eFSE animals demonstrate deficits in this task by failing to reach criterion due to an apparent inability to clear the shock zone [Barry *et al.*, 2015; Barry *et al.*, 2016a] or using inefficient avoidance strategies in which the animals stay too close to the shock zone [Patterson *et al.*, 2017]. As opposed to the water maze, the active avoidance task is a systems-level task that requires co-ordination between different brain regions that allow for associating a region of space with an aversive stimulus. Inactivation of the hippocampus and basolateral amygdala have shown these two structures to be necessary for active avoidance on the rotating arena [Cimadevilla *et al.*, 2000a; Cimadevilla *et al.*, 2000b; Vafaei *et al.*, 2007]. In addition, the task places greater demands on attention as the rat must regularly update its position in the room frame so as not to be moved into the shock zone [Kelemen and Fenton, 2010].

Over the course of their lifetime, animals that have experienced ELS may exhibit an attenuation of cognitive deficits. In postnatal day (P)35 rats subjected to kainic acid-induced status epilepticus were tested in the MWM at P46–49 or P60–63 and spatial deficits were noted, whereas at older ages (P74–77 and P91–94) no deficits were seen [Mikati *et al.*, 2001]. Likewise, following lithium-pilocarpine-induced status epilepticus at P20, rats showed increasing improvement in the MWM with age [Rutten *et al.*, 2002]. Similarly, flurothyl-induced seizures in adult rats showed that adverse seizure effects on the performance of a hidden goal task dissipates with time [Lin *et al.*, 2009]. Similarly, one study that used multiple behavioral tasks has shown that some aspects of spatial deficits diminish with age and others do not. Rats with early-life seizures tested as adults did not differ from control rats in the water maze, and although these animals showed some evidence of learning the active avoidance task, they received significantly more shocks in later training trials than controls. This was particularly evident during the second training day [Barry *et al.*, 2016a].

As mentioned above, ELS is also known to have detrimental effects on working memory in pediatric patients [Fuentes and Kerr, 2017; Protopapa *et al.*, 2016]. The task more commonly used to assess deficits in this faculty is the delayed non-match-to-sample (DNMS) task. In this task a series of trials are run where a sample phase is separated from a choice phase for several seconds and the animal has to make the opposite choice from the sample phase in order to receive a food reward. For example, Kleen and colleagues [Kleen *et al.*, 2011b] found that ELS animals had difficulty reaching task criterion on a DNMS task when randomly presented with a lever to the right or left and then having to select the opposite lever when there was a delay between sampling and choice phases between 1 and 30 seconds. Remarkably, these animals were able to perform the DNMS at the same level as control animals with remedial DNMS training trials. However, ELS animals that were able to reach criterion also exhibited significant accompanying shifts in the balance of communication between the dorsal hippocampus and prefrontal cortex during increased memory demand. The authors propose that these changes constitute compensatory network changes in the interconnected circuits of both brain regions that may underpin cognitive rehabilitation.

Finally, while not commonly considered an aspect of cognition per se, ELS have also been associated with decreased sociability [Holmes *et al.*, 2015; Lugo *et al.*, 2014]. When given the choice between interacting with a familiar or novel rat in one chamber or an object in another chamber, ELS animals frequently spent more time in the chamber with the object. As with tests of working memory [Kleen *et al.*, 2011a], this phenotype of decreased sociability was also found to correlate with altered communication between the prefrontal cortex and dorsal hippocampus [Holmes, 2015]. This finding raises the possibility that while this electrophysiological network signature may represent a compensation that correlates with improved response to memory demands, it may come at the cost of reduced sociability.

13.2.1 *Physiological alterations underpinning cognitive deficits*

A simultaneous advantage and challenge of studying the relationship between ELS and cognition in relation to physiology is that, unlike other models that are better suited toward the generation of spontaneous seizures [Curia *et al.*, 2008], neither the RFS [de Rogalski Landrot *et al.*, 2001; Riviello *et al.*, 2002] or eFSE [Bender *et al.*, 2004a; Toth *et al.*, 1998] animal models directly result in cell death. While cognitive deficits cannot be simply attributed to brain trauma, considerable evidence suggests altered physiology in both ELS models. With regard to RFS, there is synaptic reorganization indicated by sprouting in CA3 [Holmes *et al.*, 1998; Holmes *et al.*, 1999] as well as reduced neurogenesis [McCabe *et al.*, 2001]. The eFSE model has been found to provoke the attenuation of dendrites in the CA1 field of the hippocampus as well as the maintenance of immature basal dendrites and exaggeration of apical dendritic complexes in dentate gyrus granule cells [Patterson *et al.*, 2017]. These alterations in the dentate gyrus in particular, given its proposed role as both a critical gate that filters inputs [Krook-Magnuson *et al.*, 2015] and a pattern separator [Leutgeb *et al.*, 2007], may be sufficient to induce changes in functional connectivity in the hippocampal circuit that ultimately lead to performance deficits on the active avoidance task in the eFSE model [Patterson *et al.*, 2017]. In an animal model of temporal sclerosis, dentate gyrus mossy cells in particular have been shown to govern both the spread of ictal activity within the hippocampal circuit as well as the encoding of spatial context memory [Bui *et al.*, 2018]. However, the mechanisms by which dendritic alterations of granule cells change hippocampal circuit dynamics remain unknown. It may be a mistake to assume that increased length and complexity of dendritic granule cells would simply lead to an increased density of dendritic synapses that could lower the threshold of excitability as a given dendrite may have a fixed number of axonal terminal projections. For example, while the *Pten* knockout (KO) animal model of autism is associated with significant increases in the length and arborization of granule cell dendrites, accompanying changes in cell excitability may have been largely due to increased synaptic density proximal to the soma [Williams *et al.*, 2015].

Similarly, functional changes in excitability have been reported in both ELS models. For example, RFS causes persistent decreases in GABA currents in the hippocampus [Isaeva *et al.*, 2006] and neocortex [Isaeva *et al.*, 2009; Isaeva, 2009], enhanced excitation in the neocortex [Isaeva *et al.*, 2010], impairment in spike frequency adaptation [Villeneuve *et al.*, 2000], enhanced short-term plasticity in the prefrontal cortex [Hernan *et al.*, 2013], and alterations in long-term potentiation [Isaeva *et al.*, 2013; Karnam *et al.*, 2009a]. Likewise, in the eFSE model, many studies have reported increases in neuronal or network excitability [Bender *et al.*, 2003a; Bender *et al.*, 2003b; Bender *et al.*, 2004a; Bender *et al.*, 2004b; Brewster *et al.*, 2002; Brewster *et al.*, 2005; Chen *et al.*, 2001; Dube *et al.*, 2000; Dube *et al.*, 2005]. In both models, hyperexcitability is indicative of a change in the excitatory and inhibitory (E/I) balance in the brain. In particular, the eFSE model has been found to induce cell hyperexcitability through increased I_h current in hippocampal pyramidal cells [Chen *et al.*, 1999; Chen *et al.*, 2001; Dyhrfjeld-Johnsen *et al.*, 2009]. Specifically, the increased h-current leads to a greater probability of excitatory rebound by pyramidal cells. This was found to be particularly evident during trains of IPSPs that were introduced at a similar rate to those that occur naturally during the theta rhythm [Chen *et al.*, 2001]. How such changes in I_h current alter network activity in eFSE animals is unknown, yet recent efforts have explored the role of I_h current in determining oscillatory control through a multiscale computer model of hippocampal microcircuitry that included pyramidal cells, basket cell interneurons and oriens-lacunosum moleculare interneurons [Neymotin *et al.*, 2013]. While other processes may also have important modulatory influences, the model demonstrates that I_h current has a substantial influence over both theta and slow gamma frequency and amplitude. In particular, matching increases in I_h current in both pyramidal cells and basket cell interneurons was found to lead to an increase in peak theta frequency and theta power as well as a decreased slow gamma frequency and increased slow gamma power. Remarkably, such alterations in slow gamma have recently been described in a subset of eFSE animals [Barry *et al.*, 2016]. In addition, any disruption in the inherent non-uniform density of I_h current along the apical dendrites of CA1 pyramidal cells may interrupt the "democracy of synapses" that normalizes the influence of each of the major synapses along the dendrite regardless of its proximity to the soma. In normal circumstances, I_h channel distribution along the dendrite allows for temporal summation at the soma of CA1 pyramidal cells in a manner that is independent of input location [Magee, 1999]. If the distribution of I_h channels is altered, as is often the case following eFSE [Chen *et al.*, 1999, 2001], the amount of temporal summation occurring at the soma might be more related to the location of the input and lead to more of an "autocracy of synapses" along the dendrite. Taken together, the results of several studies [Chen *et al.*, 2001; Dyhrfjeld-Johnsen *et al.*, 2008] suggest that I_h-mediated current alterations across cell types could be the root of network oscillation changes in FSE animals that might ultimately influence cognitive outcomes. How these changes in cell morphology and ion channel distribution alter the temporal structure of neuronal activity, where synchronized network oscillations are critical for a variety of physiological phenomena that underpin cognition, is still unknown. However, clear changes in the brain following ELS result in the functional alteration of neural circuits that directly affect the processing of task-relevant information.

13.2.2 *Coding mechanisms bridging physiology and cognition*

Alterations in the efficacy of neural circuits following ELS are thought to fundamentally alter rate coding mechanisms [Barry *et al.*, 2015; Dube *et al.*, 2009; Karnam *et al.*, 2009b] where information is conveyed through the firing frequency of single neurons, as well as temporal coding mechanisms [Barry *et al.*, 2016a] where the transfer of information is achieved through the organization of neuronal firing within specific phases of local field potentials (LFPs), particularly in relation to phase of theta [Hasselmo and Stern, 2014]. Temporal coding in particular encourages coordination both within and between neural circuits in a manner that increases the likelihood that excitation from downstream targets will be appropriately timed to arrive at their terminal synapses in order to allow for the ordered transfer of information [Barry *et al.*, 2016a; Barry and Holmes, 2016]. Therefore, temporal coordination represents an essential part of the physiological underpinnings of ordered cognition by improving throughput of specific circuits. There is increasing evidence that one of the neurobiological consequences of repetitive or prolonged seizure activity is impairment in both rate and temporal coding of action potentials (APs), also termed units or spikes, within and between neural circuits.

An example of impaired rate coding in ELS is aberrant firing of place cells. A subset of pyramidal neurons in the hippocampus elicits APs that correspond to an animal's location within its environment [Muller, 1996; O'Keefe, 1976; O'Keefe and Dostrovsky, 1971]. Specifically, these place cells selectively discharge when the animal enters certain locations of the environment, called the cell's firing field. Since there is a close relationship between place cell activity and the ongoing spatial behavior of rats [Lenck-Santini *et al.*, 2002] as well as what spatial stimuli are encoded in the hippocampus [Barry and Muller, 2011], such signals provide the animal with a cognitive map of space that is thought to guide navigation [O'Keefe and Nadel, 1978]. Field location, size and shape are specific to each cell and each environment, and fields tend to cover the surface of the environment homogeneously when a large number of neurons are recorded simultaneously. For a given environment, in normal rats, place fields remain unchanged even between exposures separated by hours [Barry and Muller, 2011; Barry *et al.*, 2012]. The stability of place fields in familiar environments as well the phenomenon of place cell orthogonalization between environments, called remapping [Muller and Kubie, 1987] make these units of the "cognitive map" a very useful surrogate of spatial memory [O'Keefe and Conway, 1978; O'Keefe and Nadel, 1978] for both basic and translational scientists.

Place cells occur in rat pups as early as 2 ½ weeks old but continue to evolve with development, becoming more like adult neurons after P30 [Langston *et al.*, 2010; Scott *et al.*, 2011; Wills *et al.*, 2010]. Adult rats experiencing status epilepticus (SE) exhibit altered rate coding and impaired learning in the water maze [Liu *et al.*, 2003]. The hippocampal neurons of SE animals also exhibit excessive synchrony and less reactivation during rest. These features also tend to predict the rat's performance in a spatial memory task [Tyler *et al.*, 2012]. Likewise, ELS result in rate coding abnormalities. RFS during the first weeks of life cause impairment in spatial cognition with impaired place cell precision and stability [Karnam *et al.*, 2009b]. In the eFSE model, place cells from rats with impaired spatial cognition exhibit larger firing fields and faster firing rates [Barry *et al.*, 2015]. Taken together, these studies indicate that rate coding can be impaired in both seizure models and that abnormalities in excitability at the level of single cells as well as networks may contribute to impaired spatial cognition.

Rate coding of place cells does not occur in isolation and is affected by local field potentials (LFPs). In the hippocampus, place cells are not only characterized by their location-specific rate firing but also by their precise temporal firing relationship within hippocampal theta oscillations [Lenck-Santini and Holmes, 2008; Skaggs *et al.*, 1996]. When the rat enters the cell's firing field, APs will fire preferentially on the rising phase of the CA1 theta cycle. As the rat crosses the field, the cells fire earlier on successive theta cycles, a phenomenon called phase precession [O'Keefe and Recce, 1993]. Following SE in adult rats, there are marked abnormalities in phase precession of APs among pairs of neurons with parallel deficits in the Morris water maze task [Lenck-Santini and Holmes, 2008]. While theta phase precession of spike timing is one measure of temporal coding, measuring it may require methodological constraints such as restraining the rat's movements to linear tracks. This is largely because the quantification of precession is easier during controlled passes through a firing field rather than random passes at differing angles and speeds through a firing field [Huxter *et al.*, 2008; Jeewajee *et al.*, 2014]. It is also less useful for providing information concerning the organization of dynamic spike timing in circuits, particularly as a function of cognitive demand.

An additional measure of spike timing within theta that is more conducive to these questions is phase preference, or the calculation of spike probability relative to phase of theta [Barry *et al.*, 2016a; Douchamps *et al.*, 2013; Fernandez-Ruiz *et al.*, 2017; Mizuseki *et al.*, 2009; Robbe and Buzsaki, 2009; Schomburg *et al.*, 2014; Siegle and Wilson, 2014]. The preferred phase of firing in CA1 is believed to play an important role in the encoding and recall of spatial information [Hasselmo and Stern, 2014]. Input from the entorhinal cortex, a major source of cortical projections to the hippocampus, is highest at the peak of local theta and likely encodes sensory information from the environment. At this same phase, the hippocampus is more susceptible to LTP [Holscher *et al.*, 1997; Huerta and Lisman, 1995], which is consistent with the idea that this phase is optimized for encoding new information. At the trough of local theta, CA1 cells receive greater input from CA3 cells. At this phase, stimulation of Schaffer collateral or temporo-ammonic inputs induces long-term depression (LTD), which could suppress information storage during memory retrieval [Hasselmo, 2005; Hasselmo and Stern, 2014]. Because of these phase-specific physiological changes, hippocampal networks may regulate the behavioral impact of different types of information as a function of context. While spatial firing of place cells may not be dependent upon hippocampal theta oscillations [Brandon *et al.*, 2014], memory-related ensemble activity of place cells may be generated through temporal coding within theta [Wang *et al.*, 2015]. Thus, while a spatial map may be generated by the hippocampus in response to sensory information, theta may be necessary to read the spatial information from the map in order to guide behavior. The relevance of phase with encoding and recall has also been demonstrated through optogenetic inhibition of pyramidal cells in CA1 at the peak and trough of theta in animals undergoing behavioral training. Using closed-loop stimulation, inhibition triggered at the peak or trough of local theta stimulation differentially affected encoding and retrieval of spatial information, indicating that the processes related to the encoding and retrieval of task-relevant information are preferentially active at distinct phases of theta [Siegle and Wilson, 2014].

An example of phase preference is illustrated in Figure 13.1. We created both rate and phase maps for CA1 cellular APs during

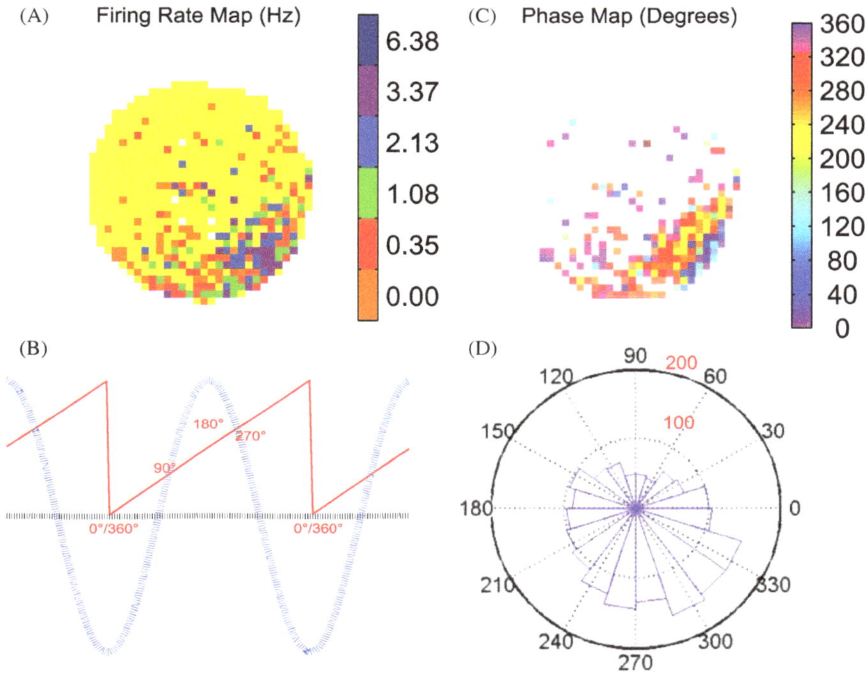

Figure 13.1. Illustration of place cell APs relative to space and theta phase preference. (A) Place cell firing rate map indicating median firing rate per pixel over the entire recording session. Darker colored pixels indicate a higher firing rate while yellow pixels indicate that the cell did not fire. (B) Illustration of the Hilbert transform (red) that was used to derive an analytic representation of the filtered theta signal (blue). The trough of the theta signal is represented at 0/360° and the peak at 180°. (C) Phase map indicating the median phase of local theta for APs in each pixel. The color code for the phase map is indicated to the right of the plot. The apparent bands of color in the firing field indicate that the APs of the place cell tend to cycle through all phases of the theta cycle and may be indicative of phase precession. (D) Rose plot circular histogram indicating the place cell's preferred firing phase with regard to local theta. The number of APs are binned by 20 18° bins (0 – 360°) where the circular dashed lines indicate the number of APs (shown in red) per bin. The pixels in the center of the firing field (A), where the majority of the APs occur, correspond to phases between 240°–320°. This is consistent with the roseplot histogram in D and suggests that phase precession and phase preference are not mutually exclusive concepts. Reprinted with permission from Barry *et al.*, 2016a.

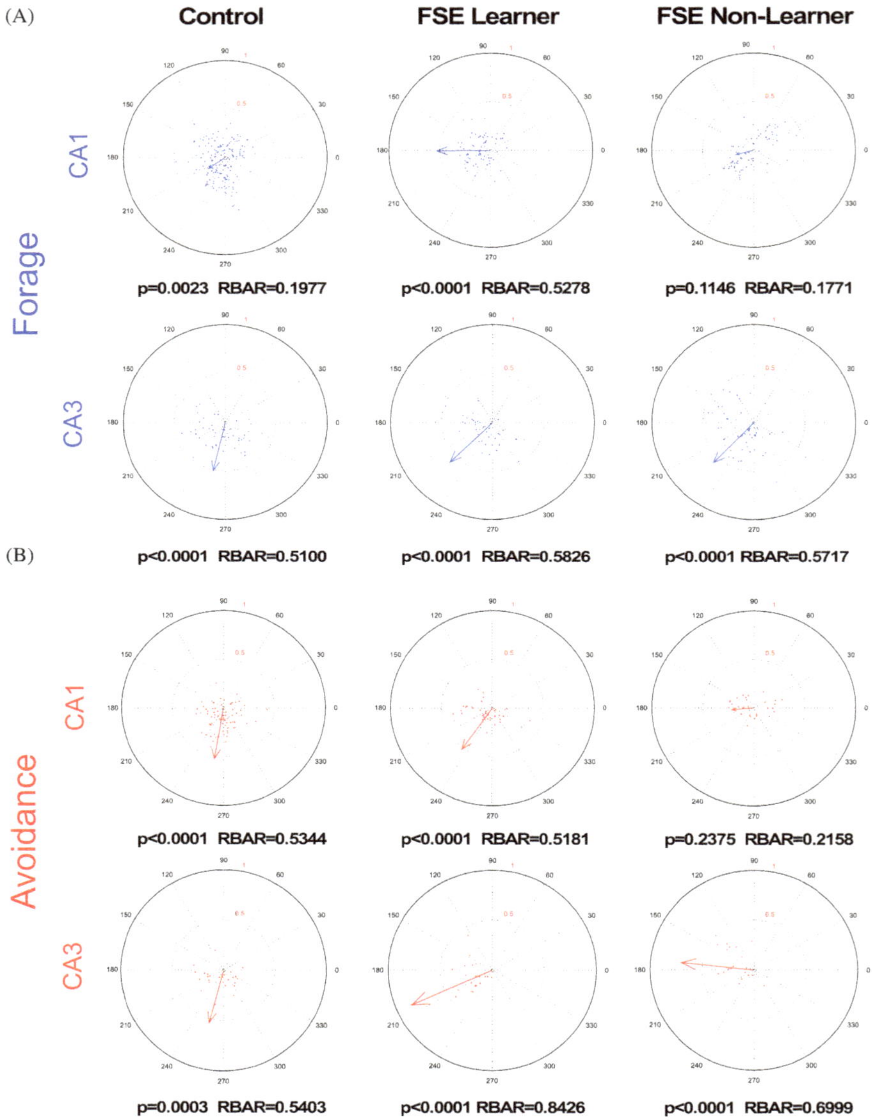

Figure 13.2. (*Continued*)

Figure 13.2. Temporal coordination of CA1 and CA3 place cells relative to local theta in response to changes in cognitive demand in control (Cont) and febrile animals that could (FSE-L) and could not (FSE-NL) meet criterion in an active avoidance task. (A) Distribution of CA1 place cell phase preference during foraging sessions from Cont (Left), FSE-L (Middle), FSE-NL (Right). Cells recorded from Cont were distributed throughout the theta cycle but showed a significant phase preference at 214°. Cells recorded from FSE-L were more likely to show phase preference at the peak of local theta at 180° than animals from the other 2 groups. While place cells recorded from FSE-NL had a mean angle of 194°, they showed no significant phase preference. The distribution of preferred firing phases for cells recorded in layer CA3 from Cont (257°, Bottom Left), FSE-L (225°, Bottom Middle), FSE-NL (226°, Bottom Right) all exhibited significant phase preference and no group differences were found in the distribution of phase preference. (B) Distribution of preferred phase of firing for place cells during avoidance sessions in layer CA1 from Cont (Left), FSE-L (Middle), FSE-NL (Right). Cells from Cont significantly shifted firing preference to the descending theta phase at 260°. Cells from FSE-L also shifted phase toward the descending phase of local theta and exhibited a preference at 234°. Again, FSE-NL displayed non-significant phase preference with respect to local theta but had a mean firing phase at 184°. Significantly more place cells displayed a phase preference between 180–270° in Cont and FSE-L than FSE-NL. As in the foraging context, the distribution of preferred firing phase for cells recorded in layer CA3 from Cont (255°, Bottom Left), FSE-L (205°, Bottom Middle), FSE-NL (174°, Bottom Right) showed significant phase preference. No significant differences were found in the distribution of phase preference between the 3 groups in CA3 during avoidance. Taken together, the preferred firing phases in CA3 are significant for all 3 groups and remain relatively constant in both contexts. The shift away from a preferred firing phase at the peak of local theta to the descending phase seen in both Cont and FSE-L would put active cells in each cell layer in alignment with regard to local theta and may indicate network alterations to adjust for increased cognitive demand. That FSE-NL CA1 place cell phase preference was non-significant and did not shift during active avoidance may therefore be indicative of network malfunction. Reprinted with permission from Barry *et al.*, 2016a.

foraging for food pellets and during performance of the active avoidance spatial task. The spatial AP information from a rate map (Figure 13.1A) and the extracted phase of local theta (Figure 13.1B) can be combined to create a phase map (Figure 13.1C). The phase map indicates that, averaged over the 30 min recording session, the APs of the cell tend to fire at the later phases of theta at the periphery of the field and then precess to earlier phases of theta as the animal moves through the field. Taken together, the firing rate map and the phase map illustrate that APs in the center of the field, where the majority of the APs occur, tend to fire in a phase range between 240 degrees and 320 degrees. This is in good agreement with the rose plot histogram (Figure 13.1D) that shows binned APs predominantly falling within this phase range.

A recent experiment has shown that eFSE impairs temporal coordination of CA1 neurons and the corresponding theta phase relationship of place cell APs within the hippocampal CA1 and CA3 circuit [Barry *et al.*, 2016a]. Remarkably, control CA1 place cell phase preference shifted significantly between a foraging task and an active avoidance task. Place cells shifted their preferred firing near the peak of local theta to a later phase of theta that was more in line with a static Θ phase preference in CA3. Similar results were found for eFSE animals that were able to meet task criterion. CA1 place cells from eFSE animals that were unable to meet active avoidance task criterion did not exhibit a preferred phase of firing in either context (Figure 13.2). AP coordination relative to theta phase between CA3 and CA1 was therefore greater in the eFSE learners and controls than in the eFSE non-learners. Thus, the absence of phase preference in these animals in CA1 as well as the corresponding absence of the shift in phase preference that aligns APs in both circuits suggest that insufficient coordination between both components of the hippocampal circuit by theta oscillations may prevent the eFSE non-learners from accurately calculating their position on the rotating arena. This causes the animals to make more errors and prevents them from meeting criterion in the avoidance task. The temporal discoordination of place cells may explain both network adaptation and network malfunction in eFSE animals with regard to cognitive outcome in the active avoidance task. While this recent work provided the first evidence that ELS impairs temporal coding of APs, further work is necessary to provide mechanistic proof that temporal coding abnormalities, or corresponding rate coding abnormalities, are sufficient to cause deficits in spatial cognition. In addition, it is not yet known whether the observed temporal discoordination of CA1 APs occurs in other models of ELS.

Finally, while not neatly falling into the realm of temporal or rate coding mechanisms, there is also a robust phenomenon of both cell firing frequency and theta frequency increasing in a linear manner with animal movement speed [Hinman *et al.*, 2011; Hinman *et al.*, 2016; Richard *et al.*, 2013; Vanderwolf, 1969]. Speed and theta frequency correlation coefficients and regression slopes were found to be abnormal and correlative with poor task performance in rats following pilocarpine-induced SE [Richard *et al.*, 2013] as well as animals with eFSE [Barry *et al.*, 2016a; Patterson *et al.*, 2017] (Figure 13.3). While the mechanism is not yet known for this discoordination between animal speed and theta frequency after SE or eFSE, it may be rooted in the same physiological alterations that lead to the temporal discoordination of APs within theta.

13.2.3 *Effect of interictal spikes (IS) on cognition*

In addition to seizures, there is compelling evidence that IS in both animals and humans can result in cognitive impairment. In both children and adults IS can cause transitory cognitive impairment [Aarts *et al.*, 1984; Binnie *et al.*, 1987; Binnie *et al.*, 1991; Shewmon and Erwin, 1988a; Shewmon and Erwin, 1988b; Shewmon and Erwin, 1988c; Shewmon and Erwin, 1989; Ung *et al.*, 2017; Xiao *et al.*, 2016]. Aarts and co-workers [Aarts *et al.*, 1984] found that IS can briefly disrupt neural processes affecting localized function within the brain region where they occur. There is an IS effect on both verbal and non-verbal short-term memory in patients with epilepsy, while there are no clear clinical manifestations during these discharges. In right-handed individuals, right hemisphere IS were associated with errors in a non-verbal task whereas left hemisphere IS resulted mainly in errors in verbal tasks. EEG discharges interfered primarily when occurring simultaneously with the presentation of the stimulus, corresponding with the encoding phase of the task. Shewmon and Erwin, in a series of carefully performed studies [Shewmon and Erwin, 1988a; Shewmon and Erwin, 1988b; Shewmon and Erwin, 1988c; Shewmon and Erwin, 1989] found that occipital IS could disrupt visual perception. IS in the occipital region caused transitory deficits with stimuli presented in the contralateral visual field. Deficits were most pronounced when they occurred during the slow wave following the IS.

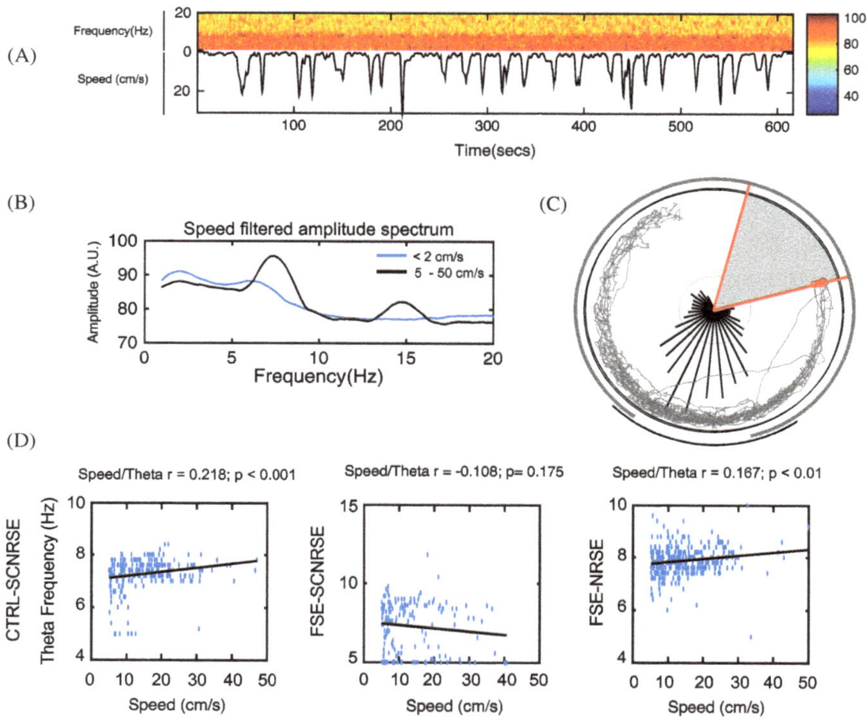

Figure 13.3. eFSE alters the linear relationship between hippocampal theta oscillations and speed in adult rats and may be corrected by peri eFSE intracranial injections of the oligonucleotide NRSE. (A) Relationship of movement-speed and spectrogram illustrating hippocampal signal amplitude and frequency changes during a 10 min active avoidance session in a control rat (CTL-SCR). Theta oscillations (5–12 Hz) increase in frequency and power relative to movement speed (Bottom). (B) As in A, speed-filtered amplitude of showing the increased theta signal amplitude when the rat is moving > 5 cm/s as compared to < 2 cm/s during. (C) As in A, polar analysis of spatial sampling during active avoidance where the vector, angle and length of the black lines emanating from the plot center indicate the proportion of time spent at each angle of the arena (0–360° in 10° bins). The outside arc (thin black line) for each plot indicates the distribution of the longest vector lengths that account for at least 50% of the session duration. The gray sector indicates the shock zone and red circles where the animal received shocks. (D) Relationship between speed and frequency (blue dots) throughout an active avoidance session in a representative rat from a control group and each eFSE group The line of best fit (black line) and the corresponding correlation coefficient between frequency and speed indicates a significant linear relationship for the control group and the treated eFSE group and a non-significant relationship for the untreated eFSE group. Adapted from Patterson *et al.*, 2017.

To study the effects of IS on memory and reaction time in animal models of SE, Kleen and colleagues [Kleen *et al.*, 2010] studied rats that developed chronic IS following intrahippocampal pilocarpine in a hippocampal-dependent operant behavioral task, delayed-match-to-sample. Hippocampal IS that occurred during memory retrieval strongly impaired performance while IS that occurred during memory encoding or memory maintenance did not affect performance in those trials. There is a significant and sustained reduction of APs for up to two seconds following the IS; when occurring in flurries, IS reduced APs firing for up to six seconds [Zhou *et al.*, 2007a]. In addition to affecting APs, the widespread inhibitory wave immediately after IS can dramatically reduce the power of gamma oscillations and other oscillatory signals in the hippocampus [Urrestarazu *et al.*, 2006]. Since, as described above, oscillations are intimately linked to ongoing learning and memory functions, this disruption in oscillations may contribute in complex ways to cognitive deficits [Halasz *et al.*, 2005; Kleen *et al.*, 2010]. However, animals that experienced eFSE, regardless of cognitive outcome on the active avoidance task, exhibited similar IS rates during the task. This reinforces the notion that the occurrence of IS may not necessarily cause cognitive deficits, as there are other network alterations that may compensate for them. This has been proposed to be the case given alterations to both spike timing within theta as well as slow gamma frequency alterations for many eFSE animals that do not exhibit cognitive deficits [Barry *et al.*, 2016].

Patients with temporal lobe epilepsy and IS have also been shown to exhibit declines in working memory during periods of IS [Krauss *et al.*, 1997]. Using similar methodology to that used in rats, Kleen and colleagues [Kleen *et al.*, 2013] investigated whether IS in patients with temporal lobe epilepsy resulted in memory impairment. Ten patients with intra-hippocampal depth electrodes were studied during a simple memory task, the Sternberg test, where 4 letters are presented and after a delay the patient has to determine whether a single letter was one of the 4 letters shown. Hippocampal IS occurring in the memory retrieval period decreased the likelihood of a correct response when the IS was contralateral to the seizure focus or bilateral. This study provided biological validity to animal models in the study of IS-related transient cognitive impairment.

Similarly, Ung and co-workers [Ung *et al.*, 2017] studied 67 patients with medication-refractory epilepsy undergoing continuous intracranial electroencephalography monitoring engaged in a delayed free recall task to test short-term memory. In this task, subjects were asked to memorize and recall lists of common nouns. The effect of each spike on the probability of successful recall was analysed using a generalized logistic mixed model. Patients with left lateralized seizure onset zones, spikes outside the seizure onset zone impacted memory encoding, whereas those within the seizure onset zone did not. In addition, spikes in the left inferior temporal gyrus, middle temporal gyrus, superior temporal gyrus, and fusiform gyrus during memory encoding reduced odds of recall by as much as 15% per spike. Spikes also reduced the odds of word retrieval, an effect that was stronger with spikes outside of the seizure onset zone. These results suggest that seizure onset regions are dysfunctional at baseline, and support the idea that interictal spikes disrupt cognitive processes related to the underlying tissue.

In addition to the transient effects of IS on behavior and cognition, IS can cause long-standing sequelae in developing animals. In studies of the effects of IS on striate cortex in rabbits, IS were elicited by epidural focal application of either penicillin [Baumbach and Chow, 1981; Crabtree *et al.*, 1981] or bicuculline [Campbell *et al.*, 1984; Ostrach *et al.*, 1984] in the striate cortex. IS were elicited for 6–12 hours following each drug application and drug applications were given daily from ages 8–9 days to 24–30 days. None of the rabbits had behavioral seizures. In single-unit recordings from the lateral geniculate nucleus, superior colliculus, and occipital cortex ipsilateral to the hemisphere with IS, there was an abnormal distribution of receptive field types whereas normal recordings were found from the contralateral hemisphere. This finding was age-dependent as adult rabbits with similarly induced interictal spikes had normal cell development. These studies showed that disruption of orderly neuronal activity in the geniculostriate system by interictal spikes during critical developmental periods in young animals has a detrimental effect on the development of receptive fields in the occipital cortex.

IS have also been elicited in young rats with flurothyl inhalation [Khan *et al.*, 2010]. Rat pups were given a low dose of flurothyl for four hours for 10 days during continuous electroencephalographic monitoring. Rats developed IS without seizures while age-matched controls under similar testing conditions had few IS. When rats were tested as adults, there was impairment in reference memory in the probe test of the Morris water maze, reference memory impairment in the four-trial radial-arm water maze, and impaired long-term potentiation. Early-life IS resulted in impaired neurogenesis in the dentate but did not cause an increase in apoptosis. This study demonstrated that IS in rat pups without seizures can result in long-standing spatial cognitive impairment. These findings suggest that IS may be even more detrimental to the developing brain.

Similarly, the neonatal ventral-hippocampal lesion (NVHL) model of schizophrenia has been shown to cause the occurrence of cortical spike-wave discharges in adult rats [Lee *et al.*, 2014]. Treatment with ethosuximide abolished the spike-wave activity, increased the synchrony between hippocampi, and improved measures of cognitive control in the active avoidance task. These results are noteworthy as they suggest that attenuating aberrant neural synchrony is sufficient to attenuate cognitive deficits, providing a promising framework for the treatment of cognitive deficits that result from neurodevelopmental disorders.

13.2.4 *Seeing the forest through the trees*

In this review, we have covered the complexities of ELS- and SE-associated physiological changes that may underpin a variety of cognitive deficits. These ELS induced cognitive and behavioral deficits are ultimately due to the pathological interactions between altered physiological components in key circuits and microcircuits relevant the neural coding mechanisms that bridge physiology and cognition. We described several studies that illustrate the long-term effects of seizures at multiple levels of neuronal functioning and the meso-scale interactions of these physiological levels that are dynamic as a function of both development and cognitive demand. In summary (Figure 13.4), FSE alter levels of the gene transcription factor NRSF

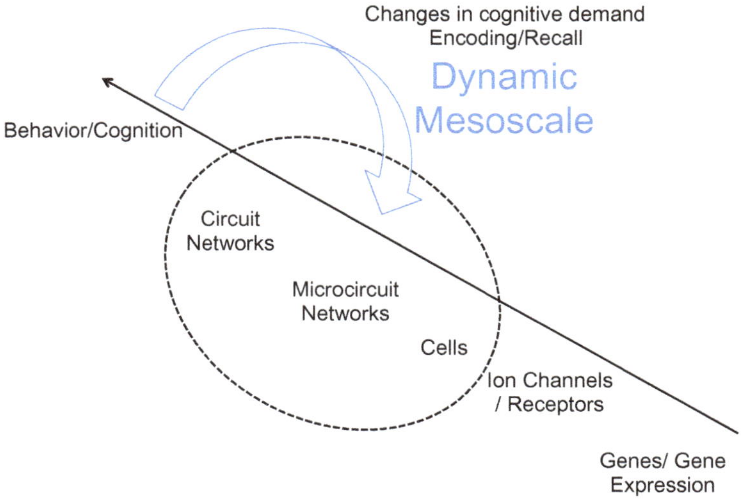

Figure 13.4. Summary of findings related to ELS induced alterations to multiple physiological scales that may account for cognitive deficits after ELS. The interaction of these physiological scales, or 'meso-scale' interactions, illustrate the importance of understanding neural coding mechanisms that are dynamic as both a function of cognitive demand and development.

(neuron-restrictive silencer factor) that can in turn alter gene expression for specific ion channels (i.e. HCN channels) and receptors [McClelland *et al.*, 2014]. It has also been shown that FSE can diminish CA1 dendrites [Patterson *et al.*, 2017]. It is possible that these alterations to dendritic morphology, a key component of the local microcircuit, would alter CA1 synaptic function that underlies the transfer of neural information between CA1 and CA3 as well as between CA1 and neocortex. While much more work needs to be done, this may explain the temporal discoordination between CA1 and CA3 cellular spike timing relative to local theta oscillations in FSE animals with spatial cognitive deficits [Barry *et al.*, 2016a]. Control animals and FSE animals without spatial deficits in this experiment not only demonstrated temporal coordination of CA1 neuronal spike timing, but that this timing was dynamic according to cognitive demand and may have allowed for improved communication between CA1 and CA3 and recall of task parameters. We therefore contend that while any exploration of ELS-induced cognitive deficits must be rooted in the resulting changes to physiology, it is these meso-scale coding mechanisms that bridge physiology and cognition that are our best hope for understanding and treating ELS-induced cognitive deficits.

Yet, how do we go about mending neural coding mechanisms that we are only beginning to understand? The ideal scenario would be to prevent the first domino from falling and avert ELS-associated physiological changes. Recent evidence indicates that the transcription factor NRSF (Neuron Restrictive Silencing Factor) significantly increases in hippocampal neurons following SE [McClelland *et al.*, 2014] or eFSE [Patterson *et al.*, 2017] and prevents the transcription of a number of genes that express many different neurotransmitters and ion channels [McClelland *et al.*, 2014]. Intracranial injections of NRSE (Neuron Restrictive Silencing Element) oligonucleotide around the time of hyperthermia induced eFSE was found to offset the increased NRSF in the hippocampus [Patterson *et al.*, 2017]. While this did not prevent the attenuation of CA1 pyramidal cell dendrites, it did appear to prevent the increased arborization and dysmaturation of dentate gyrus granule cells. NRSE appeared to alter the balance of slow and fast gamma and produce more linear speed-theta relationships in eFSE rats in comparison to the untreated eFSE animals. Remarkably, these treated eFSE rats had better cognitive outcomes on the active avoidance task than the untreated animals that exhibited inefficient avoidance strategies by staying close to the shock zone. While these results suggest that increases in the gene transcription factor NRSF after eFSE may represent the first of a cascade of falling dominos, and preventing it does appear to improve outcomes, the interpretation is still complex as it is unclear whether neural coding mechanisms are maintained after NRSE treatment. While changes to gamma oscillations and improved speed-theta relationships would suggest they are maintained, further work needs to be done. These results also raise the question as to what is the most important signal in relation to cognitive outcome — gene expression, theta activity, gamma activity, E/I balance, or some combination of these factors? How much are all of these symptoms due to physiological changes like abnormal dendrites in one or more parts of a circuit? We suggest that the proper conceptual framework is the biggest challenge to the field at present and that the best approach would be one rooted in physiology that also incorporates neural coding mechanisms.

While preventing the pathophysiological changes would be the ideal solution, the clinic often deals with cases where the last domino has fallen and the damage is already done. What is to be done then? This is the dilemma for all neurodevelopmental disorders where cognitive outcome is a major concern [Fenton, 2015; Insel, 2010] and requires addressing the very hard problem of correcting one or more neural coding mechanisms. The most likely answer to this problem requires intervention in the form of electrical or optogenetic stimulation in key neural circuits. For example, non-selective optogenetic stimulation of the medial septum (MS) has been found to influence hippocampal oscillations and improve learning in a working memory task in control animals [Blumberg *et al.*, 2016], while electrical MS stimulations in a pilocarpine model of SE were found to improve performance on a Barnes maze spatial task [Lee *et al.*, 2017]. Yet, in both these cases, the putative alterations to the coding mechanisms that drive cognition are not yet known. An alternative approach would be direct and selective manipulation of the hippocampal microcircuit in a closed-loop optogenetic system [Siegle and Wilson, 2014], although this has not yet been attempted in the context of cognitive deficits in ELS models. While it will be years until such clinical studies utilizing optogenetics are realized, a recent study has shown that 50 Hz electrical stimulation in the hippocampus, entorhinal cortex, perirhinal cortex, parahippocampal cortex, and dorsolateral prefrontal cortex of epileptic patients can improve performance in a verbal memory task [Ezzyat *et al.*, 2017]. An interesting stipulation of this finding is that stimulation was only found to have a positive influence on performance if it was delivered during trials in which specific brain regions were failing to encode information. Otherwise, the stimulation tended to have an adverse affect on performance. This finding was aided by the use of multivariate classification of signals in multiple brain regions in order to establish which classifiers accurately predicted encoding and subsequent recall.

Similarly, regression and classification models developed in rodent electrophysiology experiments have been able to reproduce spatio-temporal cellular action potential patterns from CA3 to CA1 [Song *et al.*, 2014]. This model of the multiple input/multiple output (MIMO) of spike trains is suggested to be capable of predicting and restoring regional output signals based on input. The model has successfully predicted behavioral performance on a DNMS task in rats [Song *et al.*, 2014], and has improved DMS performance in non-human primates when coupled with closed-loop stimulation [Deadwyler *et al.*, 2017a]. Preliminary evidence from studies by this group in 5 epileptic patients using MIMO derived stimulation patterns in CA1 resulted in a 15–25% improvement in working memory during DMS task performance [Deadwyler *et al.*, 2017b]. This stimulation approach therefore has great potential for acting as a neural prosthetic for the augmentation of memory.

13.3 Concluding remarks

While a complete understanding of ELS-associated cognitive impairments can seem more elusive the more we try to reach it, we are beginning to form a new framework for the multi-scalar nature of ELS. This framework requires us to learn as much as possible about the physiological basis of cognition and its underlying developmental conseequences. Ultimately, understanding the neural coding mechanisms that bridge physiology and cognition will allow us to see the forest through the trees and find effective ways of both preventing and treating ELS induced cognitive impairments.

References

Aarts, J.H., Binnie, C.D., Smit, A.M., and Wilkins, A.J. (1984). Selective cognitive impairment during focal and generalized epileptiform EEG activity, *Brain*, 107 (Pt 1), 293–308.

Bailet, L.L. and Turk, W.R. (2000). The impact of childhood epilepsy on neurocognitive and behavioral performance: a prospective longitudinal study, *Epilepsia*, 41, 426–431.

Barry, J.M. and Muller, R.U. (2011). Updating the hippocampal representation of space: place cell firing fields are controlled by a novel spatial stimulus, *Hippocampus*, 21, 481–494.

Barry, J.M., Choy, M., Dube, C., Robbins, A., Obenaus, A., Lenck-Santini, P.P., Scott, R.C., Baram, T.Z., and Holmes, G.L. (2015). T2 relaxation time post febrile status epilepticus predicts cognitive outcome, *Exp. Neurol.*, 269, 242–252.

Barry, J.M. and Holmes, G.L. (2016). Why are children with epileptic encephalopathies encephalopathic?, *J. Child Neurol.*, 31, 1495–1504.

Barry, J.M., Rivard, B., Fox, S.E., Fenton, A.A., Sacktor, T.C., and Muller, R.U. (2012). Inhibition of protein kinase Mzeta disrupts the stable spatial discharge of hippocampal place cells in a familiar environment, *J. Neurosci.*, 32, 13753–13762.

Barry, J.M., Sakkaki, S., Barriere, S.J., Patterson, K.P., Lenck-Santini, P.P., Scott, R.C., Baram, T.Z., and Holmes, G.L. (2016a). Temporal coordination of hippocampal neurons reflects cognitive outcome post-febrile status epilepticus, *EBioMedicine*, 7, 175–190.

Barry, J.M., Tian, C., Spinella, A., Page, M., and Holmes, G.L. (2016b). Spatial cognition following early-life seizures in rats: Performance deficits are dependent on task demands, *Epilepsy Behav.*, 60, 1–6.

Baumbach, H.D. and Chow, K.L. (1981). Visuocortical epileptiform discharges in rabbits: differential effects on neuronal development in the lateral geniculate nucleus and superior colliculus, *Brain Res.*, 209, 61–76.

Bender, R.A., Dube, C., and Baram, T.Z. (2004a). Febrile seizures and mechanisms of epileptogenesis: insights from an animal model, *Adv. Exp. Med. Biol.*, 548, 213–225.

Bender, R.A., Dube, C., Gonzalez-Vega, R., Mina, E.W., and Baram, T.Z. (2003a). Mossy fiber plasticity and enhanced hippocampal excitability, without hippocampal cell loss or altered neurogenesis, in an animal model of prolonged febrile seizures, *Hippocampus*, 13, 399–412.

Bender, R.A., Dubé, C., Gonzalez-Vega, R., Mina, E.W., and Baram, T.Z. (2004b). Mossy fiber plasticity and enhanced hippocampal excitability, without hippocampal cell loss or altered neurogenesis, in an animal model of prolonged febrile seizures, *Hippocampus*, 13, 399–412.

Bender, R.A., Soleymani, S.V., Brewster, A.L., Nguyen, S.T., Beck, H., Mathern, G.W., and Baram, T.Z. (2003b). Enhanced expression of a specific hyperpolarization-activated cyclic nucleotide-gated cation

channel (HCN) in surviving dentate gyrus granule cells of human and experimental epileptic hippocampus, *J. Neurosci.*, 23, 6826–6836.
Berg, A.T., Zelko, F.A., Levy, S.R., and Testa, F.M. (2012). Age at onset of epilepsy, pharmacoresistance, and cognitive outcomes: a prospective cohort study, *Neurology*, 79, 1384–1391.
Binnie, C.D., Channon, S., and Marston, D.L. (1991). Behavioral correlates of interictal spikes. *Adv. Neurol.*, 55, 113–126.
Binnie, C.D., Kasteleijn-Nolst Trenite, D.G., Smit, A.M., and Wilkins, A.J. (1987). Interactions of epileptiform EEG discharges and cognition. *Epilepsy Res.*, 1, 239–245.
Blumberg, B.J., Flynn, S.P., Barriere, S.J., Mouchati, P.R., Scott, R.C., Holmes. G.L., and Barry, J.M. (2016). Efficacy of nonselective optogenetic control of the medial septum over hippocampal oscillations: the influence of speed and implications for cognitive enhancement, *Physiol. Rep.*, 4, pii: e13048.
Bourgeois, B.D., Prensky, A.L., Palkes, H.S., Talent, B.K., and Busch, S.G. (1983). Intelligence in epilepsy: A prospective study in children, *Ann. Neurol.*, 14, 438–444.
Brandon, M.P., Koenig, J., Leutgeb, J.K., and Leutgeb, S. (2014). New and distinct hippocampal place codes are generated in a new environment during septal inactivation, *Neuron*, 82, 789–796.
Brewster, A., Bender, R.A., Chen, Y., Dube, C., Eghbal-Ahmadi, M., and Baram, T.Z. (2002). Developmental febrile seizures modulate hippocampal gene expression of hyperpolarization-activated channels in an isoform and cell-specific manner, *J. Neurosci.*, 22, 4591–4599.
Brewster, A.L., Bernard, J.A., Gall, C.M., and Baram, T.Z. (2005). Formation of heteromeric hyperpolarization-activated cyclic nucleotide-gated (HCN) channels in the hippocampus is regulated by developmental seizures, *Neurobiol. Dis.*, 19, 200–207.
Buelow, J.M., Perkins, S.M., Johnson, C.S., Byars, A.W., Fastenau, P.S., Dunn, D.W., and Austin, J.K. (2012). Adaptive functioning in children with epilepsy and learning problems, *J. Child Neurol.*, 27, 1241–1249.
Bui, A.D., Nguyen, T.M., Limouse, C., Kim, H.K., Szabo, G.G., Felong, S., Maroso, M., and Soltesz, I. (2018). Dentate gyrus mossy cells control spontaneous convulsive seizures and spatial memory, *Science*, 359, 787–790.
Campbell, B.G., Ostrach, L.H., Crabtree, J.W., and Chow, K.L. (1984). Characterization of penicillin- and bicuculline-induced epileptiform

discharges during development of striate cortex in rabbits, *Brain Res.*, 317, 125–128.

Chang, Y.C., Guo, N.W., Wang, S.T., Huang, C.C., and Tsai, J.J. (2001). Working memory of school-aged children with a history of febrile convulsions: a population study, *Neurology*, 57, 37–42.

Chen, K., Aradi, I., Thon, N., Eghbal-Ahmadi, M., Baram, T.Z., and Soltesz, I. (2001). Persistently modified h-channels after complex febrile seizures convert the seizure-induced enhancement of inhibition to hyperexcitability. *Nat. Med.*, 7, 331–337.

Chen, K., Baram, T.Z., and Soltesz, I. (1999). Febrile seizures in the immature rat model modify neuronal excitability long-term, *Nat. Med.*, 5, 888–894.

Cimadevilla, J.M., Fenton, A.A., and Bures, J. (2000a). Functional inactivation of dorsal hippocampus impairs active place avoidance in rats, *Neurosci. Lett.*, 285, 53–56.

Cimadevilla, J.M., Kaminsky, Y., Fenton, A., and Bures, J. (2000b). Passive and active place avoidance as a tool of spatial memory research in rats, *J. Neurosci. Meth.*, 102, 155–164.

Committee on the Public Health Dimensions of the Epilepsies, Board on Health Sciences Policy, Institute of Medicine (2012). *Epilepsy Across the Spectrum: Promoting Health and Understanding*. The National Academies Press.

Crabtree, J.W., Chow, K.L., Ostrach, L.H., and Baumbach, H.D. (1981). Development of receptive field properties in the visual cortex of rabbits subjected to early epileptiform cortical discharges, *Brain Res.*, 227, 269–281.

Curia, G., Longo, D., Biagini, G., Jones, R.S., and Avoli, M. (2008). The pilocarpine model of temporal lobe epilepsy, *J. Neurosci. Meth.*, 172, 143–157.

de Rogalski Landrot, I., Minokoshi, M., Silveira, D.C., Cha, B.H., and Holmes, G.L. (2001). Recurrent neonatal seizures: relationship of pathology to the electroencephalogram and cognition, *Dev. Brain Res.*, 129, 27–38.

Douchamps, V., Jeewajee, A., Blundell, P., Burgess, N., and Lever, C. (2013). Evidence for encoding versus retrieval scheduling in the hippocampus by theta phase and acetylcholine, *J. Neurosci.*, 33, 8689–8704.

Dube, C., Chen, K., Eghbal-Ahmadi, M., Brunson, K., Soltesz, I., and Baram, T.Z. (2000). Prolonged febrile seizures in the immature rat

model enhance hippocampal excitability long term, *Ann. Neurol.*, 47, 336–344.
Dube, C., Vezzani, A., Behrens, M., Bartfai, T., and Baram, T.Z. (2005). Interleukin-1beta contributes to the generation of experimental febrile seizures, *Ann. Neurol.*, 57, 152–155.
Dube, C.M., Zhou, J.L., Hamamura, M., Zhao, Q., Ring, A., Abrahams, J., McIntyre, K., Nalcioglu, O., Shatskih, T., Baram, T.Z., and Holmes, G.L. (2009) Cognitive dysfunction after experimental febrile seizures, *Exp. Neurol.*, 215, 167–177.
Dyhrfjeld-Johnsen, J., Morgan, R.J., Foldy, C., and Soltesz. I. (2008). Upregulated H-current in hyperexcitable CA1 dendrites after febrile seizures, *Front. Cell. Neurosci.*, 2, 2.
Dyhrfjeld-Johnsen, J., Morgan, R.J., and Soltesz, I. (2009). Double trouble? Potential for hyperexcitability following both channelopathic up- and downregulation of I(h) in epilepsy, *Front. Neurosci.*, 3, 25–33.
Ezzyat, Y., Kragel, J.E., Burke, J.F., Levy, D.F., Lyalenko, A., Wanda, P., O'Sullivan, L., Hurley, K.B., Busygin, S., Pedisich, I., Sperling, M.R., Worrell, G.A., Kucewicz, M.T., Davis, K.A., Lucas, T.H., Inman, C.S., Lega, B.C., Jobst, B.C., Sheth, S.A., Zaghloul, K., Jutras, M.J., Stein, J.M., Das, S.R., Gorniak, R., Rizzuto, D.S., and Kahana, M.J. (2017). Direct brain stimulation modulates encoding states and memory performance in humans, *Curr. Biol.*, 27, 1251–1258.
Farwell, J.R., Dodrill, C.B., and Batzel, L.W. (1985). Neuropsychological abilities of children with epilepsy, *Epilepsia*, 26, 395–400.
Fenton, A.A. (2015). Excitation-inhibition discoordination in rodent models of mental disorders, *Biol. Psychiatr.*, 77, 1079–1088.
Fernandez-Ruiz, A., Oliva, A., Nagy, G.A., Maurer, A.P., Berenyi, A., and Buzsaki, G. (2017). Entorhinal-CA3 dual-input control of spike timing in the hippocampus by theta-gamma coupling, *Neuron*, 93, 1213–1226.
Fuentes, A., and Kerr, E.N. (2017). Maintenance effects of working memory intervention (Cogmed) in children with symptomatic epilepsy, *Epilepsy Behav.*, 67, 51–59.
Gatt, G., Velíšková, J., Liu, Z., Moshé, S.L., and Holmes, G.L. (1993). Ontogeny of flurothyl-induced seizures: A behavioral and EEG electroencephalographic analysis, *Epilepsia*, 34(Suppl. 6), 63.
Halasz, P., Kelemen, A., Clemens, B., Saracz, J., Rosdy, B., Rasonyi, G., and Szucs, A. (2005). The perisylvian epileptic network. A unifying concept, *Ideggyogy Sz*, 58, 21–31.

Hasselmo, M.E. (2005). What is the function of hippocampal theta rhythm? Linking behavioral data to phasic properties of field potential and unit recording data, *Hippocampus*, 15, 936–949.

Hasselmo, M.E., and Stern, C.E. (2014). Theta rhythm and the encoding and retrieval of space and time, *Neuroimage*, 85 Pt 2, 656–666.

Hermann, B.P., Seidenberg, M., and Bell, B. (2002). The neurodevelopmental impact of childhood onset temporal lobe epilepsy on brain structure and function and the risk of progressive cognitive effects, *Prog. Brain Res.*, 135, 429–438.

Hernan, A.E., Holmes, G.L., Isaev, D., Scott, R.C., and Isaeva, E. (2013). Altered short-term plasticity in the prefrontal cortex after early life seizures, *Neurobiol. Dis.*, 50, 120–126.

Hinman, J.R., Brandon, M.P., Climer, J.R., Chapman, G.W., and Hasselmo, M.E. (2016). Multiple running speed signals in medial entorhinal cortex, *Neuron*, 91, 666–679.

Hinman, J.R., Penley, S.C., Long, L.L., Escabi, M.A., and Chrobak, J.J. (2011). Septotemporal variation in dynamics of theta: speed and habituation, *J. Neurophysiol.*, 105, 2675–2686.

Hoffmann, A.F., Zhao, Q., and Holmes, G.L. (2004). Cognitive impairment following status epilepticus and recurrent seizures during early development: support for the “two-hit hypothesis”, *Epilepsy Behav.*, 5, 873–877.

Holmes, G.L. (1991). The long-term effects of seizures on the developing brain: clinical and laboratory issues, *Brain Dev.*, 13, 393–409.

Holmes, G.L. (2014). What is more harmful, seizures or epileptic EEG abnormalities? Is there any clinical data?, *Epileptic Disord.*, 16 Suppl 1, 12–22.

Holmes, G.L. (2015). Cognitive impairment in epilepsy: the role of network abnormalities. *Epileptic Disord.*, 17, 101–116.

Holmes, G.L., Gairsa, J.L., Chevassus-Au-Louis, N., and Ben-Ari, Y. (1998). Consequences of neonatal seizures in the rat: morphological and behavioral effects, *Ann. Neurol.*, 44, 845–857.

Holmes, G.L., and Lenck-Santini, P.P. (2006). Role of interictal epileptiform abnormalities in cognitive impairment, *Epilepsy Behav.*, 8, 504–515.

Holmes, G.L., Sarkisian, M., Ben-Ari, Y., and Chevassus-Au-Louis, N. (1999). Mossy fiber sprouting after recurrent seizures during early development in rats, *J. Comp. Neurol.*, 404, 537–553.

Holmes, G.L., Tian, C., Hernan, A.E., Flynn, S., Camp, D., and Barry, J. (2015). Alterations in sociability and functional brain connectivity caused by early-life seizures are prevented by bumetanide, *Neurobiol. Dis.*, 77, 204–219.

Holscher, C., Anwyl, R., and Rowan, M.J. (1997). Stimulation on the positive phase of hippocampal theta rhythm induces long-term potentiation that can Be depotentiated by stimulation on the negative phase in area CAl in vivo, *J. Neurosci.*, 17, 6470–6477.

Huang, L., Cilio, M.R., Silveira, D.C., McCabe, B.K., Sogawa, Y., Stafstrom, C.E., and Holmes, G.L. (1999). Long-term effects of neonatal seizures: a behavioral, electrophysiological, and histological study, *Dev. Brain Res.*, 118, 99–107.

Huerta, P.T., and Lisman, J.E. (1995). Bidirectional synaptic plasticity induced by a single burst during cholinergic theta oscillation in CAl in vitro, *Neuron*, 15, 1053–1063.

Huxter, J.R., Senior, T.J., Allen, K., and Csicsvari, J. (2008). Theta phase-specific codes for two-dimensional position, trajectory and heading in the hippocampus, *Nat. Neurosci.*, 11, 587–594.

Insel, T.R. (2010). Rethinking schizophrenia, *Nature*, 468, 187–193.

Isaeva, E., Isaev, D., and Holmes, G.L. (2013). Alteration of synaptic plasticity by neonatal seizures in rat somatosensory cortex, *Epilepsy Res.*, 106(1–2), 280–283.

Isaeva, E., Isaev, D., Khazipov, R., and Holmes, G.L. (2006). Selective impairment of GABAergic synaptic transmission in the flurothyl model of neonatal seizures, *Eur. J. Neurosci.*, 23, 1559–1566.

Isaeva, E., Isaev, D., Khazipov, R., and Holmes, G.L. (2009). Long-term suppression of GABAergic activity by neonatal seizures in rat somatosensory cortex, *Epilepsy Res.*, 87, 286–289.

Isaeva, E., Isaev, D., Savrasova, A., Khazipov, R., and Holmes, G.L. (2010). Recurrent neonatal seizures result in long-term increases in neuronal network excitability in the rat neocortex, *Eur. J. Neurosci.*, 31, 1446–1455.

Isaeva, E.V. (2009). Mechanism of antiseizure effect of isoflurane in the immature rat hippocampus, *Fiziol. Zh.*, 55, 57–60.

Jeewajee, A., Barry, C., Douchamps, V., Manson, D., Lever, C., and Burgess, N. (2014). Theta phase precession of grid and place cell firing in open environments, *Philos. Trans. R. Soc. Lond. B Biol. Sci.*, 369, 20120532.

Karnam, H.B., Zhao, Q., Shatskikh, T., and Holmes, G.L. (2009a). Effect of age on cognitive sequelae following early life seizures in rats, *Epilepsy Res.*, 85, 221–230.

Karnam, H.B., Zhou, J.L., Huang, L.T., Zhao, Q., Shatskikh, T., and Holmes, G.L. (2009b). Early life seizures cause long-standing impairment of the hippocampal map, *Exp. Neurol.*, 217, 378–387.

Kelemen, E. and Fenton, A.A. (2010). Dynamic grouping of hippocampal neural activity during cognitive control of two spatial frames, *PLoS Biol.*, 8, e1000403.

Khan, O.I., Zhao, Q, Miller, F., and Holmes, G.L. (2010). Interictal spikes in developing rats cause long-standing cognitive deficits, *Neurobiol. Dis.*, 39, 362–371.

Kleen, J.K., Scott, R.C., Holmes, G.L., and Lenck-Santini, P.P. (2010). Hippocampal interictal spikes disrupt cognition in rats, *Ann. Neurol.*, 67, pp. 250–257.

Kleen, J.K., Scott, R.C., Holmes, G.L., Roberts, D.W., Rundle, M.M., Testorf, M., Lenck-Santini, P.P., and Jobst, B.C. (2013). Hippocampal interictal epileptiform activity disrupts cognition in humans, *Neurology*, 81, 18–24.

Kleen, J.K., Sesque, A., Wu, E.X., Miller, F.A., Hernan, A.E., Holmes, G.L., and Scott, R.C. (2011a). Early-life seizures produce lasting alterations in the structure and function of the prefrontal cortex, *Epilepsy Behav.*, 22, 214–219.

Kleen, J.K., Wu, E.X., Holmes, G.L., Scott, R.C., and Lenck-Santini, P.P. (2011b). Enhanced oscillatory activity in the hippocampal-prefrontal network is related to short-term memory function after early-life seizures, *J Neurosci.*, 31, 15397–15406.

Krauss, G.L., Summerfield, M., Brandt, J., Breiter, S., and Ruchkin, D. (1997). Mesial temporal spikes interfere with working memory, *Neurology*, 49, 975–980.

Krook-Magnuson, E., Armstrong, C., Bui, A., Lew, S., Oijala, M., and Soltesz, I. (2015). In vivo evaluation of the dentate gate theory in epilepsy, *J. Physiol.*, 593, 2379–2388.

Langston, R.F., Ainge, J.A., Couey, J.J., Canto, C.B., Bjerknes, T.L., Witter, M.P., Moser, E.I., and Moser, M.B. (2010). Development of the spatial representation system in the rat, *Science*, 328, 1576–1580.

Lee, D.J., Izadi, A., Melnik, M., Seidl, S., Echeverri, A., Shahlaie, K., and Gurkoff, G.G. (2017). Stimulation of the medial septum improves performance in spatial learning following pilocarpine-induced status epilepticus, *Epilepsy Res.*, 130, 53–63.

Lee, H., Dvorak, D., and Fenton, A.A. (2014). Targeting neural synchrony deficits is sufficient to improve cognition in a schizophrenia-related neurodevelopmental model, *Front. Psychiatr.*, 5, 15.

Lenck-Santini, P.P. and Holmes, G.L. (2008). Altered phase precession and compression of temporal sequences by place cells in epileptic rats, *J. Neurosci.*, 28, 5053–5062.

Lenck-Santini, P.P., Muller, R.U., Save, E., and Poucet, B. (2002). Relationships between place cell firing fields and navigational decisions by rats, *J. Neurosci.*, 22, 9035–9047.

Leutgeb, J.K., Leutgeb, S., Moser, M.B., and Moser, E.I. (2007). Pattern separation in the dentate gyrus and CA3 of the hippocampus, *Science*, 315, 961–966.

Lin, H., Holmes, G.L., Kubie, J.L., and Muller, R.U. (2009). Recurrent seizures induce a reversible impairment in a spatial hidden goal task, *Hippocampus*, 19, 817–827.

Liu, X., Muller, R.U., Huang, L.T., Kubie, J.L., Rotenberg, A., Rivard, B., Cilio, M.R., and Holmes, G.L. (2003). Seizure-induced changes in place cell physiology: relationship to spatial memory, *J. Neurosci.*, 23, 11505–11515.

Lucas, M.M., Lenck-Santini, P.P., Holmes, G.L., and Scott, R.C. (2011). Impaired cognition in rats with cortical dysplasia: additional impact of early-life seizures, *Brain*, 134, 1684–1693.

Lugo, J.N., Swann, J.W., and Anderson, A.E. (2014). Early-life seizures result in deficits in social behavior and learning, *Exp. Neurol.*, 256, 74–80.

Magee, J.C. (1999). Dendritic lh normalizes temporal summation in hippocampal CA1 neurons, *Nat. Neurosci.*, 2, 508–514.

Martinos, M.M., Yoong, M., Patil, S., Chin, R.F., Neville, B.G., Scott, R.C., and de Haan, M. (2012). Recognition memory is impaired in children after prolonged febrile seizures, *Brain*, 135, 3153–3164.

Martinos, M.M., Yoong, M., Patil, S., Chong, W.K., Mardari, R., Chin, R.F., Neville, B.G., de Hann, M., and Scott, R.C. (2013). Early developmental outcomes in children following convulsive status epilepticus: a longitudinal study, *Epilepsia*, 54, 1012–1019.

McCabe, B.K., Silveira, D.C., Cilio, M.R., Cha, B.H., Liu, X., Sogawa, Y., and Holmes, G.L. (2001) Reduced neurogenesis after neonatal seizures, *J. Neurosci.*, 21, 2094–2103.

McClelland, S., Brennan, G.P., Dube, C., Rajpara, S., Iyer, S., Richichi, C., Bernard, C., and Baram, T.Z. (2014). The transcription factor NRSF contributes to epileptogenesis by selective repression of a subset of target genes, *eLife*, 3, e01267.

Mikati, M.A., Tarif, S., Lteif, L., and Jawad, M.A. (2001). Time sequence and types of memory deficits after experimental status epilepticus, *Epilepsy Res.*, 43, 97–101.

Mizuseki, K., Sirota, A., Pastalkova, E., and Buzsaki, G. (2009). Theta oscillations provide temporal windows for local circuit computation in the entorhinal-hippocampal loop, *Neuron*, 64, 267–280.

Morris, R. (1984). Development of a water maze procedure for studying spatial learning in the rat, *J. Neurosci. Meth.*, 11, 47–60.

Muller, R. (1996). A quarter of a century of place cells, *Neuron*, 17, 813–822.

Muller, R.U. and Kubie, J.L. (1987). The effects of changes in the environment on the spatial firing of hippocampal complex-spike cells, *J. Neurosci.*, 7, 1951–1968.

Neill, J.C., Liu, Z., Sarkisian, M., Tandon, P., Yang, Y., Stafstrom, C.E., and Holmes, G.L. (1996). Recurrent seizures in immature rats: effect on auditory and visual discrimination, *Dev. Brain Res.*, 95, 283–292.

Neyens, L.G., Aldenkamp, A.P., and Meinardi, H.M. (1999). Prospective follow-up of intellectual development in children with a recent onset of epilepsy, *Epilepsy Res.*, 34, 85–90.

Neymotin, S.A., Hilscher, M.M., Moulin, T.C., Skolnick, Y., Lazarewicz, M.T., and Lytton, W.W. (2013). Ih tunes theta/gamma oscillations and cross-frequency coupling in an in silico CA3 model, *PLoS ONE*, 8, e76285.

O'Keefe, J. (1976). Place units in the hippocampus of the freely moving rat, *Exp. Neurol.*, 51, 78–109.

O'Keefe, J. and Conway, D.H. (1978). Hippocampal place cells in the freely moving rat: why they fire where they fire, *Exp. Brain Res.*, 31, 573–590.

O'Keefe, J. and Dostrovsky, J. (1971). The hippocampus as a spatial map: preliminary evidence from unit activity in the freely-moving rat, *Brain Res.*, 34, 171–175.

O'Keefe, J. and Nadel, L. (1978). The Hippocampus as a Cognitive Map. Oxford: Clarendon.

O'Keefe, J. and Recce, M. (1993). Phase relationships between hippocampal place units and the EEG theta rhythm, *Hippocampus*, 3, 317–330.

Ostrach, L.H., Crabtree, J.W., Campbell, B.G., and Chow, K.L. (1984). Effects of bicuculline-induced epileptiform activity on development of receptive field properties in striate cortex and lateral geniculate nucleus of the rabbit, *Brain Res.*, 317, 113–123.

Patterson, K.P., Barry, J.M., Curran, M.M., Singh-Taylor, A., Brennan, G., Rismanchi, N., Page, M., Noam, Y., Holmes, G.L., and Baram, T.Z. (2017). Enduring memory impairments provoked by developmental febrile seizures are mediated by functional and structural effects of neuronal restrictive silencing factor, *J. Neurosci.*, 37, 3799–3812.

Prasad, A.N., Burneo, J.G., and Corbett, B. (2014a). Epilepsy, comorbid conditions in Canadian children: analysis of cross-sectional data from cycle 3 of the National Longitudinal Study of Children and Youth, *Seizure*, 23, 869–873.

Prasad, C., Corbett, B.A., and Prasad, A.N. (2014b). Epilepsy, school readiness in Canadian children: data from the National Longitudinal Study of Children and Youth (NLSCY), *Seizure*, 23, 435–438.

Protopapa, F., Siettos, C.I., Myatchin, I., and Lagae, L. (2016). Children with well controlled epilepsy possess different spatio-temporal patterns of causal network connectivity during a visual working memory task, *Cogn. Neurodyn.*, 10, 99–111.

Richard, G.R., Titiz, A., Tyler, A., Holmes, G.L., Scott, R.C., and Lenck-Santini, P.P. (2013). Speed modulation of hippocampal theta frequency correlates with spatial memory performance, *Hippocampus*, 23, 1269–1279.

Riviello, P., de Rogalski Landrot, I., and Holmes, G.L. (2002). Lack of cell loss following recurrent neonatal seizures, *Dev. Brain Res.*, 135, 101–104.

Robbe, D. and Buzsaki, G. (2009). Alteration of theta timescale dynamics of hippocampal place cells by a cannabinoid is associated with memory impairment, *J. Neurosci.*, 29, 12597–12605.

Rutten, A., van Albada, M., Silveira, D.C., Cha, B.H., Liu, X., Hu, Y.N., Cilio, M.R., and Holmes, G.L. (2002). Memory impairment following status epilepticus in immature rats: time-course and environmental effects, *Eur. J. Neurosci.*, 16, 501–513.

Schomburg, E.W., Fernandez-Ruiz, A., Mizuseki, K., Berenyi, A., Anastassiou, C.A., Koch, C., and Buzsaki, G. (2014). Theta phase segregation of input-specific gamma patterns in entorhinal-hippocampal networks, *Neuron*, 84, 470–485.

Scott, R.C., Richard, G.R., Holmes, G.L., and Lenck-Santini, P.P. (2011). Maturational dynamics of hippocampal place cells in immature rats, *Hippocampus*, 21, 347–353.

Shewmon, D.A. and Erwin, R.J. (1988a). Focal spike-induced cerebral dysfunction is related to the after-coming slow wave, *Ann. Neurol.*, 23, 131–137.

Shewmon, D.A. and Erwin, R.J. (1988b). The effect of focal interictal spikes on perception and reaction time. I. General considerations, *Electroencephalogr. Clin. Neurophysiol.*, 69, 319–337.

Shewmon, D.A. and Erwin, R.J. (1988c). The effect of focal interictal spikes on perception and reaction time. II. Neuroanatomic specificity, *Electroencephalogr. Clin. Neurophysiol.*, 69, 338–352.

Shewmon, D.A. and Erwin, R.J. (1989). Transient impairment of visual perception induced by single interictal occipital spikes, *J. Clin. Exp. Neuropsychol.*, 11, 675–691.

Siegle, J.H. and Wilson, M.A. (2014). Enhancement of encoding and retrieval functions through theta phase-specific manipulation of hippocampus, *Elife*, 3, e03061.

Sillanpaa, M., Jalava, M., Kaleva, O., and Shinnar, S. (1998). Long-term prognosis of seizures with onset in childhood, *N. Engl. J. Med.*, 338, 1715–1722.

Skaggs, W.E., McNaughton, B.L., Wilson, M.A., and Barnes, C.A. (1996). Theta phase precession in hippocampal neuronal populations and the compression of temporal sequences, *Hippocampus*, 6, 149–172.

Sogawa, Y., Monokoshi, M., Silveira, D.C., Cha, B.H., Cilio, M.R., McCabe, B.K., Liu, X., Hu, Y., and Holmes, G.L. (2001). Timing of cognitive deficits following neonatal seizures: relationship to histological changes in the hippocampus, *Dev. Brain Res.*, 131, 73–83.

Song, D., Harway, M., Marmarelis, V.Z., Hampson, R.E., Deadwylerr, S.A., and Berger, T.W. (2014). Extraction and restoration of hippocampal spatial memories with non-linear dynamical modeling, *Front. Syst. Neurosci.*, 8, 97. doi: 10.3389/fnsys.2014.00097.

Toth, Z., Yan, X.X., Haftoglou, S., Ribak, C.E., and Baram, T.Z. (1998). Seizure-induced neuronal injury: vulnerability to febrile seizures in an immature rat model, *J. Neurosci.*, 18, 4285–4294.

Tyler, A.L., Mahoney, J.M., Richard, G.R., Holmes, G.L., Lenck-Santini, P.P., and Scott, R.C. (2012). Functional network changes in hippocampal CA1 after status epilepticus predict spatial memory deficits in rats, *J. Neurosci.*, 32, 11365–11376.

Ung, H., Cazares, C., Nanivadekar, A., Kini, L., Wagenaar, J., Becker, D., Krieger, A., Lucas, T., Litt, B., and Davis, K.A. (2017). Interictal epileptiform activity outside the seizure onset zone impacts cognition, *Brain*, 140, 2157–2168.

Urrestarazu, E., Jirsch, J.D., Levan, P., Hall, J., Avoli, M., Dubeau, F., and Gotman, J. (2006). High-frequency intracerebral EEG activity (100–500 Hz) following interictal spikes, *Epilepsia*, 47, 1465–1476.

Vafaei, A.A., Jezek, K., Bures, J., Fenton, A.A., and Rashidy-Pour, A. (2007). Post-training reversible inactivation of the rat's basolateral amygdala interferes with hippocampus-dependent place avoidance memory in a time-dependent manner, *Neurobiol. Learn. Mem.*, 88, 87–93.

van Esch, A., Ramlal, I.R., van Steensel-Moll, H.A., and Steyerberg, E.W. (1996). Outcome after febrile status epilepticus, *Dev. Med. Child Neurol.*, 38, 19–24.

Vanderwolf, C.H. (1969). Hippocampal electrical activity and voluntary movement in the rat, *Electroencephalogr. Clin. Neurophysiol.*, 26, 407–418.

Villeneuve, N., Ben-Ari, Y., Holmes, G.L., and Gaiarsa, J.L. (2000). Neonatal seizures induced persistent changes in intrinsic properties of CA1 rat hippocampal cells, *Ann. Neurol.*, 47, 729–738.

Wakamoto, H., Nagao, H., Hayashi, M., and Morimoto, T. (2000). Long-term medical, educational, and social prognoses of childhood-onset epilepsy: a population-based study in a rural district of Japan, *Brain Dev.*, 22, 246–255.

Wang, Y., Romani, S., Lustig, B., Leonardo, A., and Pastalkova, E. (2015). Theta sequences are essential for internally generated hippocampal firing fields, *Nat. Neurosci.*, 18, 282–288.

Weiss, E.F., Masur, D., Shinnar, S., Hesdorffer, D.C., Hinton, V.J., Bonner, M., Rinaldi, J., Van de Water, V., Culbert, J., Shinnar, R.C., Seinfeld. S., Gallentine, W., Nordli, D.R., Frank, L.M., Epstein, L., Moshe, S.L., and Sun, S. (2016). Cognitive functioning one month and one year following febrile status epilepticus, *Epilepsy Behav.*, 64, 283–288.

Williams, J., Griebel, M.L., and Dykman, R.A. (1998). Neuropsychological patterns in pediatric epilepsy, *Seizure*, 7, 223–228.

Williams, M.R., DeSpenza, T., Li, M., Gulledge, A.T., and Luikart, B.W. (2015). Hyperactivity of newborn Pten knock-out neurons results from increased excitatory synaptic drive, *J. Neurosci.*, 35, 943–959.

Wills, T.J., Cacucci, F., Burgess, N., and O'Keefe, J. (2010.) Development of the hippocampal cognitive map in preweanling rats, *Science*, 328, 1573–1576.

Wilson, M.A., Varela, C., and Remondes, M. (2015). Phase organization of network computations, *Curr. Opin. Neurobiol.*, 31, 250–253.

Xiao, F., An, D., Lei, D., Li, L., Chen, S., Wu, X., Yang, T., Ren, J., Gong, Q. and Zhou, D. (2016). Real-time effects of centrotemporal spikes on cognition in rolandic epilepsy: An EEG-fMRI study, *Neurology*, 86, 544–551.

Zhou, J.L., Lenck-Santini, P.P., Zhao, Q., and Holmes, G.L. (2007a). Effect of interictal spikes on single-cell firing patterns in the hippocampus, *Epilepsia*, 48, 720–731.

Zhou, J.L., Shatskikh, T.N., Liu, X., and Holmes, G.L. (2007b). Impaired single cell firing and long-term potentiation parallels memory impairment following recurrent seizures, *Eur. J. Neurosci.*, 25, 3667–3677.

Chapter 14
Sex Matters in Epilepsy

Jana Velíšková, MD, PhD

Departments of Cell Biology & Anatomy,
Obstetrics & Gynecology, and Neurology,
New York Medical College, Valhalla, NY, USA

14.1 Introduction

There is an increasing recognition that sex matters in all aspects of human health not only pertinent to the reproductive system but also having influence on other organs, including the brain. Sex differences involve a bias in many central nervous system (CNS) regions, which influence brain functioning and ultimately determine the outcomes of diseases affecting the brain. Thus, the presence of sexual dimorphism in the CNS determines sex differences in disease occurrence, progression and treatment. Despite these facts, sex is rarely considered in treatment strategy decisions and females are still not included equally as males in human or animal studies [Clayton and Collins, 2014; Hanamsagar and Bilbo, 2016; Zagni *et al.*, 2016].

Epidemiological studies suggest that seizures and epilepsy syndromes more likely affect men than women [Hauser *et al.*, 1996; Kotsopoulos *et al.*, 2002]. Although overall this sex difference is not significant, specific epilepsy syndromes do show a sex bias. Febrile seizures are more common in boys but girls seem to be more vulnerable to develop cognitive dysfunction when complex febrile seizures occur at very young ages compared to boys [Forsgren *et al.*, 1990;

Tsuboi, 1984; Wallace and Cull, 1979]. Higher incidences in boys than girls have been observed especially in epilepsy syndromes associated with severe encephalopathy, i.e., Ohtahara syndrome, epileptic spasms or Lennox-Gastaut syndrome [Clarke *et al.*, 1987; Luthvigsson *et al.*, 1994; Trevathan *et al.*, 1997]. On the other hand, idiopathic generalized epilepsies, especially juvenile myoclonic epilepsy, are more common in women then in men [Camfield *et al.*, 2013; Christensen *et al.*, 2005]. Sex-related differences have been described in patients with temporal lobe epilepsy, with respect to distinct regional distribution of brain dysfunction during interictal periods, seizure generalization, lateralization, as well as sensitivity to neuronal damage [Briellmann *et al.*, 2000; Helmstaedter *et al.*, 2004; Janszky *et al.*, 2004; Savic and Engel, 1998]. Here, I discuss some of the evidence from animal studies in support of these clinical observations.

14.2 The brain as a sexually dimorphic structure

To understand sex differences in the brain's health and disease, first the role of sexual dimorphism in the brain must be appreciated. Sexual dimorphism of the brain involves sex differences at microscopic as well as macroscopic levels, including but not limited to the size of neuronal nuclei and nucleoli, size of synaptic terminals and vesicles, dendritic branching, synapse organization and size of brain regions and neurotransmitter distribution [Breedlove, 1994; MacLusky and Naftolin, 1981; Toran-Allerand, 1984]. The brain's dimorphic appearance is under the influence of circulating gonadal/sex hormones, which can easily penetrate the blood-brain barrier because of their small molecular weight and lipophilic properties. The brain is sensitive to sex hormone organizational effects during critical early developmental periods [Gorski, 1971]. Original understanding of the development of sexual dimorphism in the brain assumed that feminine features are programmed to develop as the default despite the "chromosomal sex" (XX or XY). The occurrence of male features involves masculinization/defeminization of the brain under the influence of male gonadal hormones, testosterone or its metabolites estradiol and dihydrotestosterone, produced by the testis during the mid to late embryonic stage and early neonatal periods [Pilgrim and

Hutchinson, 1994]. These organizing effects on the brain during the critical differentiation period are irreversible ("imprinting effect"). In rats, male testis release testosterone during embryonic days 18–22 and the testosterone surge starts again within couple of hours after birth and continues until postnatal day (P) 6. Then the testosterone surge from developing testis is actively suppressed until the pubertal testosterone surge occurs. Since the brain is resistant to permanent organizational effects of sex hormones outside the embryonic and early life critical periods, any effects of sex hormones later in life, which may also lead to sex differences, are transient and occur only at the time when the particular hormone is present [Cooke *et al.*, 1999]. The developing female brain is somewhat protected from the effects of gonadal hormones by production of alpha-fetoprotein, which prevents the organizational effects of gonadal hormones on the brain by binding the peripheral circulating gonadal hormones. Some exceptions to this original one-sided understanding of the development of brain dimorphism need to be considered [Arnold, 2011; McCarthy and Arnold, 2011]. Recent evidence shows that certain sex differences may exist prior to the surge of gonadal hormones, e.g., a study using mesencephalic dissociated cultures showed morphological and functional differences depending on whether the cultures originated from male or female embryos taken prior to the first gonadal hormone surge by male embryonic testis [Reisert *et al.*, 1989]. Genetic mechanisms are also responsible for sex differences. Finally, the most recent studies suggest involvement of epigenetic regulation of sex differences. It seems that the sex hormones may not directly increase the gene expression but may act above the genome, at least in some brain regions. Epigenetic genome modulation is responsible for both establishment of sex differences in the brain and for the maintenance of its sexually dimorphic function, as elegantly reviewed [McCarthy, 2018].

14.3 Sex hormones, sex hormone receptors and their effects

The sex hormones are generally divided into female and male sex hormones. The female sex hormones are progesterone and estrogens (estradiol, estriol and estrone). Testosterone, androstenedione and dihydrotestosterone are the main male sex hormones, the androgens. The sex hormones, as other steroid hormones, are synthetized from cholesterol in a process called steroidogenesis [Bremer and Miller, 2014], which takes place mainly in reproductive tissues and in some specialized tissues including brain. Steroidogenesis involves downstream steroidogenic enzymes such as hydroxysteroid dehydrogenases and cytochrome P450 and is tightly regulated by various rate-limiting steps.

The classic effects of sex hormones are mediated by sex hormone receptors, which act as transcription factors by activating or repressing gene expression. Sex hormone receptors belong to the steroid hormone receptor group and when unbound, reside inside the cells within the cytoplasm. Following a ligand binding, the hormone-receptor complex forms homo- or heterodimeric receptors and leads to conformational changes to allow trans-location into the nucleus where the complex binds specific DNA sequences (sex hormone response element) of a target gene. Further interaction with additional co-factors/co-repressors, which are part of the transcriptional signaling pathways, i.e., early genes, determines whether the target gene transcription is activated, leading to new protein synthesis or repression of the gene expression. Further binding to activating proteins (AF-1 or AF-2) determines whether the transcriptional activity is ligand-independent or ligand-dependent. This classic signaling pathway is called the "genomic pathway". The genomic pathway is characterized by delayed onset (several minutes to hours), long-lasting effects (which can continue beyond the time of the ligand binding), or can be permanent.

In contrast to the "classic" genomic pathway, rapid (seconds to minutes), short-lasting effects of sex hormones, which have duration limited only to the time of ligand binding and are transient in nature, have been described recently. Further investigations into these effects uncovered a novel pathway that involves a portion of sex hormone receptors, which are nestled in the cell membrane and do not require nuclear translocation or DNA binding; thus, this signaling pathway is called the "non-genomic pathway". Sex hormone binding to these membrane-localized receptors activates different second messenger cascades; i.e., tyrosine kinase c Src (Src), protein kinase A and C (PKA and PKC), mitogen activated protein kinase (MAPK), or extracellular signal-regulated kinase (ERK). Besides sex hormone receptors, the sex hormones can directly bind to specific binding sites on various ion channels, membrane-associated kinases, and G-protein coupled receptors. Current research also suggests that binding of sex hormones to the membrane-nestled receptors may, in fact, also initiate transcription pathway signaling that does not require the classic DNA binding machinery.

It is now well established that sex hormones and their receptors act beyond the reproductive system and the brain is one of the targets of their effects.

14.4 Developmental aspects of sex differences in seizure-controlling structures

Sex differences in some brain regions develop during the embryonic period, while others are under the influence of the early postnatal testosterone surge. An example is the substantia nigra (SN). The SN is an integral part of basal ganglia, with two parts: pars compacta (SNC), which contains mainly the dopaminergic neurons and pars reticulata (SNR), which has primarily GABAergic neurons. Pathological changes in the SN lead to movement disorders, i.e., Parkinson disease, Tourette syndrome, dystonia, tardive dyskinesia, and result in extrapyramidal signs in other neurodegenerative diseases [Burns *et al.*, 2005; Davila *et al.*, 2010; Dybdal *et al.*, 2013; Lanska, 2010; Olanow and Tatton, 1999]. Animal studies show that the dopaminergic system in the SNC has sexually dimorphic features and is under the influence of sex hormones [Bottjer, 1993; Miller, 1983; Rivest *et al.*, 1995; Xu *et al.*, 1999]. This fact may give insights into the sex differences in Parkinson disease, e.g., higher incidence in men, more severe motor and cognitive symptoms, and lower life satisfaction than affected women [Buczak-Stec *et al.*, 2018; Pinares-Garcia *et al.*, 2018]. On the other hand, women have more side effects (e.g., the occurrence of dyskinesia) and an inferior response to treatment compared to men [Lyons *et al.*, 1998].

Besides movement disorders, the SN, especially the SNR GABAergic system, is an important endogenous seizure-controlling center [Iadarola and Gale, 1982; Velíšková and Moshé, 2006]. The GABAergic system in the SNR is sexually dimorphic as it shows distinct features in males and females. GABA turnover is higher in males than females [Manev and Pericic, 1987] as is the basal firing rate of the SNR GABAergic neurons [Wilson, 1993]. On the other hand, females show higher binding levels of the high-affinity GABA binding site labeled by [3H] muscimol [Canonaco *et al.*, 1996]. Also, expression of the neuronal specific potassium chloride contransporter KCC2 is higher in females compared to males, especially prepubertally [Galanopoulou *et al.*, 2003b]. Sex differences in the SNR are the result of the testosterone surge during the immediate postnatal period [Ravizza *et al.*, 2003a; Ravizza *et al.*, 2003b; Velíšková and Moshé, 2001]. Both testosterone and estrogen receptors are present in the SNR since P0 [Ravizza *et al.*, 2002].

Our functional studies showed that SNR dimorphic features are reflected by a developmentally regulated seizure-controlling function that is different in males compared to females. In male rats at P15, bilateral microinfusions of the $GABA_A$ receptor agonist muscimol into the SNR have seizure-promoting (proconvulsant) effects on flurothyl-induced seizures. At P25–30 (peripubertal period [Ojeda and Urbanski, 1994]), the SNR becomes segregated into two functionally distinct regions. SNR muscimol microinfusions have opposite effects on seizures depending on whether the microinfusions are aimed into the more frontal part of the SNR (SNRanterior) or caudal part of the SNR (SNRposterior) [Velíšková and Moshé, 2001]. In SNRanterior, muscimol has anticonvulsant effects while in SNRposterior, muscimol has proconvulsant effects on flurothyl-induced seizures. These bidirectional seizure-modulating effects within the two SNR regions persist into adulthood [Velíšková and Moshé, 2001]. These seizure-modulating effects of the two distinct SNR regions on flurothyl-induced clonic seizures have been confirmed with other GABAergic agents [Velíšková *et al.*, 1996, 1998] (Figure 14.1).

On the other hand, pharmacologic enhancement of the GABA system in females has a different outcome on seizures compared to

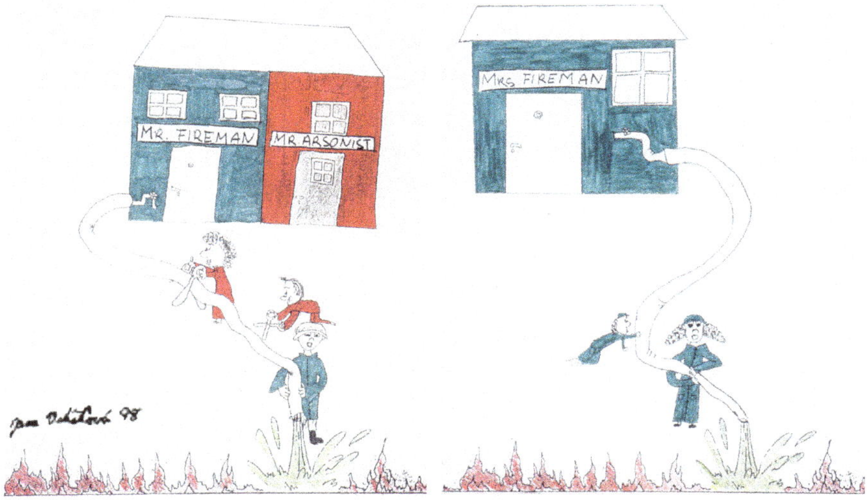

Figure 14.1. Sex- and region-specific modulation of seizure activity by the SNR depicted by my then 14-year-old daughter. See the text above and below for detailed explanation. Mr. and Mrs. Fireman with the baby girl controlling seizure activity (anticonvulsant effect) but Mr. Arsonist and his baby boy promote seizures (proconvulsant effect) [Velíšková and Moshé, 2006].

males. In P15 females, bilateral microinfusions of muscimol have no effect on flurothyl-induced seizures [Velíšková and Moshé, 2001]. The anticonvulsant effect of SNR muscimol microinfusions becomes evident earlier in female rats than in males, already between P21–25, and remains in the adulthood. Finally, microinfusions of muscimol into the SNRposterior have no effect on flurothyl-induced seizures [Velíšková and Moshé, 2001]. Thus, enhancement of the GABAergic system within the SNR in female rats has no proconvulsant effects like it has in males.

We found that the testosterone surge during the early postnatal critical period is responsible for the proconvulsant effects of muscimol microinfusions in P15 males. The role of the testosterone surge on formation of the "male" type of SNR-mediated seizure control following muscimol microinfusions has been documented by the following experiments: 1. Males were neonatally castrated (at P0) or injected with an androgen receptor antagonist flutamide on P0–P2 and then tested at P15 using flurothyl-induced seizures; muscimol microinfusions into the SNR had no effect on seizure threshold as in P15 females [Heida *et al.*, 2008; Velíšková and Moshé, 2001]. Thus, the males lost the proconvulsant response to muscimol infusions when neonatally castrated or when the androgen receptors were blocked during the early critical period for brain sexual differentiation. 2. Administration of testosterone or its metabolites, dihydrotestosterone or estrogen, to females or neonatally castrated males during the early postnatal period (P0–5) resulted in proconvulsant muscimol effects in the SNR on flurothyl-induced seizures [Velíšková and Moshé, 2001]. Interestingly, males castrated at P3 retained the proconvulsant "male type" effects of SNR muscimol infusions on flurothyl seizures.

Underlying mechanisms for the bidirectional and sex-specific effects of muscimol within the SNR on seizure control may involve a higher GABA content, mRNA levels for $\alpha 1$ subunit of the GABAA receptor or KCC2 expression [Galanopoulou *et al.*, 2003b; Ravizza *et al.*, 2003a] as well as contribution of distinct functional networks activated by SNR muscimol microinfusions in female SNR compared to males [Velíšek *et al.*, 2005].

Findings from these studies on the sex-specific properties of the GABAergic transmission within the SNR are important not only for seizure control but also for a better understanding of pathological processes in Parkinson disease. One of the common features of both pathologies is neuronal oscillations in thalamocortical circuits, which are present in Parkinson disease during tremors and during epileptic clonic seizures [Buzsaki *et al.*, 1990]. These oscillations are a result of neuronal bursting of GABAergic afferents of the thalamus originating from structures upstream regulated by the striatum, such as the SNR, and under pathological conditions may lead to rhythmic oscillations in the thalamocortical network, suggesting overlapping underlying mechanisms in both diseases [Buzsaki *et al.*, 1990]. Further, pathological processes in patients with Parkinson disease involve not only the SN dopaminergic system but also SNR GABAergic transmission [Winkler *et al.*, 1999]. These changes are especially prominent in the late stages of Parkinson disease, when patients present with akinesia and postural disturbances that do not respond to levodopa treatment but seems to be sensitive to enhancement of the SNR GABAergic system [Olanow and Tatton, 1999; Winkler *et al.*, 1999].

14.5 Sex differences in seizure susceptibility: Animal models

Only a few studies used males and females to compare possible sex differences in seizure susceptibility. Data from models of both generalized and focal seizures are discussed here.

Models of generalized seizures show that sex differences in seizure susceptibility depend on the route of administration, dose and type of convulsant agent, and species. Sensitivity to seizures induced by intraperitoneal injection of picrotoxin, an antagonist at $GABA_A$ receptors, was higher in female than in male rats and cats [Pericic and Bujas, 1997b; Pericic *et al.*, 1985, 1986; Thomas, 1990]. Similarly, intraperitoneal injection of a low dose of bicuculline, another antagonist at $GABA_A$ receptors, also showed higher seizure susceptibility in female rats compared to males [Matějovská *et al.*, 1998] However, seizure susceptibility following a high dose of bicuculline did not differ between the two sexes but priming the animals with a stressful event increased the seizure susceptibility only in male rats [Pericic and Bujas, 1997a, b]. Interestingly, intravenous injection of picrotoxin or bicuculline revealed that male rats had higher seizure susceptibility than female rats [Pericic and Bujas, 1997b]. In mice, intravenous injection of bicuculline also showed higher seizure susceptibility in male mice compared to females while no sex differences were found in seizure susceptibility to picrotoxin [Pericic and Bujas, 1997b]. In contrast to rats and cats, female mice were more resistant to picrotoxin-induced seizures compared to male mice following intraperitoneal administration [Pericic and Bujas, 1997b; Pericic *et al.*, 1986]. It can be speculated that interspecies sex variability in GABA binding, GABA content, or drug metabolism are responsible for these differences [Pericic and Bujas, 1997b].

In models of temporal lobe seizures, animal data focus mainly on generalized seizures. Using either kainic acid or pilocarpine, males showed more severe and more frequent clonic seizures compared to female rats [Mejias-Aponte *et al.*, 2002]. This accords with the clinical observation that seizure generalization in patients with temporal lobe epilepsy is more common in men [Janszky *et al.*, 2004]. Further, the increased seizure susceptibility of male rats was prevented by gonadectomy, suggesting that testosterone or its metabolites may be responsible for the heightened sensitivity to both convulsant agents in males [Mejias-Aponte *et al.*, 2002]. A clinical study found that in male patients with temporal lobe epilepsy, administration of aromatase inhibitors such as anastrazole or letrozole, which block the conversion of testosterone to β-estradiol (E2), reduced seizure frequency [Harden and MacLusky, 2005] (reviewed in detail in [Frye, 2010]). Similarly, in male rats, repeated administration of E2 accelerated pilocarpine-induced seizure onset [Galanopoulou *et al.*, 2003a] and enhanced severity of kainic acid-induced seizures in males but not in females [Nicoletti *et al.*, 1985]. An *in vitro* study showed sex-specific sensitivity within the hippocampus, a limbic structure associated with temporal lobe seizures, to circulating sex hormones [Teyler *et al.*, 1980]. Bath application of E2 to hippocampal slices from male rats increased population spike amplitudes in the CA1 region but had no effect in slices from female rats [Teyler *et al.*, 1980]. Our *in vitro* study found that E2 administration to female rats had anticonvulsant effects on low magnesium-induced epileptiform activity [Velíšková and Velíšek, 2013].

Patients with temporal lobe epilepsy commonly present with atrophy, especially in the limbic structures, suggesting that this type of seizure leads to neuronal damage. An MRI study showed that men with temporal lobe epilepsy are more sensitive to seizure-induced neuronal damage with higher structural atrophy compared to women with similar seizure frequencies [Briellmann *et al.*, 2000]. Animal studies suggest that circulating E2 plays an important role in this sex bias. In male rats, E2 administration exacerbates seizure-induced hippocampal damage [Galanopoulou *et al.*, 2003a]. In females, status epilepticus in animals without E2 (ovariectomized) leads to extensive neuronal damage in the hippocampus compared to those which experienced same seizure duration and severity but were replaced with E2 [Galanopoulou *et al.*, 2003a; Hoffman *et al.*, 2003;

Reibel *et al.*, 2000; Velíšková and Velíšek, 2007; Velíšková *et al.*, 2000] but not progesterone [Hoffman *et al.*, 2003]. These neuroprotective effects in females involve E2-mediated transcriptional regulation of gene expression, i.e., enhanced expression of neuropeptide Y [Velíšková *et al.*, 2015; Velíšková and Velíšek, 2007], an inhibitory peptide. Neuropeptide Y expressing neurons, especially those within the deep polymorphic layer of the dentate gyrus (DG) hilar region, are sensitive to seizure-induced damage [de Lanerolle *et al.*, 1989]. The DG serves as a gate by filtering the incoming activity into the hippocampus proper during physiological processes, i.e., learning [Hsu, 2007; Iijima *et al.*, 1996; Lothman *et al.*, 1992; McDermott and Schrader, 2011; Pun *et al.*, 2012]. The DG function has been compared to a context of Hebbian association and competition: the DG granule cells recognize incoming entorhinal patterns of activity, which have to be consistent and repetitive to pass through (Hebbian association), while the random patterns are blocked (non-associative Hebbian competition) [Hsu, 2007]. Once DG gating is compromised, e.g., in TLE, the patients experience learning and memory problems [Jensen, 2011; Noebels, 2011] and

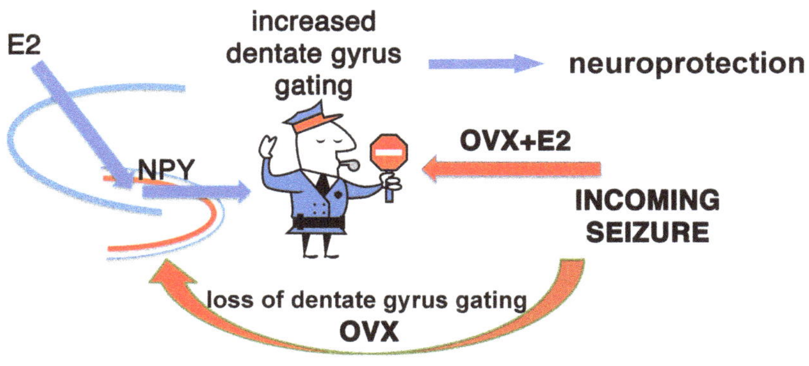

Figure 14.2. Neuroprotective effects of E2 are mediated by enhanced DG gating. E2 replacement in ovariectomized (OVX) rats increases neuropeptide Y (NPY) expression in the hilar region, which leads to selective frequency filtering of incoming activity, including seizure activity. OVX rats have low hilar NPY expression and thus, incoming seizure activity passes through the compromised DG gate and leads to neuronal damage and learning deficits [Iacobas *et al.*, 2018; Velíšková and Velíšek, 2007].

in addition seizure activity can spread throughout the hippocampus resulting in network re-modeling, abnormal function and neuronal damage [Peng and Houser, 2005; Pun *et al.*, 2012]. Our studies established that E2 mediates functional neuroprotection by preserving the DG gating properties [Iacobas *et al.*, 2018; Velíšková and Velíšek, 2007] (Figure 14.2).

14.6 Conclusions

In conclusion, clinical and animal studies show that seizure susceptibility and expression of several types of seizures are sex-dependent. These sex-specific effects are related not only to presence of sex hormones but also to sex differences in structures associated with generation or control of seizures [Velíšková and DeSantis, 2013]. These findings emphasize that each sex needs to be studied separately and that hormonal status needs to be considered especially in studies involving females during the reproductive age. Better understanding of sex and hormone-dependent influence on seizures might help to tailor sex-specific treatments with the ultimate goal of seizure control and minimal side effects.

References

Arnold, A.P. (2011). The end of gonad-centric sex determination in mammals, *Trends Genet.*, 28, 55–61.

Bottjer, S.W. (1993). The distribution of tyrosine hydroxylase immunoreactivity in the brains of male and female zebra finches, *J Neurobiol*, 24, 51–69.

Breedlove, S.M. (1994). Sexual differentiation of the human nervous system, *Annu. Rev. Psychol.*, 45, 389–418.

Bremer, A.A. and Miller, W.L. (2014). Regulation of steroidogenesis. In Cellular Endocrinology in Health and Disease, A. Ulloa-Aguirre, and P.M. Conn, eds. (Academic Press), pp. 207–227.

Briellmann, R.S., Berkovic, S.F., and Jackson, G.D. (2000). Men may be more vulnerable to seizure-associated brain damage, *Neurology*, 55, 1479–1485.

Buczak-Stec, E.W., Konig, H.H., and Hajek, A. (2018). Impact of incident Parkinson's disease on satisfaction with life, *Front. Neurol.*, 9, 589.

Burns, J.M., Galvin, J.E., Roe, C.M., Morris, J.C., and McKeel, D.W. (2005). The pathology of the substantia nigra in Alzheimer disease with extrapyramidal signs, *Neurology*, 64, 1397–1403.

Buzsaki, G., Smith, A., Berger, S., Fisher, L.J., and Gage, F.H. (1990). Petit mal epilepsy and parkinsonian tremor: hypothesis of a common pacemaker, *Neuroscience*, 36, 1–14.

Camfield, C.S., Striano, P., and Camfield, P.R. (2013). Epidemiology of juvenile myoclonic epilepsy, *Epilepsy Behav.*, 28 Suppl 1, S15–17.

Canonaco, M., Tavolaro, R., Facciolo, R.M., Carelli, A., Cagnin, M., and Cristaldi, M. (1996). Sexual dimorphism of GABAA receptor levels in subcortical brain regions of a woodland rodent (Apodemus sylvaticus), *Brain Res. Bull.*, 40, 187–194.

Christensen, J., Kjeldsen, M.J., Andersen, H., Friis, M.L., and Sidenius, P. (2005). Gender differences in epilepsy, *Epilepsia*, 46, 956–960.

Clarke, M., Gill, J., Noronha, M., and McKinlay, I. (1987). Early infantile epileptic encephalopathy with suppression burst: Ohtahara syndrome, *Dev. Med. Child. Neurol.*, 29, 520–528.

Clayton, J.A. and Collins, F.S. (2014). Policy: NIH to balance sex in cell and animal studies, *Nature*, 509, 282–283.

Cooke, B.M., Tabibnia, G., and Breedlove, S.M. (1999). A brain sexual dimorphism controlled by adult circulating androgens, *Proc. Natl. Acad. Sci. U.S.A.*, 96, 7538–7540.

Davila, G., Berthier, M.L., Kulisevsky, J., Asenjo, B., Gomez, J., Lara, J.P., Chacon, S.J., and Campos, V.M. (2010). Structural abnormalities in the substantia nigra and neighbouring nuclei in Tourette's syndrome, *J. Neural. Transm.*, 117, 481–488.

de Lanerolle, N.C., Kim, J.H., Robbins, R.J., and Spencer, D.D. (1989). Hippocampus interneuron loss and plasticity in human temporal lobe epilepsy, *Brain Res.*, 495, 387–395.

Dybdal, D., Forcelli, P.A., Dubach, M., Oppedisano, M., Holmes, A., Malkova, L., and Gale, K. (2013). Topography of dyskinesias and torticollis evoked by inhibition of substantia nigra pars reticulata, *Mov. Disord.*, 28, 460–468.

Forsgren, L., Sidenvall, R., Blomquist, H.K., and Heijbel, J. (1990). A prospective incidence study of febrile convulsions, *Acta Paediatr. Scand.*, 79, 550–557.

Frye, C.A. (2010). Effects and mechanisms of progestogens and androgens in ictal activity, *Epilepsia*, 51 Suppl 3, 135–140.

Galanopoulou, A.S., Alm, E.M., and Velíšková, J. (2003a). Estradiol reduces seizure-induced hippocampal injury in ovariectomized female but not in male rats, *Neurosci Lett.*, 342, 201–205.

Galanopoulou, A.S., Kyrozis, A., Claudio, O.I., Stanton, P.K., and Moshe, S.L. (2003b). Sex-specific KCC2 expression and GABA(A) receptor function in rat substantia nigra, *Exp. Neurol.*, 183, 628–637.

Gorski, R.A. (1971). Gonadal hormones and the perinatal development of neuroendocrine function. In Frontiers in Neuroendocrinology, L. Martini, and W.F. Ganong, eds. (New York: Oxford University Press), pp. 237–290.

Hanamsagar, R. and Bilbo, S.D. (2016). Sex differences in neurodevelopmental and neurodegenerative disorders: Focus on microglial function and neuroinflammation during development, *J. Steroid Biochem. Mol. Biol.*, 160, 127–133.

Harden, C. and MacLusky, N.J. (2005). Aromatase inhibitors as add-on treatment for men with epilepsy, *Expert Rev. Neurother.*, 5, 123–127.

Hauser, W.A., Annegers, J.F., and Rocca, W.A. (1996). Descriptive epidemiology of epilepsy: contributions of population-based studies from Rochester, Minnesota. *Mayo Clin. Proc.*, 71, 576–586.

Heida, J.G., Velíšková, J., and Moshé, S.L. (2008). Blockade of androgen receptors is sufficient to alter the sexual differentiation of the substantia nigra pars reticulata seizure-controlling network, *Epileptic Disord.*, 10, 8–12.

Helmstaedter, C., Brosch, T., Kurthen, M., and Elger, C.E. (2004). The impact of sex and language dominance on material-specific memory before and after left temporal lobe surgery, *Brain*, 127, 1518–1525.

Hoffman, G.E., Moore, N., Fiskum, G., and Murphy, A.Z. (2003). Ovarian steroid modulation of seizure severity and hippocampal cell death after kainic acid treatment, *Exp. Neurol.*, 182, 124–134.

Hsu, D. (2007). The dentate gyrus as a filter or gate: a look back and a look ahead, *Prog Brain Res.*, 163, 601–613.

Iacobas, D.A., Iacobas, S., Nebieridze, N., Velíšek, L., and Velíšková, J. (2018). Estrogen protects neurotransmission transcriptome during status epilepticus, *Front. Neurosci.* 12, 332.

Iadarola, M.J. and Gale, K. (1982). Substantia nigra: site of anticonvulsant activity mediated by γ-aminobutyric acid, *Science*, 218, 1237–1240.

Iijima, T., Witter, M.P., Ichikawa, M., Tominaga, T., Kajiwara, R., and Matsumoto, G. (1996). Entorhinal-hippocampal interactions revealed by real-time imaging, *Science*, 272, 1176–1179.

Janszky, J., Schulz, R., Janszky, I., and Ebner, A. (2004). Medial temporal lobe epilepsy: gender differences, *J. Neurol. Neurosurg. Psychiatry*, 75, 773–775.

Jensen, F.E. (2011). Epilepsy as a spectrum disorder: Implications from novel clinical and basic neuroscience, *Epilepsia*, 52 Suppl 1, 1–6.

Kotsopoulos, I.A., van Merode, T., Kessels, F.G., de Krom, M.C., and Knottnerus, J.A. (2002). Systematic review and meta-analysis of incidence studies of epilepsy and unprovoked seizures, *Epilepsia*, 43, 1402–1409.

Lanska, D.J. (2010). Chapter 33: The history of movement disorders, *Hand. Clini. Neurol.*, 95, 501–546.

Lothman, E.W., Stringer, J.L., and Bertram, E.H. (1992). The dentate gyrus as a control point for seizures in the hippocampus and beyond, *Epilepsy Res.*, Suppl 7, 301–313.

Luthvigsson, P., Olafsson, E., Sigurthardottir, S., and Hauser, W.A. (1994). Epidemiologic features of infantile spasms in Iceland, *Epilepsia*, 35, 802–805.

Lyons, K.E., Hubble, J.P., Troster, A.I., Pahwa, R., and Koller, W.C. (1998). Gender differences in Parkinson's disease, *Clin. Neuropharmacol.*, 21, 118–121.

MacLusky, N.J. and Naftolin, F. (1981). Sexual differentiation of the central nervous system, *Science*, 211, 1294–1303.

Manev, H. and Pericic, D. (1987). Sex difference in the turnover of GABA in the rat substantia nigra, *J. Neural. Transm.*, 70, 321–328.

Matějovská, I., Velíšková, J., and Velíšek, L. (1998). Bicuculline-induced rhythmic EEG episodes: gender differences and the effects of ethosuximide and baclofen treatment, *Epilepsia*, 39, 1243–1252.

McCarthy, M.M. (2018). Sex and the developing brain. In, Colloquium Digital Library of Life Sciences (Morgan & Claypool: Morgan & Claypool), pp. 1–153.

McCarthy, M.M. and Arnold, A.P. (2011). Reframing sexual differentiation of the brain, *Nat. Neurosci.*, 14, 677–683.

McDermott, C.M. and Schrader, L.A. (2011). Activation of kappa opioid receptors increases intrinsic excitability of dentate gyrus granule cells, *J. Physiol.*, 589, 3517–3532.

Mejias-Aponte, C.A., Jimenez-Rivera, C.A., and Segarra, A.C. (2002). Sex differences in models of temporal lobe epilepsy: role of testosterone, *Brain Res.*, 944, 210–218.

Miller, J.C. (1983). Sex differences in dopaminergic and cholinergic activity and function in the nigro-striatal system of the rat, *Psychoneuroendocrinology*, 8, 225–236.

Nicoletti, F., Speciale, C., Sortino, M.A., Summa, G., Caruso, G., Patti, F., and Canonico, P.L. (1985). Comparative effects of estradiol benzoate, the antiestrogen clomiphene citrate, and the progestin medroxyprogesterone acetate on kainic acid-induced seizures in male and female rats, *Epilepsia*, 26, 252–257.

Noebels, J. (2011). A perfect storm: Converging paths of epilepsy and Alzheimer's dementia intersect in the hippocampal formation, *Epilepsia*, 52 Suppl 1, 39–46.

Ojeda, S.R. and Urbanski, H.F. (1994). Puberty in the rat. In The Physiology of Reproduction, E. Knobil, and J. Neil, eds. (New York: Raven Press, Ltd.), pp. 363–409.

Olanow, C.W. and Tatton, W.G. (1999). Etiology and pathogenesis of Parkinson's disease, *Ann. Rev. Neurosci.*, 22, 123–144.

Peng, Z. and Houser, C.R. (2005). Temporal patterns of fos expression in the dentate gyrus after spontaneous seizures in a mouse model of temporal lobe epilepsy, *J. Neurosci.*, 25, 7210–7220.

Pericic, D. and Bujas, M. (1997a). Sex differences in bicuculline-induced convulsions: interaction with stress and ligands of benzodiazepine binding sites, *Brain Res.*, 752, 279–284.

Pericic, D. and Bujas, M. (1997b). Sex differences in the response to GABA antagonists depend on the route of drug administration, *Exp. Brain Res.*, 115, 187–190.

Pericic, D., Manev, H., and Geber, J. (1986). Sex-related differences in the response of mice, rats and cats to the administration of picrotoxin, *Life Sci.*, 38, 905–913.

Pericic, D., Manev, H., and Lakic, N. (1985). Sex differences in the response of rats to drugs affecting GABAergic transmission, *Life Sci.*, 36, 541–547.

Pilgrim, C. and Hutchinson, J.B. (1994). Developmental regulation of sex differences in the brain: Can the role of gonadal steroids be redefined?, *Neuroscience*, 60, 843–855.

Pinares-Garcia, P., Stratikopoulos, M., Zagato, A., Loke, H., and Lee, J. (2018). Sex: a significant risk factor for neurodevelopmental and neurodegenerative disorders, *Brain Sci*, 8, pii: E154. doi: 10.3390/brainsci8080154.

Pun, R.Y., Rolle, I.J., Lasarge, C.L., Hosford, B.E., Rosen, J.M., Uhl, J.D., Schmeltzer, S.N., Faulkner, C., Bronson, S.L., Murphy, B.L., Richards, D.A., Holland, K.D., and Danzer, S.C. (2012). Excessive activation of

mTOR in postnatally ggenerated granule cells is sufficient to cause epilepsy, *Neuron*, 75, 1022–1034.
Ravizza, T., Friedman, L.K., Moshé, S.L., and Velíšková, J. (2003a). Sex differences in GABA(A)ergic system in rat substantia nigra pars reticulata, *Int. J. Dev. Neurosci.*, 21, 245–254.
Ravizza, T., Galanopoulou, A.S., Velíšková , J., and Moshé, S.L. (2002). Sex differences in androgen and estrogen receptor expression in rat substantia nigra during development: an immunohistochemical study, *Neuroscience*, 115, 685–696.
Ravizza, T., Velísková, J., and Moshé, S.L. (2003b). Testosterone regulates androgen and estrogen receptor immunoreactivity in rat substantia nigra pars reticulata, *Neurosci. Lett.*, 338, 57–61.
Reibel, S., Andre, V., Chassagnon, S., Andre, G., Marescaux, C., Nehlig, A., and Depaulis, A. (2000). Neuroprotective effects of chronic estradiol benzoate treatment on hippocampal cell loss induced by status epilepticus in the female rat, *Neurosci. Lett.*, 281, 79–82.
Reisert, I., Engele, J., and Pilgrim, C. (1989). Early sexual differentiation of diencephalic dopaminergic neurons of the rat in vitro, *Cell Tissue Res.*, 255, 411–417.
Rivest, R., Falardeau, P., and Di Paolo, T. (1995). Brain dopamine transporter: gender differences and effect of chronic haloperidol, *Brain Res.*, 692, 269–272.
Savic, I. and Engel, J., Jr. (1998). Sex differences in patients with mesial temporal lobe epilepsy, *J. Neurol. Neurosurg. Psychiatry*, 65, 910–912.
Teyler, T.J., Vardaris, R.M., Lewis, D., and Rawitch, A.B. (1980). Gonadal steroids: Effects on excitability of hippocampal pyramidal cells, *Science*, 209, 1017–1019.
Thomas, J. (1990). Gender difference in susceptibility to picrotoxin-induced seizures is seizure- and stimulation-dependent, *Brain Res. Bull.*, 24, 7–10.
Toran-Allerand, C.D. (1984). Gonadal hormones and brain development: implications for the genesis of sexual differentiation. *Ann. N.Y. Acad. Sci.*, 435, 101–111.
Trevathan, E., Murphy, C.C., and Yeargin-Allsopp, M. (1997). Prevalence and descriptive epidemiology of Lennox-Gastaut syndrome among Atlanta children, *Epilepsia*, 38, 1283–1288.
Tsuboi, T. (1984). Epidemiology of febrile and afebrile convulsions in children in Japan, *Neurology*, 34, 175–181.
Velíšek, L., Velíšková, J., Ravizza, T., Giorgi, F.S., and Moshé, S.L. (2005). Circling behavior and [14C]2-deoxyglucose mapping in rats: possible

implications for autistic repetitive behaviors, *Neurobiol. Dis.*, 18, 346–355.
Velíšková, J. and DeSantis, K.A. (2013). Sex and hormonal influences on seizures and epilepsy, *Horm. Behav.*, 63, 267–277.
Velíšková, J., Iacobas, D., Iacobas, S., Sidyelyeva, G., Chachua, T., and Velíšek, L. (2015). Oestradiol Regulates Neuropeptide Y Release and Gene Coupling with the GABAergic and Glutamatergic Synapses in the Adult Female Rat Dentate Gyrus, *J. Neuroendocrinol.*, 27, 911–920.
Velíšková, J., Löscher, W., and Moshé, S.L. (1998). Regional and age specific effects of zolpidem microinfusions in the substantia nigra on seizures, *Epilepsy Res.*, 30, 107–114.
Velíšková, J. and Moshé, S.L. (2001). Sexual dimorphism and developmental regulation of substantia nigra function, *Ann. Neurol.*, 50, 596–601.
Velíšková, J. and Moshé, S.L. (2006). Update on the role of substantia nigra pars reticulata in the regulation of seizures, *Epilepsy Curr.*, 6, 83–87.
Velíšková, J. and Velíšek, L. (2007). β-Estradiol increases dentate gyrus inhibition in female rats via augmentation of hilar neuropeptide Y, *J. Neurosci.*, 27, 6054–6063.
Velíšková, J. and Velíšek, L. (2013). Gonadal status-dependent effects of in vivo beta-estradiol administration to female rats on in vitro epileptiform activity induced by low [Mg] in combined hippocampus-entorhinal cortex slices, *Epilepsy Res.*, 107, 297–301.
Velíšková, J., Velíšek, L., Galanopoulou, A.S., and Sperber, E.F. (2000). Neuroprotective effects of estrogens on hippocampal cells in adult female rats after status epilepticus, *Epilepsia*, 41, S30–35.
Velíšková, J., Velíšek, L., Nunes, M.L., and Moshé, S.L. (1996). Developmental regulation of regional functionality of substantia nigra $GABA_A$ receptors involved in seizures, *Eur. J. Pharmacol.*, 309, 167–173.
Wallace, S.J. and Cull, A.M. (1979). Long-term psychological outlook for children whose first fit occurs with fever, *Dev. Med. Child Neurol.*, 21, 28–40.
Wilson, M.A. (1993). Gonadectomy and sex modulate spontaneous activity of substantia nigra pars reticulata neurons without modifying GABA/benzodiazepine responsiveness, *Life Sci.*, 53, 217–225.
Winkler, C., Bentlage, C., Nikkhah, G., Samii, M., and Bjorklund, A. (1999). Intranigral transplants of GABA-rich striatal tissue induce behavioral recovery in the rat Parkinson model and promote the effects obtained by intrastriatal dopaminergic transplants, *Exp. Neurol.*, 155, 165–186.

Xu, Z.C., Chwang, W., Li, X., Chen, X., and He, P. (1999). Gender difference in dopamine concentration and postischemic neuronal damage in neostriatum after unilateral dopamine depletion, *Exp. Neurol.*, 158, 182–191.
Zagni, E., Simoni, L., and Colombo, D. (2016). Sex and gender differences in central nervous system-related disorders, *Neurosci. J.*, 2016, 2827090.

Index

Lightning Source UK Ltd.
Milton Keynes UK
UKHW020249250921
391114UK00001B/39

9 789813 277724